Arthroplasty: Biomechanics and Clinical Techniques

Arthroplasty: Biomechanics and Clinical Techniques

Editor: Gordon Shaw

MURPHY & MOORE
www.murphy-moorepublishing.com

www.murphy-moorepublishing.com

MURPHY & MOORE

Cataloging-in-Publication Data

Arthroplasty : biomechanics and clinical techniques / edited by Gordon Shaw.
p. cm.
Includes bibliographical references and index.
ISBN 978-1-63987-058-5
1. Arthroplasty. 2. Joints--Surgery. 3. Surgery, Plastic. 4. Human mechanics. I. Shaw, Gordon.
RD686 .A78 2022
617.472 059 7--dc23

Murphy & Moore Publishing,
1 Rockefeller Plaza,
New York City, NY 10020, USA

ISBN 978-1-63987-058-5 (Hardback)

Contents

Preface

This book has been an outcome of determined endeavour from a group of educationists in the field. The primary objective was to involve a broad spectrum of professionals from diverse cultural background involved in the field for developing new researches. The book not only targets students but also scholars pursuing higher research for further enhancement of the theoretical and practical applications of the subject.

The surgical procedure in orthopedics wherein the articular surface of a musculoskeletal joint is replaced or realigned is termed as arthroplasty. Some of the major types of procedures in arthroplasty are joint replacement, resurfacing arthroplasty and resectional arthroplasty. Joint replacement involves replacing a joint or joint surface with a prosthesis through surgery. A single or both bone surfaces are shaved off and replaced by a metal covering in resurfacing arthroplasty. Resectional arthroplasty seeks to remove bone and joint surface, and join the remaining ends. There are also techniques and procedures which fall under the umbrella of arthroplasty such as silicone replacement arthroplasty, mold arthroplasty and osteotomy. This book unfolds the innovative aspects of arthroplasty which will be crucial for the progress of this field in the future. Also included herein is a detailed explanation of the biomechanics and clinical techniques in the field of arthroplasty. This book will help the readers in keeping pace with the rapid changes in this field.

It was an honour to edit such a profound book and also a challenging task to compile and examine all the relevant data for accuracy and originality. I wish to acknowledge the efforts of the contributors for submitting such brilliant and diverse chapters in the field and for endlessly working for the completion of the book. Last, but not the least; I thank my family for being a constant source of support in all my research endeavours.

Editor

1

Anterior Primary Total Hip Arthroplasty

Ulrich Bechler, Bernhard Springer and
Friedrich Boettner

Abstract

Total hip arthroplasty (THA) is the preferred treatment for end-stage osteoarthritis of the hip. The posterior, posterolateral, direct lateral, anterolateral, or the anterior approaches are the currently established surgical approaches for THA. Over the last decade, the anterior approach has gained increasing popularity. Its muscle-sparing nature and flu oroscopy-guided component positioning are the most important benefits. It has been suggested that postoperative recovery is facilitated by an anterior approach. Patients do not need to follow hip precautions, and can return to driving after 1 week. The anterior approach uses a muscle interval between the tensor fasciae latae and the rectus femoris to open the capsule without detachment of muscles. Especially, the external rotators and posterior capsule remain intact and reduce the risk of posterior dislocation. Accuracy of acetabular component positioning has an impact on postoperative dislocation rates, polyethylene wear, and impingement. When the operation is done in a supine position, fluoroscopy is available to check the acetabular component inclination and anteversion during THA as well as leg length and offset. The current chapter reports on the surgical approach, surgical technique, and results of anterior THA.

Keywords: primary total hip arthroplasty, minimally invasive surgery, anterior approach, osteoarthritis, intraoperative fluoroscopy, outcome

1. Introduction

THA is used to treat a variety of primary and secondary end-stage osteoarthritis, and has the primary goal to decrease pain, restore function, and increase joint mobility [1]. Depending on the specific patient there are various surgical techniques described to perform a THA. The general goal is to have an accurate and reproducible procedure and to avoid complications. Younger and more active patients have increased functional demands during early recovery. Utilizing an intramuscular approach allows for a faster return to activities of daily living, reduced pain, shortened recovery, and reduced costs [1].

The various available approaches are characterized by their own distinct advantages and risks. Extensions to these approaches have been described and allow for more extensive exposure and revision procedures.

In the USA, the most frequently used approach is the posterior approach. It provides easy access to the hip joint and minimizes the trauma to the hip abductor muscles. However, detachment of external rotator muscles and a complete capsulectomy results in an increased dislocation rate [2, 3]. Therefore, the repair of the external rotators and the capsule is of great importance in posterior THA [4]. In addition, the posterior approach is associated with an increased variance of acetabular component positioning [5–7]. Poor component positioning increases the risk of dislocation, facilitates increased polyethylene wear, and impingement [5, 8, 9]. Variations in the lateral patient position and the lack of intraoperative fluoroscopy might explain the less predictable cup positioning [10].

The lateral approach (anterolateral) with the patient lying in a supine position is a popular approach in Europe. The posterior part of the gluteus medius insertion can be preserved. However, injury or release of its anterior portion can result in limping [11]. Fractures of the greater trochanter are more likely using the lateral approach compared to the posterior approach [12, 13]. Postoperative patient-reported limping occurs twice as often using the lateral approach compared to the anterior approach [14]. Limping may be caused by trochanteric pain, leg length discrepancy, lack of offset restoration, nerve injury, or insufficiency of the gluteal muscles [15].

The anterior THA is unique because of its intramuscular and internervous exposure of the hip joint. A release of major muscular stabilizers is not necessary for most patients. First described by Smith-Peterson in 1949, the anterior approach became more popular in the USA over the last decade [16]. Rapid recovery, decreased dislocation rate, fluoroscopy controlled restoration of leg length, and offset as well as component position are its main benefits.

2. History

In 1881, Carl Hueter was the first surgeon to describe the anterior approach for resection of the femoral head. Smith-Peterson further developed the approach and described the extended exposure of the pelvis to perform a hip replacement. In 1978, Wagner preferred the approach for hip resurfacing procedures due to its preservation of the femoral blood supply and intermuscular dissection [17]. In 1947, the Judet table was developed and predominantly used in France. Ten years later, a special table was developed to optimize and ease the positioning of the operated leg in order to decrease injury to muscles and bone.

In the US, the anterior approach was originally combined with a lateral incision to facilitate the insertion of the femoral component and was marketed by Zimmer Biomet (Warsaw, IN, USA) in conjunction with Richard Berger as a "two incision" THA [1, 18]. Because of the higher complication rate, especially on the femoral side (fracture), the approach fell out of favor in the beginning of the twenty-first century [19]. At the same time, Joel Matta promoted an anterior approach without a second incision [20]. Matta soon realized that a special table similar to the Judet table was needed to improve exposure of the femur and provide elevation of the femur. Since the Judet table was not available in the USA, he pursued the development of the Hana® table (Mizuho OSI, Union City, CA, USA).

In 2004, large studies [20, 21] showed encouraging outcomes with low dislocation rate (<1%) and improved component positioning, but above all faster recovery pushed the interest in the anterior approach.

3. Anatomy and approach

The anterior approach classically described as Smith-Peterson approach uses an incision proximal and distal to the anterior superior iliac spine (ASIS) along the tensor fasciae latae [16]. While the proximal portion of the Smith-Peterson approach facilitates exposure of the pelvis, the distal portion is used during a direct anterior THA to expose the hip joint. The groin area usually has less subcutaneous fat than the lateral thigh, and therefore an anterior approach often has a more direct access to the fascial layer. The ASIS and greater trochanter are used as bony landmarks to guide placement of the incision. The incision usually starts

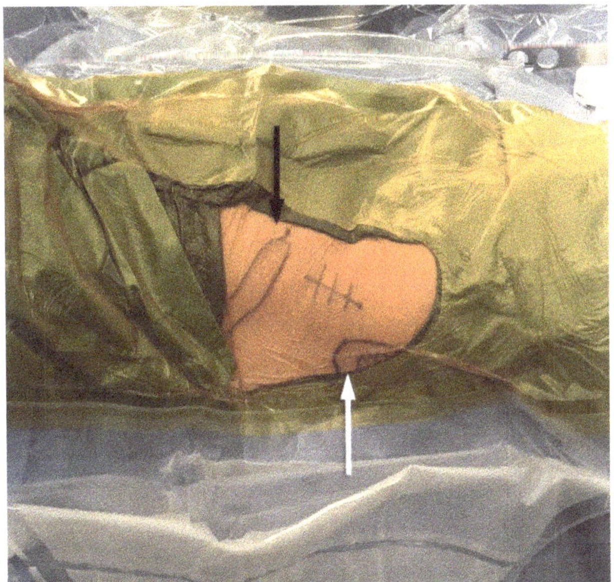

Figure 1. Patient in a supine position on a Hana® table. The skin incision, the anterior superior iliac spine (black arrow), and greater trochanter (white arrow) are marked.

two fingerbreadths lateral and distal of the ASIS and extends distally and posteriorly in line with the tensor fasciae latae muscle [20]. A slightly more lateral position can help to avoid the lateral femoral cutaneous nerve (LFCN) that enters the thigh medially to the ASIS (**Figure 1**).

The approach uses an intermuscular plane and does not require muscle releases. Medially, the interval borders to the Sartorius muscle (innervated by the femoral nerve) and laterally to the tensor fasciae latae muscle (innervated by the superior gluteal nerve) [22]. While the original Smith-Petersen approach entered between the sartorius muscle and the tensor fasciae latae, the modern anterior approach usually stays inside the fascia of the tensor fasciae latae to minimize the risk to injure the LFCN (**Figure 2**) [22]. Care should be taken not to confuse the medial located sartorius muscle and the more lateral tensor fasciae latae. Both can usually, easily be separated by the direction of the fibers. The tensor fasciae latae muscle fibers ran toward the lateral thigh in contrast to the sartorius muscle fibers, which run medially. After skin incision, the fascia of the tensor is split followed by deep finger dissection to separate the overlying fascia and the muscle belly of the tensor fasciae latae and progress toward its medial borders.

The deep intermuscular fat tissue between tensor and rectus femoris muscle contains the ascending branch of the lateral circumflex artery just proximal to the vastus lateralis muscle. At the level of the capsule, the interval is bordered by the gluteus medius (superior gluteal nerve) and medially by the rectus femoris muscle (femoral nerve). Ligations of the branches of the circumflex vessels are necessary to prevent perioperative bleeding and postoperative hematoma formation (**Figure 3**).

A Hohmann retractor is used to expose the anterior hip capsule. It is placed underneath the rectus muscle. A second blunt retractor is placed around the lateral femoral neck. The reflected head of the rectus femoris muscle is elevated and released to expose the capsule entirely. The released tendon can be marked to facilitate its identification and repair at the end of the procedure.

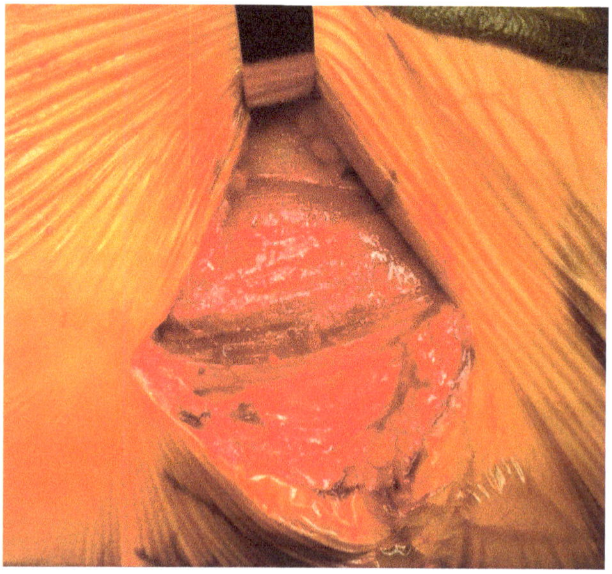

Figure 2. Incision of the fascia of the tensor fasciae latae muscle.

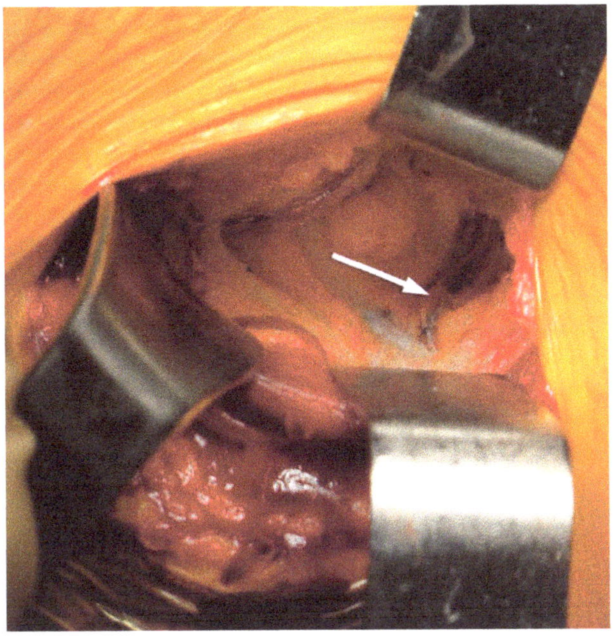

Figure 3. Image of the deep interval bordered laterally by the gluteus medius (superior gluteal nerve) and medially by the rectus femoris muscle (femoral nerve). The lateral femoral circumflex vessels (arrow) are visualized proximal to the vastus lateralis muscle.

4. Surgical technique

The procedure is performed under general or regional anesthesia. It can be performed with a standard operating table with an Omni-Tract® femur elevating system (Integra, Plainsboro, NJ, USA) or a specialized orthopedic table (Hana®, Mizuho OSI, Union City, CA, USA). The latter helps to control hip rotation, abduction, flexion, and traction of the affected extremity and facilitates exposure of the proximal femur for femoral component insertion. However, the costs, fracture risk, and limited ability to intraoperatively test the range of motion (ROM) are its main disadvantages. A number of alternative tables are currently available by other manufactures.

The authors recommend careful templating and implant selection. The primary goal of the templating is to guide acetabular reaming toward the most appropriate reamer size. On the femoral side, depending on the type of femur, shorter implants with less sizable distal dimensions might be preferred in a Dorr Type A Femur, while compression broaching for a longer implant with a collar might be preferred for a Dorr Type C femur [23]. In addition, careful planning of the femoral neck resection can help intraoperatively to restore the leg length.

The patient is lying supine on the table with a perineal post and both legs secured with the feet in boots. The pelvis and the nonsurgical hip are placed in a neutral position. After the standard anterior approach, as described above, a T-shaped capsulotomy is performed with medial and lateral extension at the level of the intertrochanteric ridge (**Figure 4**). The capsule can be tagged and preserved for later repair. Two Hohmann retractors are now placed within the capsule around the lateral and medial femoral neck. A napkin ring double osteotomy of the femoral neck is performed to ease removal of the head (**Figure 5**). The femoral head is removed with a corkscrew extractor. Additional traction and external rotation on the operated

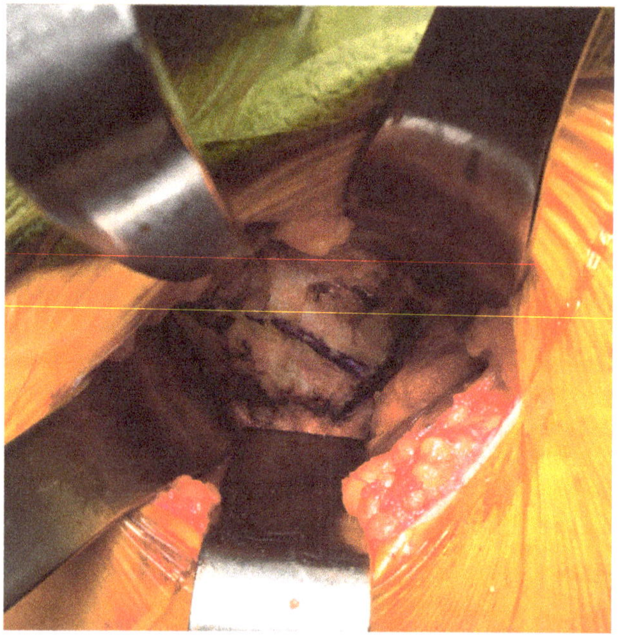

Figure 4. Markings for the T-shaped capsulotomy with medial and lateral extension.

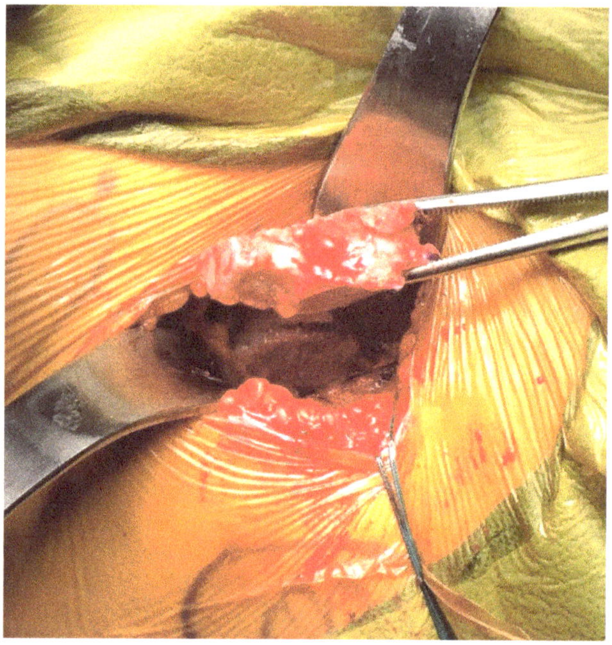

Figure 5. Photograph of a napkin ring double osteotomy of the femoral neck.

leg supports removal of the napkin ring and exposure of the acetabulum. Alternatively, to the *in situ* neck osteotomy, the hip can be dislocated using a corkscrew. The capsular releases are completed with the hip dislocated before the hip is reduced, the neck is cut, and the head removed (technique according to Matta et al. [20]).

Multiple retractors are used to facilitate acetabular exposure. First, an acetabular retractor is placed inferiorly to the fovea against the transverse acetabular ligament. This usually requires a short incision of the medial capsule. This is, followed by an anterior retractor, placed between the anterior labrum and capsule. A posterior retractor can be placed between the posterior labrum and capsule. The foveal tissue and labrum are removed. The acetabulum is either reamed under direct visualization or under fluoroscopy guidance. A press fit cup is placed and impacted (**Figure 6**). To facilitate cup alignment under the anterior acetabular bone, an implant less hemispherical then 180° is preferred. It also helps to medialize the center of rotation in comparison to a hemispherical cup.

The C-arm is used to guide intraoperative component positioning. An alternative to this technique is the use of intraoperative navigation. Because of the supine position and easy access to the iliac crest intraoperative navigation is usually fairly straightforward in anterior THA. Other techniques available for optimized cup position are based on C-arm images and include software programs like Radlink® (Radlink, El Segundo, CA, USA) and Jointpoint® (Jointpoint Inc., Belleair Bluffs, FL, USA).

The C-arm is positioned in 90° to the supine patient and centered over the pelvis to make sure the pelvis is in a neutral position (**Figure 7**). A neutral pelvis position is the requirement for any of the described C-arm based algorithms. If no software is available, the cup inclination can be checked with the C-arm centered in the middle of the pelvis. After reaching the target inclination of the acetabular component, the C-arm is moved over the operated hip. After estimating the cup anteversion based on the opening ellipse, the cup anteversion can be determined based on the C-arm tilt angle described by Boettner et al. and Zingg et al. [6, 24] (**Figure 8**). When aligned perfectly the elliptical shape of the cup presents as a line. The tilt angle can be measured on the C-arm and used to calculate the acetabular anteversion. Following correct acetabular implant positioning, the final liner is inserted and osteophytes are removed.

Exposure of the proximal femur can be facilitated by a standard release to minimize traction forces on the greater trochanter. This prevents intraoperative complications like fractures

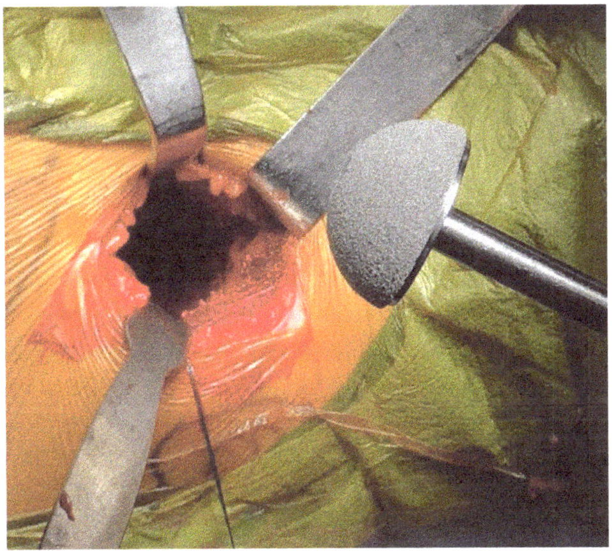

Figure 6. A press fit cup is placed and impacted into the reamed acetabulum.

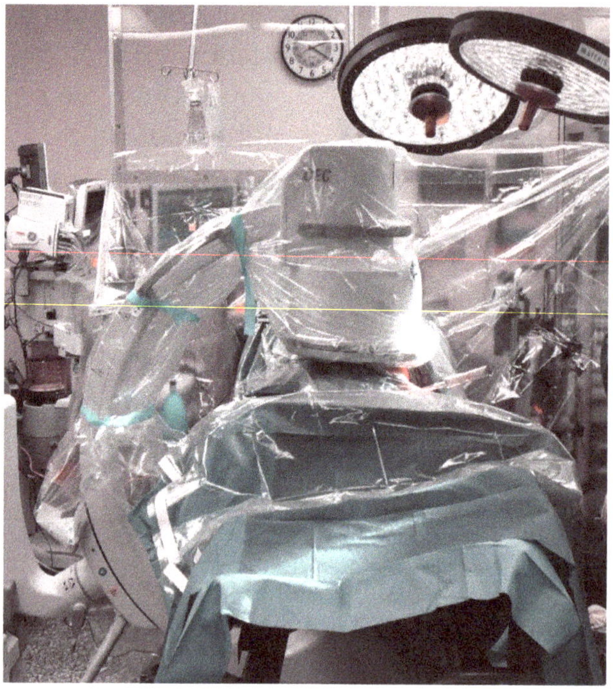

Figure 7. C-arm position in a 90° angle to the supine patient. The beam is centered over the neutral pelvis to assess inclination of the cup.

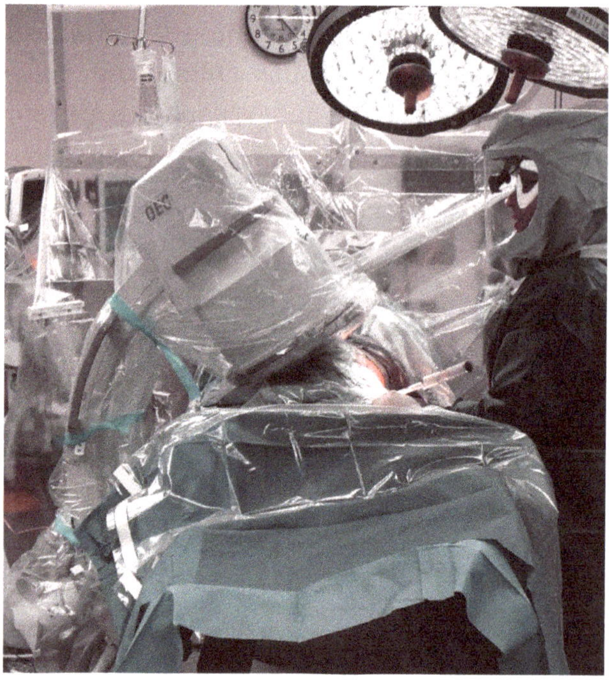

Figure 8. C-arm is tilted away from the operated hip until the ellipse of the positioned acetabular component is a straight line. The tilt angle is measured on the C-arm.

during anterior mobilization of the femur. The gluteus minimus muscle is elevated of the lateral capsule. The operated leg is positioned in extension, 90° external rotation and 20° adduction. In flexible patients adequate exposure might be possible without further releases;

however, the senior author favors the release of the conjoined tendon. The piriformis muscle insertion is preserved together with the posterior capsule, obturator externus muscle, and quadratus femoris muscle.

The Hana table® or Omni-tract® retractor provides a hook attached to a connector arm of the table. In combination with maximum extension of the leg, the hook elevates the femur anteriorly and provides better exposure for the preparation of the femoral component (**Figure 9**). Offset handles facilitate the broaching of the femur. Femoral preparation and broaching the femoral canal is done in a standardized fashion (**Figure 10**). The final trial stem is impacted into the femur with a trial head and neck.

Care should be taken not to injure the tensor fasciae latae. Good exposure to the femoral canal eases preparation and broaching. After adding the trial neck and head, the surgeon can reduce the dislocate hip with gentle traction and internal rotation. The surgeon guides the femoral head into the socket. Fluoroscopy can be used to assess leg length discrepancy, offset, and implant alignment.

For measurements of the leg length discrepancy, the inter-teardrop line is used as horizontal reference of the fluoroscopy image. The difference between the vertical distances from the reference line to the most prominent point on each lesser trochanter defines the leg length discrepancy with reference to the contralateral hip. Neutral pelvis position and equal leg abduction and rotation are required for accurate measurements. Alternatively, leg length and offset can be determined by overlaying two print-out images and comparing the contour of the operated hip to either the opposite normal or the preoperative image. Finally, the definite femoral component is implanted. The wound is irrigated and the anterior capsule closed using Vicryl #0 suture (**Figure 11**). The reflected head of the rectus can be repaired. Finally, the fascia of the tensor fasciae latae muscle is closed with #0 Vicryl sutures (**Figure 12**).

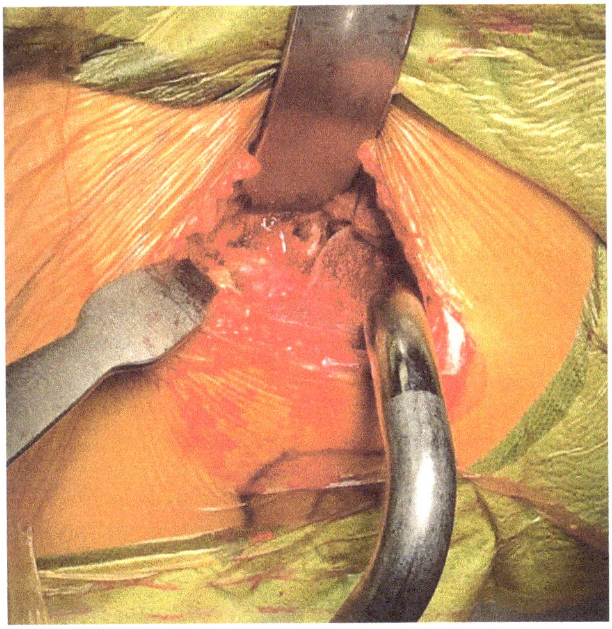

Figure 9. A hook attached to a connector arm of the table facilitates femoral exposure.

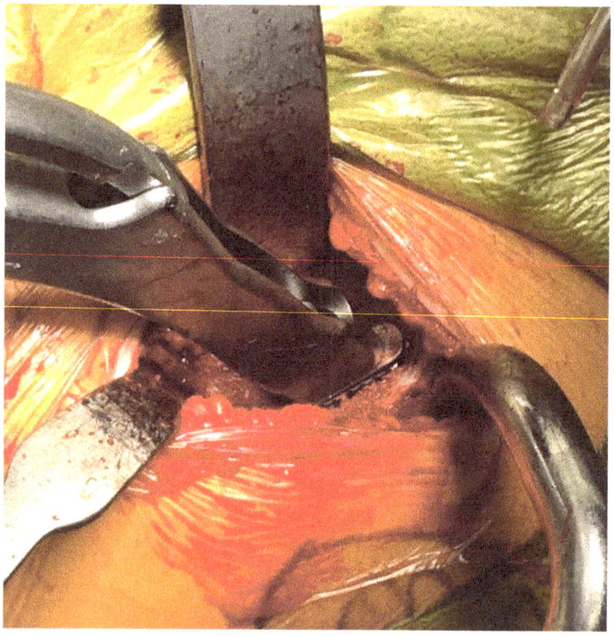

Figure 10. Photograph shows broaching of the femoral component.

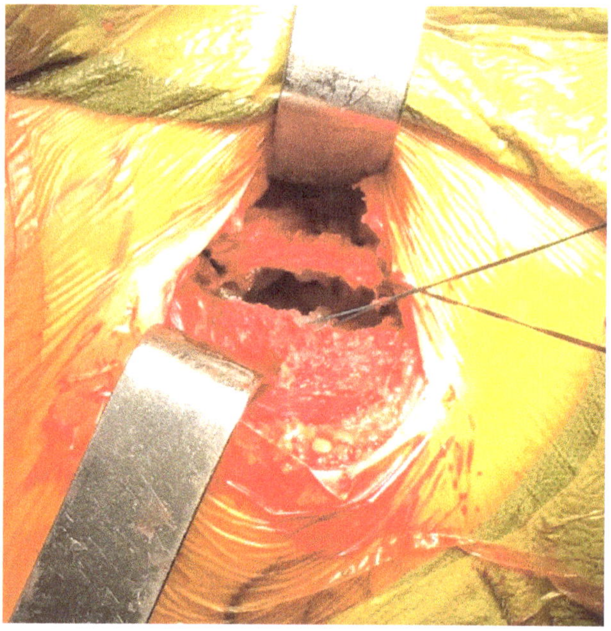

Figure 11. Tagging sutures in the medial and lateral capsular sleeve.

Many surgeons prefer a curved "Banana Type" stem for the anterior approach. Straight stem designs with a lateral shoulder require more aggressive releases including the piriformis tendon. There have been some concerns about increased femoral loosening rates and continued efforts are made to improve and develop femoral implant design. Due to the missing lateral shoulder, the curved stem provides no lateral support. As a result, lateralization and subsidence

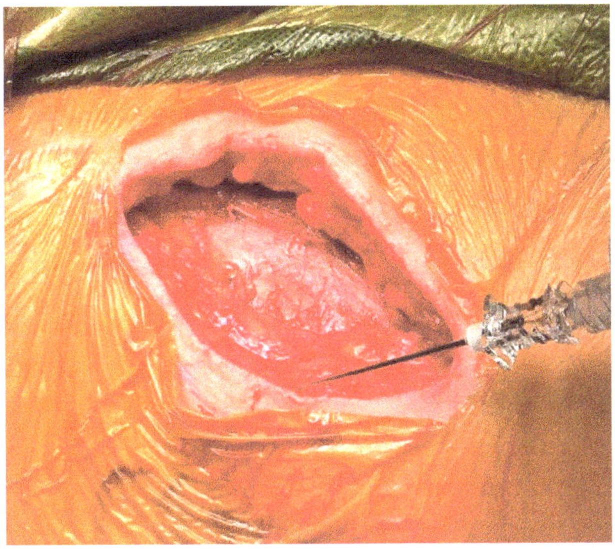

Figure 12. Photograph of the closed fascia of the tensor fasciae latae. A local anesthetic is injected into the subcutaneous layer.

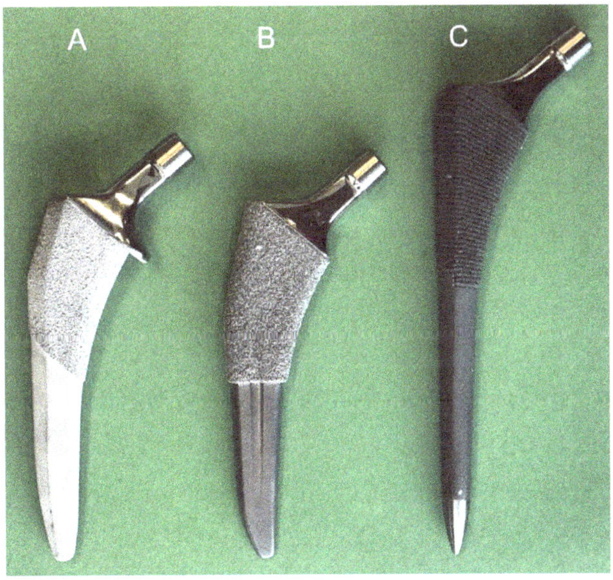

Figure 13. DePuy Synthes, Warsaw, IN, USA: (A) Medial collar and triple tapered ACTIS® Total Hip System. (B) Tapered-wedge TRI-LOCK® Bone Preservation Stem. (C) SUMMIT® Tapered Hip System.

with weight bearing can occur. The new stem designs often add a medial collar to augment primary stability for immediate weight bearing and reduced risk of subsidence (**Figure 13**).

To increase short and long-term stability, fully coated stems are preferred to achieve more reliable fixation. In addition, an overall more canal filling proximal stem design provides more proximal bone fixation compared to blade shaped medial-lateral implant fixation.

5. Standard table

Several advantages exist for the standard table in comparison to the Hana table. The ability to maneuver the legs allow for intraoperative assessment of leg length. The surgeon can directly manage the leg and no additional assistance is required to manage the table. In general, any operative table can be used that is radiolucent and allows for extension of the legs at the level of the hip joint. Regarding the surgical technique, there is no difference in the type of soft tissue releases between a standard or specialized table. The patient is positioned in a supine position with the hip joint at the level of the table break. It is necessary to hyperextend the operated hip during femoral preparation. Draping both lower extremities in a sterile fashion allows an intraoperative crossover of the operated leg for femoral exposure. The leg length discrepancy can be measured manually.

If an anterior retractor is used, the bone hook is inserted with the femur in neutral rotation. Afterward the leg is placed in a figure 4 position (external rotation) to release the medial capsule down to the lesser trochanter. There is no difference in the soft tissue release technique; however, the piriformis usually has to be released in heavy male patients. The distal part of the standard table is extended to 40° allowing hyperextension of the operated hip as well as adduction and external rotation while positioning the limb crossing under the contralateral side.

6. Outcome

Over the last couple of years, the anterior approach has become increasingly popular. Many advantages are described in comparison to the other approaches mentioned at the beginning of this chapter. Patients treated with the minimal invasive approach suffer less pain and consume fewer narcotics [25, 26]. This is usually explained by less soft-tissue damage while avoiding muscle splitting and detachment in comparison to the posterior or anterolateral approach.

An improved hip function and earlier return to normal gait are attributed to using an intermuscular and internervous interval [27, 28]. Rodriguez et al. have shown that patients reach certain milestones after an anterior THA earlier compared to a posterior THA. However, patients with a posterior approach had a similar result after 12 weeks [29].

The possibility of using intraoperative fluoroscopy when performing an anterior THA offers advantages over a posterior THA. The percentage of cup placed in the safe zone increases when using fluoroscopy routinely [6]. A higher precision and increased accuracy when implanting cup components can lead to a decreased dislocation rate [6, 21]. The anterior approach also improves relation of leg length and offset [7].

The majority of hip dislocations occur during the first 3 months after surgery. The healing of the posterior capsule and external rotator muscles release during a conventional posterior approach is considered the reason for early dislocation [30]. Hip precautions are recommended for 4–12 weeks to prevent any flexion and internal rotation after posterior THA [31].

The muscle sparing anterior approach avoids release of the piriformis and obturator externus tendon. No specific hip precautions are needed and the patient is able to return to his or her normal activities after surgery without limitations [32]. The dislocation rate for the anterior THA is described in literature ranges between 0.6 and 0.9% [20, 21]. It is lower in comparison to those reported for other approaches; however, comparative studies have failed to show a consistent benefit [33, 34]. The senior author has no reported dislocations at all after performing more than 500 THAs using an anterior approach.

7. Challenges with the anterior approach

Switching the surgical approach to an anterior THA is associated with a learning curve within the first 40–100 cases [35, 36]. Improvements in surgical and fluoroscopy times as well as differences in leg length have been reported during the learning curve [37, 38]. During the learning curve, it is recommended to carefully select patients. In general, preferred patients are thin and younger females with elongated femoral necks and a type B Dorr Femur.

The anterior approach has some specific complications. These include LFCN injury and greater trochanteric fracture. Injury of LFCN is most commonly encountered during exposure and retraction. The nerve is located in the intermuscular-internervous interval between the sartorius and tensor fasciae latae muscle and is at risk if the incision is extended distally. Its course varies in different branching patterns and is at risk in approximately one-third of the patients during an anterior approach [39]. The risk of an injury can be minimized when staying inside the tensor fascia rather than the interval between the tensor and sartorius muscle [40]. LCFN neurapraxia occurs in approximately 0–5% of patients [41, 42]. None of the patients experienced any hip-related functional limitations, while most symptoms resolving after 6–24 months [37, 43, 44].

Muscle damage has not been considered a major problem due to the intermuscular nature of the approach [45]. Nevertheless, incorrect placement or retraction may cause damage. During capsular exposure the rectus femoris muscle is elevated and at risk. Attention while placing the retractors or using specialized retractors developed for the anterior THA can reduce the risk of soft-tissue damage. During femoral exposure the tensor is at risk for injury as well.

Cup alignment is challenging when performing an anterior THA due to limited view of the anterior acetabular wall. When inserting the reamer into the acetabulum, the anterior aspect of the femur might block its entrance. This may lead to an anterior shift of the reamer and can violate the anterior wall. Careful retractor placement and use of intraoperative fluoroscopy can minimize the risk associated with reaming.

Fractures might occur during femoral preparation, while manipulating on a specialized table [20]. Aggressive extension and external rotation of the femur using the table can result in a fracture of the tip of the greater trochanter secondary to tension of the conjoined tendon. Calcar fractures are the results of medial force on the calcar during broaching and can be fixed with cerclages (**Figure 14**). A rare complication, which might only occur when using a specialized

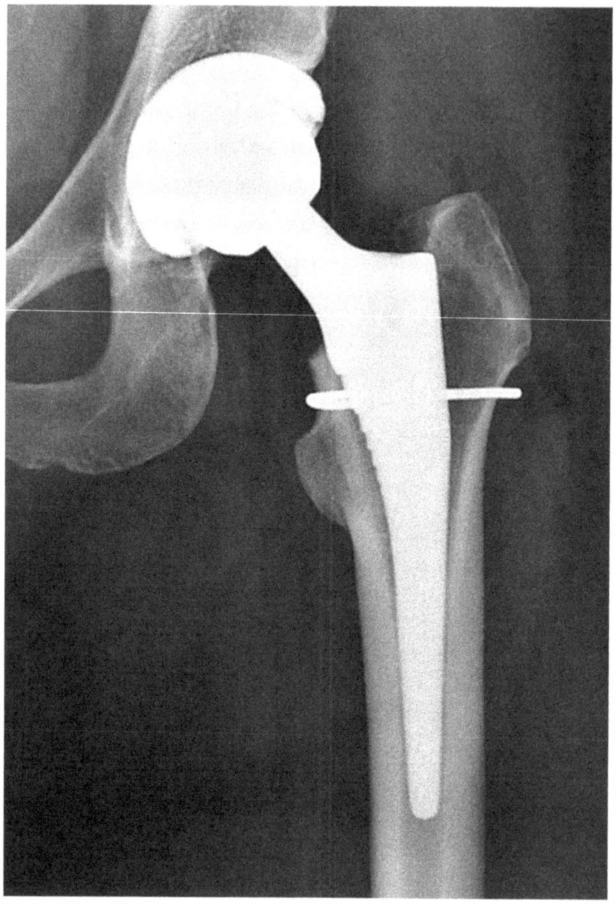

Figure 14. Intraoperative complication: calcar fracture fixed with two cerclages.

table, is a fracture of the ankle while performing external rotation in order to dislocate the operated hip. This is why close monitoring of the torque applied to the fixed leg is necessary.

In general, straight access to the femoral canal is limited in an anterior approach. The correct implant design and broaching instruments are essential and avoid malpositioning or fractures [46]. Perforation of the femur can occur when the direction of the femoral canal is not respected. The risk of postoperative complications in the hand of an experienced surgeon performing an anterior approach is comparable to other approaches.

The dislocation rate for the anterior THA is lower compared to the anterolateral and posterior approach [47]. Preserving the piriformis tendon, obturator externus tendon, and posterior capsule increases the stability when using the anterior approach. Therefore, the routine use of hip precautions for the anterior approach is not recommended [32].

The risk of postoperative hematoma can be minimized by routine exposure and proper ligation of the ascending branches of the lateral femoral circumflex vessels. The vessels are variable in number, location, and extend, but are usually found underneath the deep fascial layer of the tensor fasciae latae. At the end of the procedure, care should be taken for hemostasis. The risk of postoperative drainage can be reduced by meticulous capsular and tensor fasciae closure. Kasparek et al. describes the topical use of tranexamic acid (TXA) to reduce transfusion rates and increase postoperative Hb-levels [48]. For all patients undergoing anterior THA, intravenous TXA should be used as part of blood management. The location of the wound in the groin close to a natural skin fold can result in wound dehiscence and infections in patients with a larger soft tissue pannus overlaying the incision.

8. Conclusion

The popularity of the anterior approach has increased in the last decade. Its soft tissue sparing nature results in a faster recovery and a more stable hip joint. Postoperative precautions are not routinely applied. The use of intraoperative fluoroscopy has improved cup positioning and restoration of the leg length and offset.

Contribution statement

I attest to the fact that all authors have participated in the research, read the manuscript, attest to the validity and legitimacy of the data and its interpretation, and agree to its submission.

Author details

Ulrich Bechler, Bernhard Springer and Friedrich Boettner*

*Address all correspondence to: boettnerf@hss.edu

Adult Reconstruction and Joint Replacement Division, Hospital for Special Surgery, New York, NY, USA

References

[1] Berry DJ, Berger RA, Callaghan JJ, Dorr LD, Duwelius PJ, Hartzband MA, et al. Minimally invasive total hip arthroplasty. Development, early results, and a critical analysis. Presented at the Annual Meeting of the American Orthopaedic Association, Charleston, South Carolina, USA, June 14, 2003. The Journal of Bone and Joint Surgery. American Volume. 2003;**85-a**(11):2235-2246

[2] Woolson ST, Rahimtoola ZO. Risk factors for dislocation during the first 3 months after primary total hip replacement. The Journal of Arthroplasty. 1999;**14**(6):662-668

[3] L'Hommedieu CE, Gera JJ, Rupp G, Salin JW, Cox JS, Duwelius PJ. Impact of anterior vs posterior approach for total hip arthroplasty on post-acute care service utilization. The Journal of Arthroplasty. 2016;**31**(9 Suppl):73-77

[4] Kwon MS, Kuskowski M, Mulhall KJ, Macaulay W, Brown TE, Saleh KJ. Does surgical approach affect total hip arthroplasty dislocation rates? Clinical Orthopaedics and Related Research. 2006;**447**:34-38

[5] Lewinnek GE, Lewis JL, Tarr R, Compere CL, Zimmerman JR. Dislocations after total hip-replacement arthroplasties. The Journal of Bone and Joint Surgery. American Volume. 1978;**60**(2):217-220

[6] Boettner F, Zingg M, Emara AK, Waldstein W, Faschingbauer M, Kasparek MF. The accuracy of acetabular component position using a novel method to determine anteversion. The Journal of Arthroplasty. 2016;**32**(4):1180-1185

[7] Lin TJ, Bendich I, Ha AS, Keeney BJ, Moschetti WE, Tomek IM. A comparison of radiographic outcomes after total hip arthroplasty between the posterior approach and direct anterior approach with intraoperative fluoroscopy. The Journal of Arthroplasty. 2016

[8] Little NJ, Busch CA, Gallagher JA, Rorabeck CH, Bourne RB. Acetabular polyethylene wear and acetabular inclination and femoral offset. Clinical Orthopaedics and Related Research. 2009;**467**(11):2895-2900

[9] Malik A, Maheshwari A, Dorr LD. Impingement with total hip replacement. The Journal of Bone and Joint Surgery. American Volume. 2007;**89**(8):1832-1842

[10] Rathod PA, Bhalla S, Deshmukh AJ, Rodriguez JA. Does fluoroscopy with anterior hip arthroplasty decrease acetabular cup variability compared with a nonguided posterior approach? Clinical Orthopaedics and Related Research. 2014;**472**(6):1877-1885

[11] Hardinge K. The direct lateral approach to the hip. The Journal of Bone and Joint Surgery. British Volume. 1982;**64**(1):17-19

[12] Nakai T, Liu N, Fudo K, Mohri T, Kakiuchi M. Early complications of primary total hip arthroplasty in the supine position with a modified Watson-Jones anterolateral approach. Journal of Orthopaedics. 2014;**11**(4):166-169

[13] Hendel D, Yasin M, Garti A, Weisbort M, Beloosesky Y. Fracture of the greater trochanter during hip replacement: A retrospective analysis of 21/372 cases. Acta Orthopaedica Scandinavica. 2002;**73**(3):295-297

[14] Amlie E, Havelin LI, Furnes O, Baste V, Nordsletten L, Hovik O, et al. Worse patient-reported outcome after lateral approach than after anterior and posterolateral approach in primary hip arthroplasty. A cross-sectional questionnaire study of 1,476 patients 1-3 years after surgery. Acta Orthopaedica. 2014;**85**(5):463-469

[15] Sueyoshi T, Meding JB, Davis KE, Lackey WG, Malinzak RA, Ritter MA. Clinical predictors for possible failure after total hip arthroplasty. Hip International: The Journal of Clinical and Experimental Research on Hip Pathology and Therapy. 2016;**26**(6):531-536

[16] Smith-Petersen MN. Approach to and exposure of the hip joint for mold arthroplasty. The Journal of Bone and Joint Surgery. American Volume. 1949;**31a**(1):40-46

[17] Wagner H. Surface replacement arthroplasty of the hip. Clinical Orthopaedics and Related Research. 1978;**134**:102-130

[18] Berger RA. Total hip arthroplasty using the minimally invasive two-incision approach. Clinical Orthopaedics and Related Research. 2003;**417**:232-241

[19] Desser DR, Mitrick MF, Ulrich SD, Delanois RE, Mont MA. Total hip arthroplasty: Comparison of two-incision and standard techniques at an AOA-accredited community hospital. The Journal of the American Osteopathic Association. 2010;**110**(1):12-15

[20] Matta JM, Shahrdar C, Ferguson T. Single-incision anterior approach for total hip arthroplasty on an orthopaedic table. Clinical Orthopaedics and Related Research. 2005;**441**:115-124

[21] Siguier T, Siguier M, Brumpt B. Mini-incision anterior approach does not increase dislocation rate: A study of 1037 total hip replacements. Clinical Orthopaedics and Related Research. 2004;**426**:164-173

[22] Unger AS, Stronach BM, Bergin PF, Nogler M. Direct anterior total hip arthroplasty. Instructional Course Lectures. 2014;**63**:227-238

[23] McLaughlin JR, Lee KR. Long-term results of uncemented total hip arthroplasty with the Taperloc femoral component in patients with Dorr type C proximal femoral morphology. The Bone & Joint Journal. 2016;**98-b**(5):595-600

[24] Zingg M, Boudabbous S, Hannouche D, Montet X, Boettner F. Standardized fluoroscopy-based technique to measure intraoperative cup anteversion. Journal of Orthopaedic Research: Official Publication of the Orthopaedic Research Society. 2017;**35**(10):2307-2312

[25] Alecci V, Valente M, Crucil M, Minerva M, Pellegrino CM, Sabbadini DD. Comparison of primary total hip replacements performed with a direct anterior approach versus the standard lateral approach: Perioperative findings. Journal of Orthopaedics and Traumatology: Official Journal of the Italian Society of Orthopaedics and Traumatology. 2011;**12**(3):123-129

[26] Miller LE, Gondusky JS, Bhattacharyya S, Kamath AF, Boettner F, Wright J. Does surgical approach affect outcomes in total hip arthroplasty through 90 days of follow-up? A systematic review with meta-analysis. The Journal of Arthroplasty. 2017;**33**(4):1296-1302

[27] Mayr E, Nogler M, Benedetti MG, Kessler O, Reinthaler A, Krismer M, et al. A prospective randomized assessment of earlier functional recovery in THA patients treated by minimally invasive direct anterior approach: A gait analysis study. Clinical Biomechanics. 2009;**24**(10):812-818

[28] Nakata K, Nishikawa M, Yamamoto K, Hirota S, Yoshikawa H. A clinical comparative study of the direct anterior with mini-posterior approach: Two consecutive series. The Journal of Arthroplasty. 2009;**24**(5):698-704

[29] Rodriguez JA, Deshmukh AJ, Rathod PA, Greiz ML, Deshmane PP, Hepinstall MS, et al. Does the direct anterior approach in THA offer faster rehabilitation and compa-

rable safety to the posterior approach? Clinical Orthopaedics and Related Research. 2014;**472**(2):455-463

[30] Prietzel T, Hammer N, Schleifenbaum S, Adler D, Pretzsch M, Kohler L, et al. The impact of capsular repair on the dislocation rate after primary total hip arthroplasty: A retrospective analysis of 1972 cases. Zeitschrift für Orthopädie und Unfallchirurgie. 2014;**152**(2):130-143

[31] Schmidt-Braekling T, Waldstein W, Akalin E, Benavente P, Frykberg B, Boettner F. Minimal invasive posterior total hip arthroplasty: Are 6 weeks of hip precautions really necessary? Archives of Orthopaedic and Trauma Surgery. 2015;**135**(2):271-274

[32] Restrepo C, Mortazavi SM, Brothers J, Parvizi J, Rothman RH. Hip dislocation: Are hip precautions necessary in anterior approaches? Clinical Orthopaedics and Related Research. 2011;**469**(2):417-422

[33] Maratt JD, Gagnier JJ, Butler PD, Hallstrom BR, Urquhart AG, Roberts KC. No difference in dislocation seen in anterior vs posterior approach total hip arthroplasty. The Journal of Arthroplasty. 2016;**31**(9 Suppl):127-130

[34] Tamaki T, Oinuma K, Miura Y, Higashi H, Kaneyama R, Shiratsuchi H. Epidemiology of dislocation following direct anterior total hip arthroplasty: A minimum 5-year follow-up study. The Journal of Arthroplasty. 2016;**31**(12):2886-2888

[35] de Steiger RN, Lorimer M, Solomon M. What is the learning curve for the anterior approach for total hip arthroplasty? Clinical Orthopaedics and Related Research. 2015;**473**(12):3860-3866

[36] Goytia RN, Jones LC, Hungerford MW. Learning curve for the anterior approach total hip arthroplasty. Journal of Surgical Orthopaedic Advances. 2012;**21**(2):78-83

[37] Seng BE, Berend KR, Ajluni AF, Lombardi AV Jr. Anterior-supine minimally invasive total hip arthroplasty: Defining the learning curve. The Orthopedic Clinics of North America. 2009;**40**(3):343-350

[38] Masonis J, Thompson C, Odum S. Safe and accurate: Learning the direct anterior total hip arthroplasty. Orthopedics. 2008;**31**(12 Suppl 2):129-143

[39] Rudin D, Manestar M, Ullrich O, Erhardt J, Grob K. The anatomical course of the lateral femoral cutaneous nerve with special attention to the anterior approach to the hip joint. The Journal of Bone and Joint Surgery. American Volume. 2016;**98**(7):561-567

[40] Homma Y, Baba T, Kobayashi H, Desroches A, Ozaki Y, Ochi H, et al. Safety in early experience with a direct anterior approach using fluoroscopic guidance with manual leg control for primary total hip arthroplasty: A consecutive one hundred and twenty case series. International Orthopaedics. 2016;**40**(12):2487-2494

[41] Lovell TP. Single-incision direct anterior approach for total hip arthroplasty using a standard operating table. The Journal of Arthroplasty. 2008;**23**(7 Suppl):64-68

[42] Restrepo C, Parvizi J, Pour AE, Hozack WJ. Prospective randomized study of two surgical approaches for total hip arthroplasty. The Journal of Arthroplasty. 2010;**25**(5):671.e1-679.e1

[43] Bhargava T, Goytia RN, Jones LC, Hungerford MW. Lateral femoral cutaneous nerve impairment after direct anterior approach for total hip arthroplasty. Orthopedics. 2010;**33**(7):472

[44] Goulding K, Beaule PE, Kim PR, Fazekas A. Incidence of lateral femoral cutaneous nerve neuropraxia after anterior approach hip arthroplasty. Clinical Orthopaedics and Related Research. 2010;**468**(9):2397-2404

[45] Agten CA, Sutter R, Dora C, Pfirrmann CW. MR imaging of soft tissue alterations after total hip arthroplasty: Comparison of classic surgical approaches. European Radiology. 2017;**27**(3):1312-1321

[46] Homma Y, Baba T, Ochi H, Ozaki Y, Kobayashi H, Matsumoto M, et al. Greater trochanter chip fractures in the direct anterior approach for total hip arthroplasty. European Journal of Orthopaedic Surgery & Traumatology: Orthopedie Traumatologie. 2016;**26**(6):605-611

[47] Higgins BT, Barlow DR, Heagerty NE, Lin TJ. Anterior vs. posterior approach for total hip arthroplasty, a systematic review and meta-analysis. The Journal of Arthroplasty. 2015;**30**(3):419-434

[48] Kasparek MF, Faschingbauer M, Waldstein W, Boettner CS, Boettner F. Topical tranexamic acid is equivalent to targeted preoperative autologous blood donation in total hip arthroplasty. The Journal of Arthroplasty. 2016;**32**(4):1176-1179

2

The Current Trend of Total Ankle Replacement

Binghua Zhou and Kanglai Tang

Abstract

Total ankle replacement (TAR) was introduced for end-stage arthritis of the ankle joint in the 1970s. TAR is becoming the modality of choice and offers better mobility, improved gait, and reduces the development of subsequent subtalar joint arthritis when compared with ankle arthrodesis. To maintain the longest function of ankle replacements, the design of the prosthesis should allow for smooth and continuous interaction and normal gait. Improved operative techniques, the surgeon's experience, as well as appropriate patient selection can anticipate better outcomes. Deformities of the ankle and foot should be corrected before TAR is performed. Despite the functional limitations following the revision of TAR, the revision still offers a cost-effective alternative to ankle arthrodesis. The decision to treat with TAR depends on the surgeon's technique, as well as on the patient's condition.

Keywords: Ankle, Prosthesis, Kinematics, Replacement, Complication

1. Introduction

1.1. Back ground and history

Total ankle replacement (TAR) was introduced for end-stage arthritis of the ankle joint in the 1970s. Initial poor clinical results due to imperfect prosthesis design and our incomplete knowledge of the biomechanics of the foot and ankle limited the using of TAR. Despite high numbers of failures in early generations of ankle prostheses, there has been a continued and increasing interest in TAR for end-stage arthritis. Nowadays, scientists are working on fourth-generation ankle prostheses, which are characterized by three-part, mobile-bearing, uncemented design. The STARTM ankle prosthesis was one of these fourth-generation ankle prostheses, which was approved for use by the United States Food and Drug Administration (FDA) in May 2009. The clinical outcomes of TAR have been increasing in terms of progress.

Newer studies suggested that implant survival rates were 70% to 95% during follow-up periods that ranged from 2 to 12 years. TAR is increasingly used as an alternative to arthrodesis.

The ankle joint is subjected to more weight-bearing force per square centimeter and is more commonly injured than any other joint in the body. Approximately 6% to 13% of all cases of osteoarthritis (OA) involve the ankle joint. While the incidence of severe ankle arthritis is clearly less than that of the hip or knee, OA of the ankle is a main cause of disability, which impairs functional mobility and leads to poor quality of life. Unlike the hip and knee joints, in which the primary causes of degeneration are primary OA and inflammatory diseases, 70–80% of ankle arthritis is post-traumatic and the remaining cases are related to primary OA and rheumatoid arthritis [1, 2, 3].

The treatment options for severe ankle arthritis have changed during the past 10 to 15 years. Currently, treatment options include ankle arthrodesis and TAR. There remains considerable controversy surrounding the benefits of each procedure and treatment option, especially concerning the idea that patients might benefit from one approach more than the other. TAR has some disadvantages such as expensive cost, implant loosening, ankle instability, higher infection rate, and higher re-operation rate [6–9]. TAR remains a less satisfactory solution when compared to other joint replacements; however, TAR offers greater range of motion in the ankle with improved gait kinematics, reduced stress, and potentially causes less arthritis in adjacent joints [3]. In addition, with regards to cost-effectiveness analysis, TAR has better quality-adjusted life years when compared to arthrodesis, albeit at a higher cost [10].

In this chart, we will introduce the decision-making process of whether to use TAR or arthrodesis, as well as discuss the history of TAR, the characteristics of different prosthesis designs, their clinical outcome, and the complications and revisions associated with TAR.

2. Prosthesis design

Lord and Marotte introduced an inverted hip prosthesis as a disappointing solution for ankle replacement in 1970 [4]. The original first-generation TAP was non-anatomical, cemented, and restrictive. It is not surprising then that the original first-generation TAP prostheses are associated with severe osteolysis, component loosening, impingement, infection, and soft-tissue breakdown; this has led many surgeons to discredit this procedure. For these reasons, there has been a continuous effort to develop a safe, stable, and long-lasting ankle prosthesis that could replicate the complex anatomy of the ankle joint and better mimic ankle biomechanics.

Implant design played a large role in the effect of loading direction on the magnitude and direction of the joint's motion. Bone–implant displacements occurred along the directions expected on the basis of the implant interface geometries. Various ankle designs are available, including two-component and three-component systems [5]. After unacceptably high failure rates had been published for the first generation of implants [1–5], the second generation of implants achieved marked improvements in clinical outcomes [6–8]. Second- and third-generation prostheses followed these first implants, and interest in this procedure has resurged in the past decade. These new designs include changes in the geometry and design of the components, as well as the use or non-use of polymethylmethacrylate bone cement, which is termed a two- or three-component design. The third-generation prosthesis is characterized by the non-use of cement, accurate anatomy, and better ROM of the ankle joint. Mobile-bearing implants are designed without constraint to reduce meniscal wear and to increase the longevity of the implant, which features mobile PE inlays. The stability of the bone–implant interface has been explored in an unconstrained, three-piece mobile-bearing implant using the concepts of implant migration and inducible displacement. Fixed-bearing designs, in contrast, are designed to increase stability, reduce micromotion at the bone–implant interface, and decrease bearing dislocation. In addition, the surgical instrumentation and technique are improved and redesigned for the new prosthesis.

The third-generation of ankle prostheses includes the HINTEGRA ankle (New deal, Lyon, France/Integra, Plainsboro, NJ, USA), the INBONE TAR implant (Wright Medical Technology, Arlington, TN, USA), the Agility prosthesis (DePuy Orthopaedic, Warsaw, IN, USA), the STAR prosthesis (Scandinavian TAR), the Mobility prosthesis (DePuy, Leeds, United Kingdom), and the Salto Talaris (Tornier, Edina, MN, USA).

2.1. HINTEGRA ankle prosthesis

The HINTEGRA prosthesis is a three-component, mobile-bearing ankle replacement with cobalt–chromium tibial and talar components [6]. The polyethylene mobile-bearing element provides axial rotation, physiological flexion, and extension mobility, and it also provides inversion and eversion stability [7, 8]. The HINTEGRA, which is a flat, anatomically shaped component, fully contacts the resected area with fixation of its tibial component. All inserted components have locking pegs on the talar component. The tibial component consists of a flat tray with raised spikes for bone fixation. The anterior side has a flange with holes for screw fixation. The talar component has medial and lateral walls and two fixation pegs; two screws may be used for added fixation, if appropriate. The ingrowth surface is plasma-sprayed titanium with a hydroxyapatite coat [9, 10]. Therefore, the HINTEGRA ankle prosthesis may be used for the treatment of major coronal plane deformities and as a salvage of failed ankle replacements.

2.2. INBONE ankle prosthesis

Amongst the third-generation ankle implants approved by the US FDA, the INBONE TAR implant employs a fixed-bearing design with a modular stem system for both the tibial and the talar components. The INBONE system features a technique that offers potential advantages in improved stem fixation and a unique intramedullary alignment system. It has a broader polyethylene component that conforms to the saddle ankle geometry, and it also provides a large surface area that spreads out stress gradients, leading to possible decreased wear [11]. A. Datir found that only the lateral talar component angle and the mean difference between the pre- and postoperative tibial slope had significant correlations with postsurgical outcomes in INBONE ankle replacement [11].

2.3. Agility ankle prosthesis

The Agility TAR System, which is almost exclusively without polymethylmethacrylate cement fixation, was the most commonly used implant in the United States from 1998 to 2007. The design process started in 1978, with prototype completion and cadaver implantation occurring in 1981 [12, 13]. It was first implanted in a patient in 1985 and subsequently marketed in 1992 as the "DePuy Alvine Total Ankle Prosthesis". From 1985 to 2007, the implant went through a total of four generations and seven phases of implant improvement [13, 14]. The US FDA has cleared it for use only with polymethylmethacrylate cement fixation [15]. The Agility prosthesis is a semi-constrained ankle replacement with a cobalt–chromium talar component, a titanium tibial component, and a fixed polyethylene bearing [16]. It is characterized by a tibial component, which provides a talar component with a larger surface area. The talar component of the Agility system was prone to shift forward and backward along the talar groove during plantar flexion–dorsiflexion loading, and it would also rock about its long axis in inversion–eversion loading. The ingrowth surface consists of cobalt–chromium sintered beads. Fixation on the tibial side is aided by syndesmotic arthrodesis. Fixation on the talar side is achieved with the use of a keel under a flat-cut component.

2.4. STAR ankle prosthesis

The STARTM ankle was first approved by the US FDA in 1998 [17]. It was a three-part, mobile-bearing, uncemented ankle replacement. The STAR prosthesis featured a cementless design with a plasma-sprayed titanium coat [18]. Fixation on the tibia was achieved with use of two barrels on the flat tibial component. The talar component was fixed with the use of two sidewalls and a fin on the inferior surface. The tibial component of the STAR was most susceptible to normal motion on the bone surface, especially in plantar flexion–dorsiflexion and inversion–eversion loading. On average, of the three loading directions, the internal–external rotation resulted in the smallest relative motions of both of the STAR components since the device allowed for unconstrained rotation about this axis [19].

2.5. Mobility ankle prosthesis

The Mobility prosthesis is a mobile-bearing ankle replacement with cobalt–chromium components on the tibial and talar sides, and it also features a sintered bead ingrowth surface [20]. The tibial component has a stem placed into the tibia with an anterior bone window. The talar component has two fins on the inferior surface; no sidewalls are present on the talar component. The talar cut has three surfaces. The prosthesis has not undergone design changes during the course of the study.

2.6. Salto Talaris Ankle prosthesis

The Salto Talaris TAP, with design and instrumentation based on the Salto mobile-bearing TAP, was approved for use by the US FDA in 2006. Although it is a fixed-bearing device, the instrumentation and component trialing incorporate a rotationally mobile tibial trial component that allows for self-alignment on the resected surface of the distal aspect of the tibia, which is determined by the talar component. The final implant has a polyethylene insert that is rigidly fixed to the tibial component and does not allow for rotational or translational motion between the two surfaces.

3. Kinematics

Normal ankle kinematics attenuates ground reaction impact forces and impact loading on the subtalar joint. The importance of achieving normal ankle kinematics during stance is very important for both function of the ankle and long survivorship of the prosthesis. During a normal gait cycle, the talus has a continuously changing axis of rotation against the tibia as well as a gliding motion against the calcaneus, respectively. The talus and mortise widen slightly anatomically from posterior to anterior. Following talus plantar flexion, the narrowest portion of the talus sits in the ankle mortise and allows for rotational movement between the talus and mortise. When the talus is maximally dorsiflexed, the wider portion of the talar articular surface locks into the ankle mortise, allowing for little or no rotation between the talus and the mortise [21, 22].

Compared to a normal ankle, ankle OA shows a significant deficiency in triplanar ankle movement, the second active maximal vertical and maximal medial ground reaction force, sagittal and transverse ankle joint moments, and ankle joint power [2]. However, J.F. Baumhauer reported that ankle arthrodesis results in a normal gait postoperatively, especially when there is a normal subtalar joint and talonavicular joint [23].

S. Singer reported that TAR with first-generation TAP resulted in increasingly normal gait mechanics during sagittal joint motion, which was maintained, and it also resulted in more normal ankle kinematics when compared with those following arthrodesis [24]. The gait patterns of TAR with the third-ankle prosthesis more closely resembled normal gait during sagittal plane motion and dorsiflexion, and it also resulted in a normal range of tibial tilt when compared with the gait patterns of patients following arthrodesis [24]. Peak plantar flexor moment increased in arthrodesis patients and decreased in TAR patients. TAR appears to regain more natural ankle joint function. R.M. Queen compared the kinetics of TAR with that of the INBONETM or Salto Talaris, as well as that of the normal contralateral ankle in bilateral patients; the results showed that walking speed, step time, step and stride length, and propulsion ground reaction forces improved following TAR. However, peak dorsiflexion did not change. At the same time, the dorsiflexion angle during heel strike was increased on the nonsurgical side [25].

A. Rosello Anon et al. reported that kinetic gait parameters were similar to those of a healthy ankle following TAR with HINTEGRA [26]. M.E. Hahn reported that both arthrodesis and TAR patients were similar in terms of demographics and anthropometrics. Neither group increased their average daily step count [27]. Gait patterns in both treatment groups were not completely normalized [24]; however, both treatment groups did not exhibit equivalent to normal plantar flexion motion, ankle moments, and power when compared with the normal group. Further investigation is needed to determine why patients who have undergone TAR do not use the plantar flexion motion in the terminal-stance phase, as well as to explain the limited increase in power generation at toe-off after replacement [24].

In addition, walking speed, step, and stride length improves from the preoperative phase to each postoperative time point. Peak dorsiflexion did not changed over time or between sides; however, the dorsiflexion angle during heel strike was increased on the nonsurgical side. Peak plantar flexion moment, stance, step time, weight acceptance, and propulsion ground reaction forces improved from the preoperative period to 1 year postsurgery on the surgical side. These results indicated that fixed-bearing TAR was effective at improving gait mechanics in patients with painful end-stage ankle arthritis. In addition, TAR resulted in the maintenance of ankle dorsiflexion during the stance phase; however, a decrease in dorsiflexion angle was present during heel strike on the operative side when compared with the nonoperative side up to 2 years following TAR. Finally, following TAR, the asymmetry in temporal gait variables and peak plantar flexion moment were improved, although differences did remain between the operative and nonoperative limbs for stance, step, and swing time, as well as for the peak plantar flexion moment 2 years following TAR. This remaining gait asymmetry is of potential concern because of the possibility that the patient might overload the contralateral limb and engage compensatory walking mechanics that could lead to secondary injuries following TAR [25].

4. Indication and contraindication

If adequate conservative measures for the treatment of end-stage ankle osteoarthritis have failed, surgery may be taken into consideration. M.R. McGuire reported that TAR is indicated in rheumatoid patients with severe ankle involvement who have not responded to medical management. TAR is especially suitable for those patients who will place minimal stress on the ankle, those for whom no destruction of the hip or knee joint is found, and for those who are 65 years of age or older. The elderly may not tolerate the prolonged immobilization or repeated operations that arthrodesis may require. TAR should not be used in young patients with post-traumatic arthritis [28]. J.R. Ramaskandhan found that early outcomes following TAR for patients with post-traumatic OA are comparable with those for patients with OA and rheumatoid arthritis [29]. More importantly, patients whose lifestyle or employment requires them to walk down ramps may have an advantage with TAR when compared with an arthrodesis. In addition, I. Hetsroni reported that TAR has better quality-adjusted life years when compared to arthrodesis, albeit at a higher cost [10].

TAR improves clinical and functional outcomes independent of preoperative tibiotalar alignment when postoperative alignment is restored to neutral at the time of replacement. Therefore, one of the keys to success may be to achieve coronal plane balance by performing additional osseous and soft- tissue procedures in patients with coronal plane deformity [30]. Preoperative talar varus deformity increases the technical difficulty of TAR and is associated with an increased failure rate. Deformity of >20° has been reported to be a contraindication to replacement. T. Trajkovski determined whether clinical outcomes of TAR in patients with ankle arthritis and a preoperative talar varus deformity of 10° were comparable with those of patients with a varus deformity of <10°. Satisfactory results can be achieved in patients with varus malalignment of 10°, which should not be considered a contraindication to TAR [31].

With the population ageing, the absolute number of patients affected by ankle OA is likely to increase, which means that there are more and more potential candidates for TAR. For this reason, there is a trend of increasing indications; as such, clinical guidelines regarding implant migration must be established to ensure successful outcomes [3]. On the other hand, some patients might be younger and have higher physical demands, placing the damaged joint under increased stress [32]. Based on this, young age and high physical demand are currently considered contraindications for TAR.

Taking into account numerous individual criteria, the most appropriate indication substantially influences the outcome of patients with end-stage ankle arthritis who are treated by ankle TAR.

5. Technique of TAR

We present a typical case who underwent TAR. She was a 59-years-old woman and had a severe pain on her left ankle. She failed to respond to a trial of conservative treatment for ≥6 months.

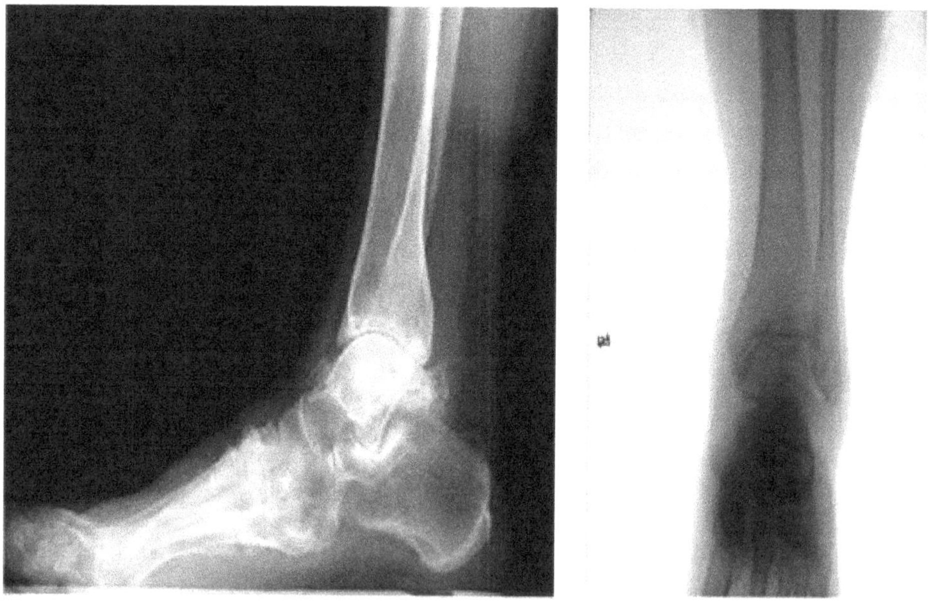

Figure 1. The preoperative X ray images showed a severe osteoarthritis in the left ankle.

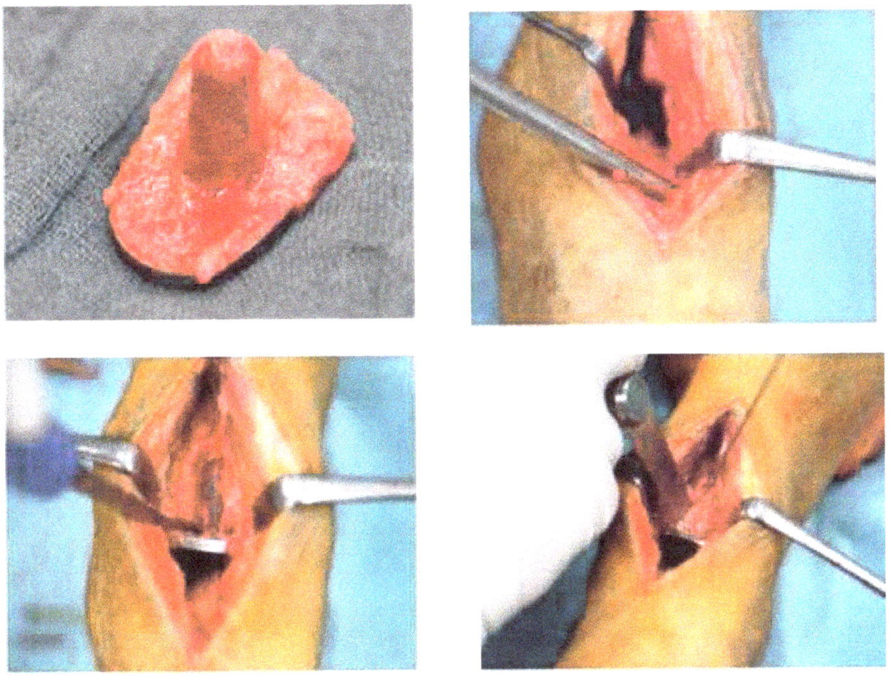

Figure 2. The picture showed incision and the osteotomy.

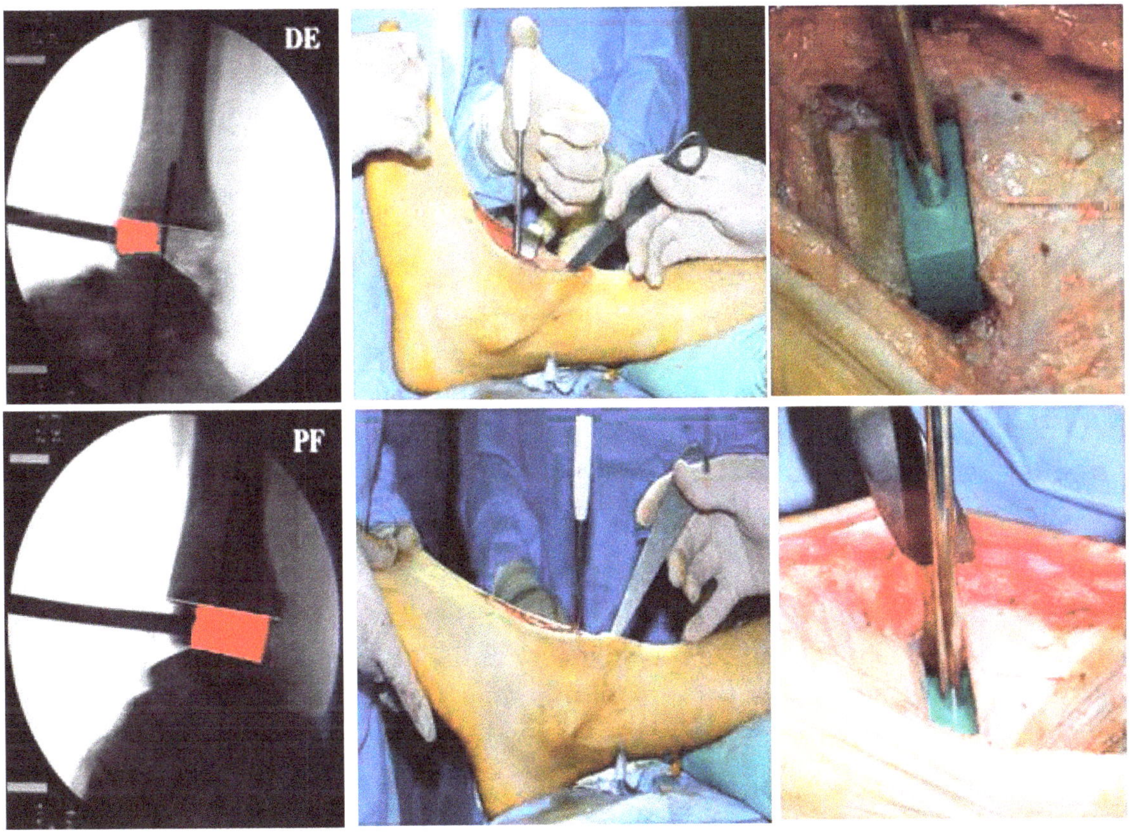

Figure 3. The pictures showed that the ankle joint is in a good alignment with the template.

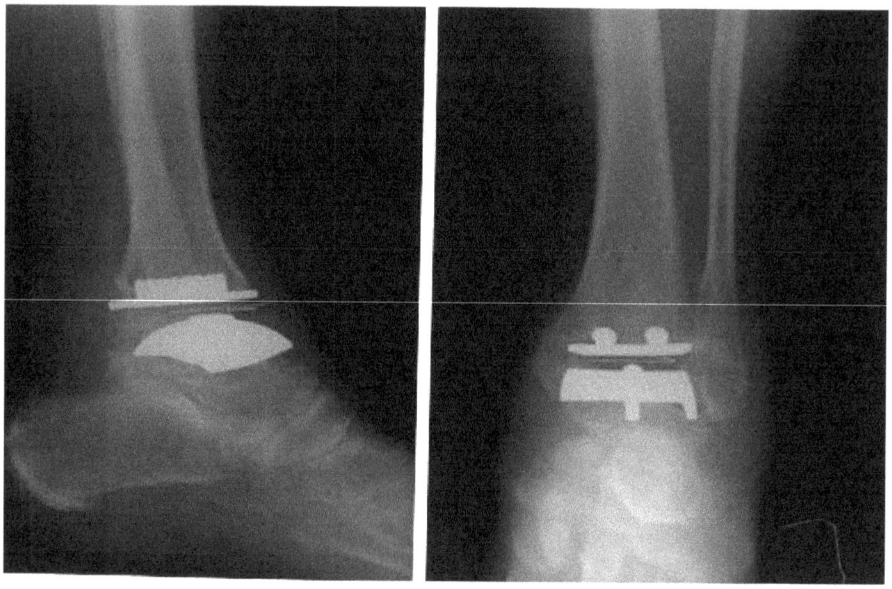

Figure 4. The pictures showed the X rays image of ankle joint after TAR 2 years postoperatively.

6. Outcomes of TAR

Modern TAR systems have either a fixed-bearing or a mobile-bearing design. In the United States, fixed-bearing, two-component designs are more commonly used. S. Noelle reported that STAR prostheses achieved a high satisfaction rate following TAR, and exhibited clear pain relief in patients between March 2005 and May 2010 [33]. J.R. Jastifer reported that the overall implant survival of STAR prosthesis was 94.4% at a minimum of 10 years of follow-up. A total of 39% of patients required additional surgical procedures, most of which were performed more than 9 years postoperatively, and one patient required a revision of the prosthesis. Preoperative VAS pain scale scores, Mean Buechel–Pappas Scale scores, and mean AOFAS Ankle–Hindfoot Scale scores improved from 8.1 to 2.1, from 32.8 to 82.1, and from 32.8 to 78.1 at the latest follow-up, respectively. All patients reported their outcomes as good or excellent. In the current cohort of STAR ankle patients, implant survival, patient satisfaction, pain relief, and function ratings were high. However, the rate of additional procedures was also high, which highlights the need for patient follow-up and additional long-term outcome studies on TAR [17].

Early clinical results indicate that the Salto Talaris fixed-bearing TAR system can provide significant improvements in terms of pain, quality of life, and standard functional measures in patients with end-stage ankle arthritis [34]. Implant survival at a mean follow-up time of 2.8 years was 96% when metallic component revision, removal, or impending failure was used as the endpoint. For the Salto Talaris total ankle implant, a high incidence of bony overgrowth occurs at the margins of the tibial tray. The frequency and amount of overgrowth were directly related to the amount of cortical coverage at the bone–implant interface [35]. Patients who underwent TAR with the INBONETM or Salto Talaris prosthesis demonstrated that they were able to walk faster, and they also exhibited an improvement in gait symmetry. However, this improvement did not appear to return the patient to a symmetric walking pattern by 2 years post-TAR [25].

The Agility prosthesis typically exhibited greater relative motion than did the STAR, with significant differences observed for both the tibial component in inversion–eversion rotation and for the talar component in internal–external rotation. The magnitudes of the relative motions were affected by the loading direction and compression. The motion magnitudes were quite large, with values exceeding 1, 000 mm for the Agility talar component in plantar flexion–dorsiflexion and in inversion–eversion. Large motions at the bone–implant interface, resulting from weak initial fixation, may inhibit implant osseointegration early in the healing process, and it may also contribute to the overall likelihood of implant failure resulting from aseptic loosening [19].

The overall survival rates of the HINTEGRA implant were 94% and 84% after 5 and 10 years, respectively. The mid-term survivorship of the HINTEGRA implant was comparable with that of other third-generation TARs [36]. The mid-term to long-term survivorship of a TAR in which a HINTEGRA implant was used is promising, and it is in agreement with the survivorship findings for other third-generation total ankle implants. There were no polyethylene failures and amputations. The generation category of the prosthesis, the cause of ankle OA, and the age of the patient were identified as independent risk factors for prosthesis failure.

There is a concern that placing a TAP in the setting of a fused hindfoot will create abnormal stresses on the ankle joint and will thus lead to increased early wear or degeneration of the implant. Ipsilateral hindfoot arthrodesis in combination with TAR may diminish functional outcome and prosthesis survivorship when compared to isolated TAR. J.S. Lewis reported that TAR with the STAR performed with ipsilateral hindfoot arthrodesis resulted in significant improvements in pain and functional outcomes, which was in contrast to prior studies; however, overall outcomes were inferior to those observed for isolated TAR [37]. The authors of this study have speculated that the mobile-bearing design may play an important role in the transfer of rotational movement from the tibia into calcaneal inversion/eversion in patients with a fused hindfoot [37].

Future work could examine the effect of normalizing gait asymmetry on long-term outcomes following TAR. Additional work should focus on gait changes following TAR, as well as on gait symmetry results when comparing fixed and mobile-bearing implants to better assess the overall viability of modern TAR prostheses as a long-term solution for the treatment of severe, painful ankle OA.

7. Complications

The first- and second-generation ankle prostheses were cemented and constrained, which led to higher failure rates [11, 12]. With continuously improving design and fewer constraints, third-generation ankle implants are increasingly favored; however, the technical demands of

TAR are substantial. There are still some complications that the surgeon should treat carefully. The recorded complication rate of TAR was 23%, while intraoperative bone fracture and wound healing had a failure rate of at least 50% [38]. The short-term complications of TAR included intraoperative malleolar fractures and skin necrosis. The mid-term clinical outcomes showed a 41% complication rate including instability, infections, subtalar arthritis, malalignment, and one tibial bone cyst, which led to the need for subsequent surgery. Adequate patient selection and a thorough knowledge of associated complications are mandatory to reduce the number of complications and increase the rates of ankle replacement survivorship [39, 40].

M.A. Glazebrook classified the complications following TAR into three tiers: high-grade, medium-grade, and low-grade. High-grade complications result in a greater than 50% failure rate in TAR, including deep infection, aseptic loosening, and implant failure. Medium-grade complications are defined as technical error, subsidence, and postoperative bone fracture. Finally, low-grade complications are defined as intraoperative bone fractures and wound healing problems, which should be considered [41]. Recently, R.J. Gad thought that the three-grade classification system of complications did not reliably reflect practitioners' experiences, and they thus categorized complications as either high or low risk for the early failure of TAR [38].

7.1. Loosening of the prosthesis

Initial clinical results were poor, largely because of early loosening [42, 43]. Aseptic loosening is the predominant failure mechanism in TAR; in fact, A. Henricson reported that about 40% of revision cases are due to aseptic loosening [44]. Primary stability may be affected by the initial implant fixation; in addition, known uncemented talar designs rely on bone ingrowth for fixation, which requires minimal relative motion between the implant and the host bone.

The greater magnitudes of relative motion in the Agility prosthesis suggest that primary instability of the implant may contribute to its higher clinically observed aseptic loosening rate. However, large motions at the bone–implant interface, resulting from a weak initial fixation, may inhibit implant osseointegration early in the healing process and contribute to the overall likelihood of failure resulting from aseptic loosening [19]. Future TAR designs will require better fixation to improve outcomes.

Implant migration is a good clinical evaluation tool for the loosening of prosthesis following TAR. Implant migration was defined as a change in implant location from the immediate postoperative radiograph. J.W.-Y. Fong designed a radiostereometric analysis marker insertion protocol to evaluate the stability of the migration of a fixed-bearing design following TAR [45]. The results showed that the migration of a fixed-bearing design was within the normal range.

S.A. Brigido presented a measurement technique to assess implant migration, which was supported by the high level of inter-rater reliability and intraclass correlation. The results showed that the mean INBONETM implant migration was 0.7 mm at 1 year and 1.0 mm at 2 years. Time and sex were significant predictors of implant migration [3].

Although talar subsidence and migration are recognized complications, empirical observations of postoperative patients with a Salto Talaris ankle replacement have suggested a high rate of posterior bony overhang and resultant overgrowth. In addition, it has been noted that a relatively high percentage of these implants were inserted at an angle other than perpendicular to the anatomic axis of the tibia. Specifically, the implants were usually placed in varus and with a positive slope [35].

7.2. Periprosthetic fracture

Inlay fractures are relatively common, which indicates potential for the improvement of implants. The documentation of intraoperative surgical errors leading to revision surgery varies significantly among registers [46]. The results of the present study indicate a high incidence of hypertrophic bone proliferation when the dimensions of the tibial component do not match the anteroposterior depth of the tibia at the plane of resection. Despite the high occurrence rate, the clinical relevance of hypertrophic bone is obscure. After insertion, the position of the components is not expected to change. Disruption of the extraosseous talar blood supply at the time of ankle replacement may be a factor contributing to talar component subsidence—a common mechanism of early failure following ankle replacement [39].

The stable biological coating of prosthesis components and high initial structural stability is critical for successful TAR. Continuing observation of patients who have undergone TAR is warranted for the purpose of conducting long-term analysis of prosthesis failures in order to improve the outcomes associated with this surgical technique.

7.3. Infection

Deep infection rates following TAR have been reported to be as high as 4.6% [47]. M.S. Myerson retrospectively reported on the patient- and prosthesis-associated demographics of infected TAR and the outcomes following treatment. The results showed that the treatment of deep infections following TAR is dependent on an accurate and timely diagnosis. A more uniform diagnostic approach, including immediate ankle joint aspiration and the evaluation of inflammatory markers before starting antibiotics, may allow for early surgical intervention, as well as for improved monitoring of a patient's response to treatment. Only a limited number of patients who develop a deep infection following primary or revision TAR can expect to undergo successful joint-preserving revision arthroplasty. However, hindfoot arthrodesis with intramedullary fixation and structural allograft may be a reliable alternative [48].

Patients with a body mass index higher than 30 showed a higher rate of complications after TAR. Cardiovascular and peripheral vascular disease, smoking, osteoporosis, and overweight are risk factors for a worse survival rate. Preoperative MRI and long-leg X-rays to evaluate any angular deformities of other joints are recommended. Additionally, angiography and neurological examination is recommended for selected patients.

In conclusion, adequate patient selection and thorough knowledge of the surgical technique used are mandatory to reduce the number of complications and to increase ankle replacement survivorship.

8. Revision of TAR

Design improvements have increased the success of TAR; revision rates of TAR are higher than those for hip and knee replacement. The revision rates of TAR are approximately 10%–17% at 5 years [38, 40]. In the current cohort of STAR patients, implant survival at a minimum of 10 years of follow-up was high. However, 39% of patients required some sort of secondary procedure, most of which occurred after 9 years of follow-up [17]. A. Henricson et al. defined ankle replacement revision as the extraction of one or more bone-incorporated components or the exchange of a broken plastic component without any known trauma' [49, 50]. Based on the definition, the authors classified the revision of TAR as having either mechanical causes or nonmechanical causes.

8.1. Mechanical causes of revision

Malalignment and periprosthetic fracture are the major sources of mechanical failure in TAR [23]. S. Manegold et al. classified periprosthetic ankle fractures following TAR into three different types, which are based on three items: the cause of the fracture, the anatomic location of the fracture, and prosthesis stability.

The first parameter evaluates the fracture cause—Type 1: an intraoperative fracture; Type 2: a postoperative traumatic fracture; and Type 3: a postoperative stress fracture. The second parameter is the anatomic location of the periprosthetic fracture. The fracture is assigned a letter (A through D). Concomitant injuries involving bimalleolar fractures and diaphyseal lower-leg fractures are classified as AB and BC, respectively. The third parameter involved the stability of the implanted components. If there are no clinical or radiographic signs of implant loosening, or if the fracture does not reach the prosthesis, the implant can be considered stable. In the presence of periprosthetic osteolysis or fracture-related implant loosening, the prosthesis is classified as unstable. This classification is relatively clear and can be conducted on the basis of the treatment options used. However, the effectiveness of the classification system still needs to be confirmed by the treatment results [51].

Coronal plane malalignment at the level of the tibiotalar joint is not uncommon in end-stage ankle arthritis. Restoration of neutral coronal plane alignment is important in TAR. If an ankle joint prosthesis is not well balanced and edge loading occurs, increased contact stresses on the polyethylene insert can result in accelerated polyethylene wear and premature implant failure. Ancillary procedures performed before, during, or after TAR to correct deformities are thus important in preventing failure due to instability in the varus ankle [31].

There are limited choices currently available in the revision of ankle replacements due to the need to correct osteotomy for alignment. However, the "salvage" can be challenging because a lot of bone has been lost. Alternative approaches include direct arthrodesis with shortening, arthrodesis with interposition graft (autograft, allograft, or shape porous metals), or revision ankle replacement with a larger replacement.

8.2. Nonmechanical causes revision

The most prevalent cause of non-mechanical revision involves aseptic loosening. Ellington and Myerson provided a grading system that ranged from 1 to 3 to define the severity of talar component subsidence and to predict the outcomes following revision. In grade 1, the subsidence of the talar component is minimal. In grade 2, the talar component has subsided into the talar body, but it has not violated the subtalar joint. In grade 3, the talar component has migrated onto or through the subtalar joint [15, 52].

M.A. Prissel et al. described a technique for the management of extensive talar aseptic osteolysis for the revision of Agility systems with the use of geometric metal-reinforced polymethylmethacrylate cement augmentation. This technique preserves the subtalar joint, provides immediate component stability, and restores component alignment and height [15]. The authors used three or four titanium plasma-coated triangular metallic arthrodesis rods (3 mm or 7 mm) or large-diameter acetabular screws placed in a triangular or quadrangular orientation around the periphery of the remaining talus and the body of the calcaneus. The superior aspects of the rods or screws should create a parallel surface, allowing the talar component to reside at the proper level to restore the anatomic height of the hindfoot and mechanical function of the ankle joint [15].

Collectively, the classification of periprosthetic fractures and the grading system used for component subsidence can facilitate therapeutic decision making, as they allows for the differential analysis of the causes of these conditions; they can also serve as a guide when making the choice between operative and nonoperative treatment options. There were still obvious functional limitations following the revision of TAR, with fewer than half of the patients returning to previous activity levels. However, the revision of TAR is still a cost-effective alternative to other available options and it still allows for additional revision should late failure occur.

9. Decision-making process of using arthrodesis or TAR

Patients with ankle arthritis and deformity who experience severe pain and functional disability, and do not respond to nonoperative treatment modalities, are candidates for TAR [53]. Currently, there is no consensus regarding which treatment, arthrodesis or replacement, is better for end-stage ankle arthritis.

Ankle arthrodesis is still considered to be the gold standard for the treatment of end-stage ankle arthritis. Ankle arthrodesis yielded good radiographic and functional outcomes in primary arthrodesis [54, 55], bilateral ankle arthrodesis [56], or combined ankle and hindfoot arthrodesis, even in revision cases following TAR [57]. Arthroscopic ankle arthrodesis provides not only an alternative to traditional open techniques but also an obvious advantage including decreased complications, reduced postoperative pain, and shorter hospital stays [58, 59, 60, 61]. There exists fair evidence-based literature (grade B) to support a recommendation for the use of ankle arthroscopy for ankle arthrodesis [62].

Ankle arthrodesis has an approximately 10%–40% nonunion rate [23, 53]. Osteonecrosis of the talus and smoking are known risk factors for nonunion [53]. Risk factors associated with prolonged hospital stay were advanced age, female sex, diabetes mellitus, and more than one general or surgery-related complication [63]. The published literature on the long-term follow-up of modern TAR achieved significantly higher implant survival rates, patient satisfaction, pain relief, and range of motion (ROM) and American Orthopaedic Foot and Ankle Society (AOFAS) scores following the third ankle prosthesis [29, 64]. Complication and survivorship rates were comparable between both groups [65]. Compared to arthrodesis, the primary advantages of TAR include maintenance of motion of the ankle and reduced risk of developing adjacent joint arthritis. J.J. Jiang reported that TAR was independently associated with a lower risk of blood transfusion, non-home discharge, and overall complications when compared to ankle arthrodesis during the index hospitalization period. TAR was also independently associated with a higher hospitalization charge, but the length of stay was similar between the two groups [66]. S. Singer reported that improvement in patient-reported Ankle Osteoarthritis Scale and Short Form-36 scores were similar for both arthrodesis and TAR groups [24]. In addition, R. Rodrigues-Pinto reported that complication and survivorship rates were comparable between both TAR arthrodesis groups [65]. A multicenter study showed that the intermediate-term clinical outcomes of TAR with third-generation prostheses were comparable in a diverse cohort in which treatment was tailored to patient presentation; the rates of reoperation and major complications were higher following ankle replacement when compared with arthrodesis [67].

Although the AOFAS hindfoot scale is the most frequently used outcome instrument in TAR studies, its score has been under recent scrutiny with respect to its moderate level of correlation, its satisfactory degree of reliability, and its degree of responsiveness [68, 69, 70]. The SF-36 and Visual Analog Scale (VAS) pain scoring systems are generic, but validated, outcome measures. Therefore, it will be essential to standardize data collection, evaluation, publication, and the assessment of register data in TAR. TAR outcome measurement by means of registers has several specific requirements necessitating additional documentation beyond the basic dataset [46].

In conclusion, the current investigation demonstrated that neither arthrodesis nor TAR replicated normal ankle function, and there were no differences in ankle power, moments, or temporal gait parameters between the two patient groups. Both arthrodesis and TAR achieved good clinical outcomes. Compared with ankle arthrodesis, the rates of complication with TAR are comparable. Although complications following TAR are frequent, the results of TAR are improving and promising; TAR can reliably improve a person's quality of life. Nevertheless, patient selection and education are essential.

10. Conclusion

TAR is becoming the modality of choice for the treatment of end-stage degenerative joint disease of the ankle. To maintain the longest function of ankle replacements, the design of the prosthesis should allow for smooth and continuous interaction and normal gait. TAR offers better mobility, improved gait, and reduces the development of subsequent subtalar joint arthritis when compared with ankle arthrodesis. The decision to treat with TAR or ankle arthrodesis depends on the surgeon's technique, as well as on the patient's condition. Improved operative techniques, the surgeon's experience, as well as appropriate patient selection can anticipate better outcomes. Deformities of the ankle and foot should be corrected before TAR is performed. The revision of a replacement is ultimately inevitable due to aseptic loosening and infection. Despite the functional limitations following the revision of TAR, the revision still offers a cost-effective alternative to ankle arthrodesis.

Author details

Binghua Zhou* and Kanglai Tang*

*Address all correspondence to: binghua1979@gmail.com; kanglaitang@hotmail.com

Department of Orthopedic Surgery, China

References

[1] C.L. Saltzman, M.L. Salamon, G.M. Blanchard, T. Huff, A. Hayes, J.A. Buckwalter, A. Amendola. Epidemiology of ankle arthritis: report of a consecutive series of 639 patients from a tertiary orthopaedic center. Iowa Orthopaed J 2005;25:44.

[2] V. Valderrabano, B.M. Nigg, V. von Tscharner, D.J. Stefanyshyn, B. Goepfert, B. Hintermann. Gait analysis in ankle osteoarthritis and total ankle replacement. Clin Biomech 2007;22:894–904.

[3] S.A. Brigido, G.M. Wobst, M.M. Galli, S.T. Bleazey, N.M. Protzman. Evaluating component migration after modular stem fixed-bearing total ankle replacement. J Foot Ankle Surg 2015;54(3):326-31.

[4] G. Lord, J. Marotte. Total ankle prosthesis. Technic and 1st results. Apropos of 12 cases, Revue de chirurgie orthopédique et réparatrice de l'appareil moteur 1973;59:139.

[5] N.E. Gougoulias, A. Khanna, N. Maffulli. History and evolution in total ankle arthroplasty, Br Med Bull 2009;89:111–51.

[6] B. Hintermann, V. Valderrabano. Total ankle replacement. Foot Ankle Clin 2003;8:375–405.

[7] A. Cracchiolo, J.K. DeOrio. Design features of current total ankle replacements: implants and instrumentation. J Am Acad Orthopaed Surgeons 2008;16:530–40.

[8] H. Kofoed. Scandinavian total ankle replacement (STAR). Clin Orthopaed Related Res 2004;424:73–9.

[9] B. Hintermann. Current designs of total ankle prostheses, Total Ankle Arthroplasty: Historical Overview, Current Concepts and Future Perspectives 2005;59–89.

[10] B. Hintermann. History of total ankle arthroplasty, Total Ankle Arthroplasty: Historical Overview, Current Concepts and Future Perspectives 2005;43–57.

[11] A. Datir, M. Xing, A. Kakarala, M.R. Terk, S.A. Labib. Radiographic evaluation of in-bone total ankle arthroplasty: a retrospective analysis of 30 cases. Skel Radiol 2013;42:1693–701.

[12] F. Alvine. Design and development of the Agility ankle. Foot Ankle Specialist 2009;2:45–50.

[13] F. Alvine. Total ankle arthroplasty: new concepts and approaches. Contemp Orthopaed 1991;22:397–403.

[14] F.G. Alvine. The Agility ankle replacement: the good and the bad. Foot Ankle Clin 2002;7:737–53.

[15] M.A. Prissel, T.S. Roukis. Management of extensive tibial osteolysis with the Agility™ total ankle replacement systems using geometric metal-reinforced polymethylmethacrylate cement augmentation. J Foot Ankle Surg 2014;53:101–7.

[16] M.T. Pyevich, C.L. Saltzman, J.J. Callaghan, F.G. Alvine. Total ankle arthroplasty: a unique design. Two to twelve-year follow-up*. J Bone Joint Surg 1998;80:1410–20.

[17] J.R. Jastifer, M.J. Coughlin. Long-term follow-up of mobile bearing total ankle arthroplasty in the United States. Foot Ankle Int 2014; 1071100714550654.

[18] J. Gittins, R.A. Mann. The history of the STAR total ankle arthroplasty. Foot Ankle Clin 2002;7:809–16.

[19] K.A. McInnes, A.S. Younger, T.R. Oxland. Initial instability in total ankle replacement: a cadaveric biomechanical investigation of the STAR and agility prostheses. J Bone Joint Surg 2014;96:e147.

[20] P. Wood, M. Karski, P. Watmough. Total ankle replacement. The results of 100 mobility total ankle replacements. J Bone Joint Surg British Volume 2010;92:958–62.

[21] J.J. Yu, S. Sheskier. Total ankle replacement – evolution of the technology and future applications. Bull Hosp Jt Dis 2013;72(2014):120–8.

[22] I. Hetsroni, M. Nyska, G. Mann, G. Rozenfeld, M. Ayalon. Subtalar kinematics following resection of tarsal coalition. Foot Ankle Int 2008;29:1088–94.

[23] J.F. Baumhauer. Ankle arthrodesis versus ankle replacement for ankle arthritis. Clin Orthop Relat Res 2013;471:2439–42.

[24] S. Singer, S. Klejman, E. Pinsker, J. Houck, T. Daniels. Ankle arthroplasty and ankle arthrodesis: gait analysis compared with normal controls. J Bone Joint Surg 2013;95:e191 191–110.

[25] R.M. Queen, R.J. Butler, S.B. Adams Jr, J.K. DeOrio, M.E. Easley, J.A. Nunley. Bilateral differences in gait mechanics following total ankle replacement: a two year longitudinal study. Clin Biomech 2014;29:418–22.

[26] A. Rosello Anon, I. Martinez Garrido, J. Cervera Deval, D. Herrero Mediavilla, M. Sanchez Gonzalez, V. Vicent Carsi. Total ankle replacement in patients with end-stage ankle osteoarthritis: clinical results and kinetic gait analysis. Foot Ankle Surg 2014;20:195–200.

[27] M.E. Hahn, E.S. Wright, A.D. Segal, M.S. Orendurff, W.R. Ledoux, B.J. Sangeorzan. Comparative gait analysis of ankle arthrodesis and arthroplasty: initial findings of a prospective study. Foot Ankle Int 2012;33:282–9.

[28] M.R. McGuire, R.F. Kyle, R.B. Gustilo, R.F. PREMER. Comparative analysis of ankle arthroplasty versus ankle arthrodesis. Clin Orthopaed Related Res 1988;226:174–81.

[29] J.R. Ramaskandhan, R. Kakwani, S. Kometa, K. Bettinson, M.S. Siddique. Two-year outcomes of mobility total ankle replacement. J Bone Joint Surg Am 2014;96:e53.

[30] R.M. Queen, S.B. Adams, N.A. Viens, J.K. Friend, M.E. Easley, J.K. DeOrio, J.A. Nunley. Differences in outcomes following total ankle replacement in patients with neutral alignment compared with tibiotalar joint malalignment. J Bone Joint Surg 2013;95:1927–34.

[31] T. Trajkovski, E. Pinsker, A. Cadden, T. Daniels. Outcomes of ankle arthroplasty with preoperative coronal-plane varus deformity of 10 or greater. J Bone Joint Surg 2013;95:1382–8.

[32] J.A. Buckwalter, C. Saltzman, T. Brown. The impact of osteoarthritis: implications for research. Clin Orthopaed Related Res 2004;427:S6–15.

[33] S. Noelle, C.C. Egidy, M.B. Cross, M. Gebauer, W. Klauser. Complication rates after total ankle arthroplasty in one hundred consecutive prostheses. Int Orthopaed 2013;37:1789–94.

[34] K.M. Schweitzer, S.B. Adams, N.A. Viens, R.M. Queen, M.E. Easley, J.K. DeOrio, J.A. Nunley. Early prospective clinical results of a modern fixed-bearing total ankle arthroplasty. J Bone Joint Surg 2013;95:1002–11.

[35] C.M. King, J.M. Schuberth, J.C. Christensen, K.M. Swanstrom. Relationship of alignment and tibial cortical coverage to hypertrophic bone formation in Salto Talaris< sup>®</sup> total ankle arthroplasty. J Foot Ankle Surg 2013;52:355–9.

[36] A. Barg, L. Zwicky, M. Knupp, H.B. Henninger, B. Hintermann. HINTEGRA total ankle replacement: survivorship analysis in 684 patients. J Bone Joint Surg 2013;95:1175–83.

[37] J.S. Lewis, S.B. Adams, R.M. Queen, J.K. DeOrio, J.A. Nunley, M.E. Easley. Outcomes after total ankle replacement in association with ipsilateral hindfoot arthrodesis. Foot Ankle Int 2014;35:535–42.

[38] R.J. Gadd, T.W. Barwick, E. Paling, M.B. Davies, C.M. Blundell. Assessment of a three-grade classification of complications in total ankle replacement. Foot Ankle Int 2014;1071100714524549.

[39] R. Rodrigues-Pinto, J. Muras, X. Martín Oliva, P. Amado. Functional results and complication analysis after total ankle replacement: early to medium-term results from a Portuguese and Spanish prospective multicentric study. Foot Ankle Surg 2013;19:222–8.

[40] J.K. Ellington, S. Gupta, M.S. Myerson. Management of failures of total ankle replacement with the agility total ankle arthroplasty. J Bone Joint Surg 2013;95:2112–8.

[41] M.A. Glazebrook, K. Arsenault, M. Dunbar. Evidence-based classification of complications in total ankle arthroplasty. Foot Ankle Int 2009;30:945–9.

[42] B. Bolton-Maggs, R. Sudlow, M. Freeman. Total ankle arthroplasty. A long-term review of the London Hospital experience. J Bone Joint Surg British Volume 1985;67:785–90.

[43] J.D. Demottaz, J.M. Mazur, W.H. Thomas, C.B. Sledge, S.R. Simon. Clinical study of total ankle replacement with gait analysis. A preliminary report. J Bone Joint Surg Am 1979;61:976–88.

[44] A. Henricson, J.-Å. Nilsson, Å. Carlsson. 10-year survival of total ankle arthroplasties: a report on 780 cases from the Swedish Ankle Register. Acta Orthopaed 2011;82:655–9.

[45] J.W.-Y. Fong, A. Veljkovic, M.J. Dunbar, D.A. Wilson, A.W. Hennigar, M.A. Glazebrook. Validation and precision of model-based radiostereometric analysis (MBRSA) for total ankle arthroplasty. Foot Ankle Int 2011;32:1155–63.

[46] G. Labek, S. Todorov, L. Iovanescu, C.I. Stoica, N. Böhler. Outcome after total ankle arthroplasty—results and findings from worldwide arthroplasty registers. Int Orthopaed 2013;37:1677–82.

[47] R.T. Goldman, G.R. Scuderi, J.N. Insall. 2-stage reimplantation for infected total knee replacement. Clin Orthopaed Related Res 1996;331:118–24.

[48] M.S. Myerson, R. Shariff, A.J. Zonno. The management of infection following total ankle replacement demographics and treatment. Foot Ankle Int 2014;1071100714543643.

[49] H. Kofoed. Ankle replacement revision. Foot Ankle Surg 2013;19:69.

[50] A. Henricson, A. Carlsson, U. Rydholm. What is a revision of total ankle replacement? Foot Ankle Surg 2011;17:99–102.

[51] S. Manegold, N.P. Haas, S. Tsitsilonis, A. Springer, S. Märdian, K.-D. Schaser. Periprosthetic fractures in total ankle replacement: classification system and treatment algorithm. J Bone Joint Surg 2013;95:815–20.

[52] S. Gupta, J.K. Ellington, M.S. Myerson. Management of specific complications after revision total ankle replacement. Seminars in Arthroplasty, Elsevier, 2010, pp. 310–319.

[53] N.A. Abidi, G.S. Gruen, S.F. Conti. Ankle arthrodesis: indications and techniques. J Am Acad Orthopaed Surgeons 2000;8:200–9.

[54] S. Wang, Z. Huang, G. Xiong, G. Chen, Z. Yin, H. Jiang, Modified Blair ankle fusion for ankle arthritis. Chin J Traumatol = Zhonghua chuang shang za zhi/Chinese Medical Association 2014;17:136.

[55] P.S. Cooper. Complications of ankle and tibiotalocalcaneal arthrodesis. Clin Orthopaed Related Res 2001;391:33–44.

[56] M.T. Houdek, B.K. Wilke, D.B. Ryssman, N.S. Turner. Radiographic and functional outcomes following bilateral ankle fusions. Foot Ankle Int 2014;1071100714551947.

[57] M.S. Myerson, R. Shariff, A.J. Zonno. The management of infection following total ankle replacement: demographics and treatment. Foot Ankle Int 2014;35:855–62.

[58] R.D. Ferkel, M. Hewitt. Long-term results of arthroscopic ankle arthrodesis. Foot Ankle Int 2005;26:275–80.

[59] M.S. Myerson, G. Quill. Ankle arthrodesis: a comparison of an arthroscopic and an open method of treatment. Clin Orthopaed Related Res 1991;268:84–95.

[60] I. Winson, D. Robinson, P. Allen. Arthroscopic ankle arthrodesis. J Bone Joint Surg British Volume 2005;87:343–7.

[61] D.R. Collman, M.H. Kaas, J.M. Schuberth. Arthroscopic ankle arthrodesis: factors influencing union in 39 consecutive patients. Foot Ankle Int 2006;27:1079–85.

[62] M.A. Glazebrook, V. Ganapathy, M.A. Bridge, J.W. Stone, J.P. Allard. Evidence-based indications for ankle arthroscopy. Arthroscopy 2009;25:1478–1490.

[63] M.E. Menendez, A.G. Bot, V. Neuhaus, D. Ring, A.H. Johnson. Factors influencing discharge disposition after ankle arthrodesis. Foot Ankle Int 2014;35:578–83.

[64] J.R. Jastifer, M.J. Coughlin. Long-term follow-up of mobile bearing total ankle arthroplasty in the United States. Foot Ankle Int 2015 ;36(2):143-50.

[65] R. Rodrigues-Pinto, J. Muras, X. Martín Oliva, P. Amado. Total ankle replacement in patients under the age of 50. Should the indications be revised? Foot Ankle Surg 2013;19:229–33.

[66] J.J. Jiang, O.N. Schipper, N. Whyte, J.L. Koh, B.C. Toolan. Comparison of perioperative complications and hospitalization outcomes after ankle arthrodesis versus total ankle arthroplasty from 2002 to 2011. Foot Ankle Int 2014;1071100714558511.

[67] T.R. Daniels, A.S. Younger, M. Penner, K. Wing, P.J. Dryden, H. Wong, M. Glazebrook. Intermediate-term results of total ankle replacement and ankle arthrodesis. A COFAS multicenter study. J Bone Joint Surg 2014;96:135–42.

[68] L. Bader, K. Park, Y. Gu, M.J. O'Malley. Functional outcome of endoscopic plantar fasciotomy. Foot Ankle Int 2012;33:37–43.

[69] T. Ibrahim, A. Beiri, M. Azzabi, A.J. Best, G.J. Taylor, D.K. Menon. Reliability and validity of the subjective component of the American Orthopaedic Foot and Ankle Society clinical rating scales. J Foot Ankle Surg 2007;46:65–74.

[70] H.B. Kitaoka, I.J. Alexander, R.S. Adelaar, J.A. Nunley, M.S. Myerson, M. Sanders. Clinical rating systems for the ankle-hindfoot, midfoot, hallux, and lesser toes. Foot Ankle Int 1994;15:349–53.

3

Surgical Approaches for Total Knee Arthroplasty

Stefan Cristea, Vlad Predescu, Șerban Dragosloveanu, Ștefan Cuculici and Nicholas Mărăndici

Abstract

Total knee arthroplasty surgery is a current practice in orthopedic surgery. The success of this intervention consists in part in the realignment of the lower extremity's anatomical axis, adequate implant orientation and design, good implant fixation, proper soft tissue balancing, and stability. A good exposure also allows optimal placement of the components. Our preferred approach is the median parapatellar approach in most cases. However, the orthopedic surgeon may face anatomical variants associated with knee types that may complicate the classic approach. We are reviewing multiple surgical approaches also used by us in our clinic in total knee arthroplasty, as well as additional techniques in these surgical approaches. The MIS approach can be used in many cases to reduce pain and speed the healing process. All of the total knee arthroplasty approaches are detailed with anatomical illustrations along with advantages and disadvantages of each. The ultimate goal is to restore knee function as quickly as possible and to preserve the anatomical integrity of the joint.

Keywords: Total knee arthroplasty, approaches, MIS approaches, orthopedic surgery

1. Introduction

Total knee arthroplasty surgery is indicated in primary or secondary knee osteoarthritis. The success of this intervention consists in part in the realignment of the lower extremity's anatomical axis, adequate implant orientation and design, good implant fixation, proper soft tissue balancing, and stability. A good exposure also allows optimal placement of the components.

2. Patient preparation

The patient is placed supine on the operating table. After suitable skin preparation, drapes are applied in order to leave the leg free. A pneumatic tourniquet is applied as high as possible as to minimize compression of the thigh muscles, which would otherwise restrict knee mobility. A special table support (Figure 1) allows the knee to be flexed and extended several times during the operation; another option is to add a roll support on an ordinary table (Figure 2). Included in the preoperative preparation of the leg is the administration of a short-acting, non-depolarizing muscle relaxant that should provide sufficient muscle paralysis before and during the surgery.

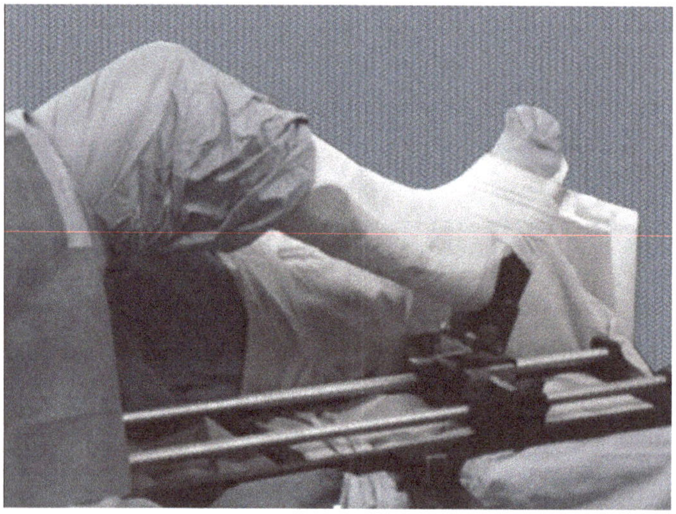

Figure 1. Special table support for TKA.

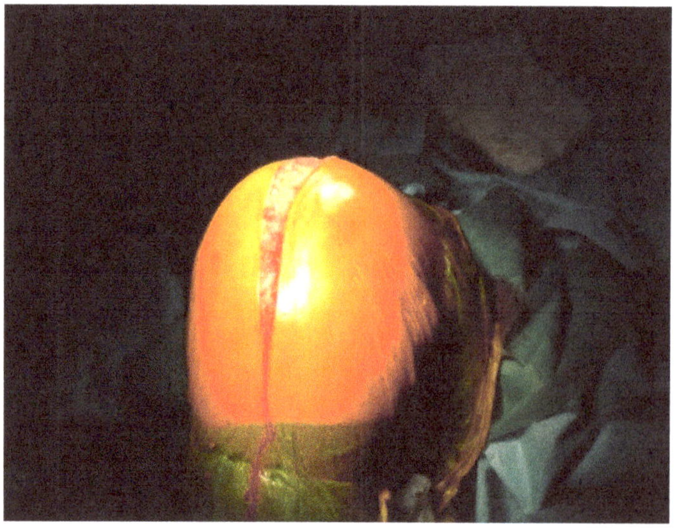

Figure 2. Position on the table.

The minimum duration needed for muscle relaxation is around 30–40 minutes. The anesthesiologist must adjust the medication dose depending on patient's habitus and weight to acquire this interval. This will ease patellar eversion if desired and minimize tension in the quadriceps distal to the level of the tourniquet. Muscle relaxant is required to be injected before the inflation of the tourniquet. As an alternative, epidural or spinal anesthesia will produce adequate muscle relaxation.

Apply a tourniquet proximally on the thigh and inflate it with the knee hyperflexed so as most part of the thigh muscles remains below the tourniquet's level. This will minimize restriction of the quadriceps and facilitate the eversion of the patella.

As soon as the patient is prepped on the operating table and the sterile drapes are applied, the landmarks for the surgical incision will be determined with the knee in extension (Figure 3).

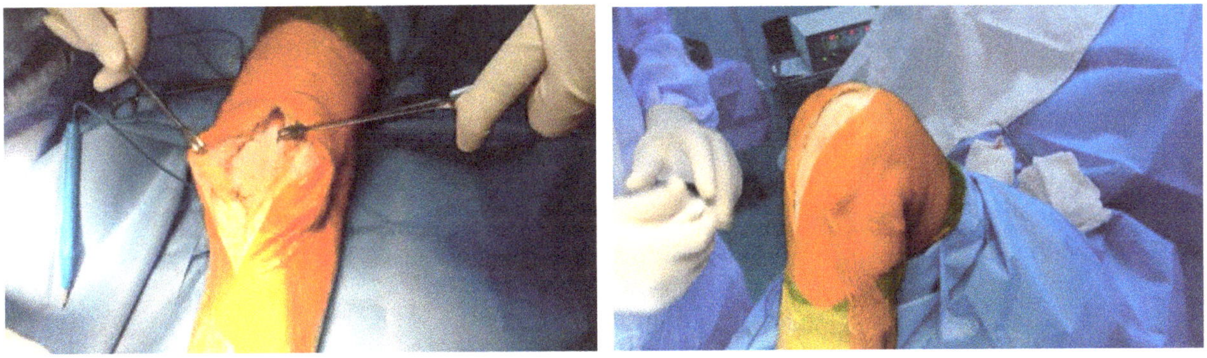

Figure 3. Position on the table.

Surgical wound healing is of utmost importance in the success of knee arthroplasty. Oftentimes, a wound healing issue may appear and lead to devastating complications; therefore, this should be avoided and treated aggressively from the beginning. There are high risk patients who tend to develop this: steroid users, obese individuals, rheumatoid arthritis patients, smokers, diabetics, methotrexate users, as well as patients suffering from hypovolemia, reduced transcutaneous oxygen levels, and scars from previous surgery.

Frequently, some patients have had previous operations, undergoing osteotomies or arthroplasties, so previous incisions may be used or incorporated to decrease the risk of skin slough. If this is not possible, the new incision must have a safe corridor of at least 5 cm from the old one. Another possibility is to incise perpendicular to the old scars, or at least at a 60° angle. If there are different longitudinal skin incisions, the most lateral should be used in order to avoid a large lateral skin flap. If the skin is too damaged, a plastic surgeon's advice should be sought, considering the option of soft tissue expanders or sham incisions.

Any approach includes removal of osteophytes from the margins of the intercondylar notch and from the tibia which may aid in identification of landmarks (Figures 4 and 5).

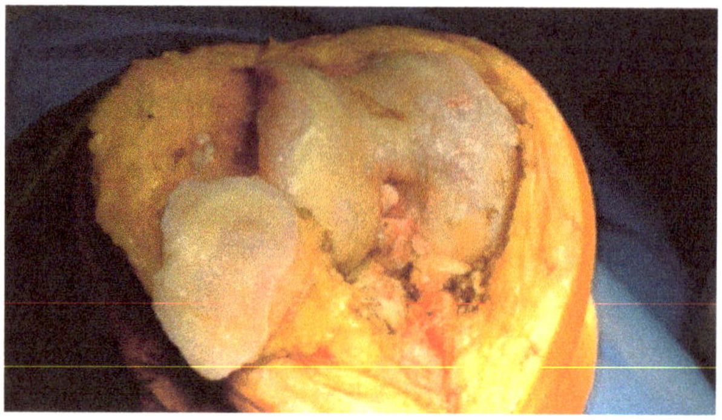

Figure 4. Knee large exposure.

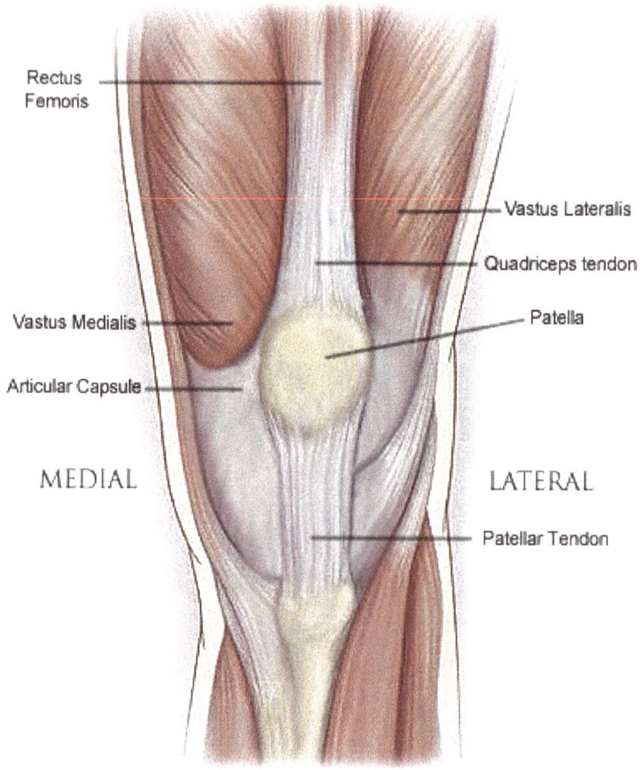

Figure 5. Anatomical landmarks.

3. Anteromedial parapatellar approach

Use a standard anterior midline incision (Figure 6) extending from a point 5 cm proximal to the apex on the patella to the tibial tubercle. Dissect subcutaneous tissues. Enter the capsule through a medial parapatellar approach approximately 1 cm from the medial border of the patella (Figure 7). Incise the quadriceps mechanism longitudinally to allow adequate patellar eversion [1] and sufficient knee flexion (Figure 8). Another variant is the Insall [2] anterior approach, in which the longitudinal fibers of the quadriceps tendon are carefully separated from the medial half of the patella preserving a substantial layer of tissue. Evert the patella laterally with the knee maintained in extension. Keeping the patella everted laterally, flex the knee to expose the knee joint. Wound closure with suture of the extensor mechanism facilitates the rapid recovery.

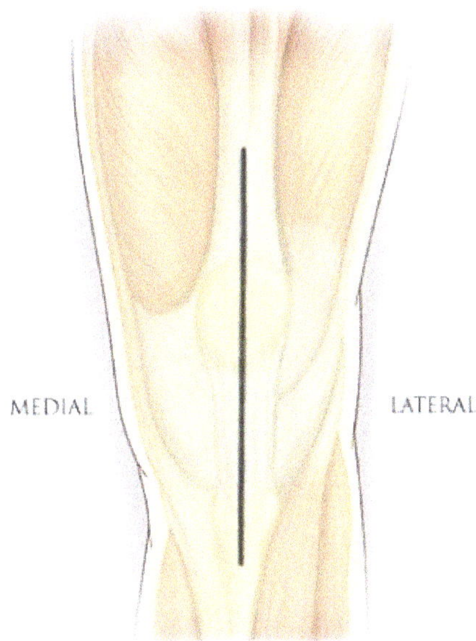

Figure 6. Standard anterior midline incision.

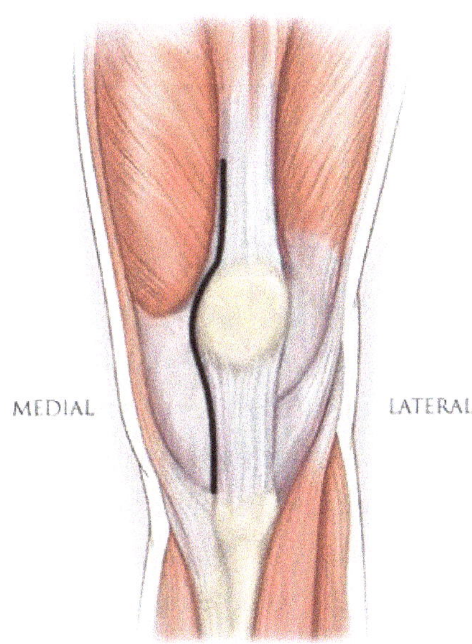

Figure 7. Medial parapatellar approach.

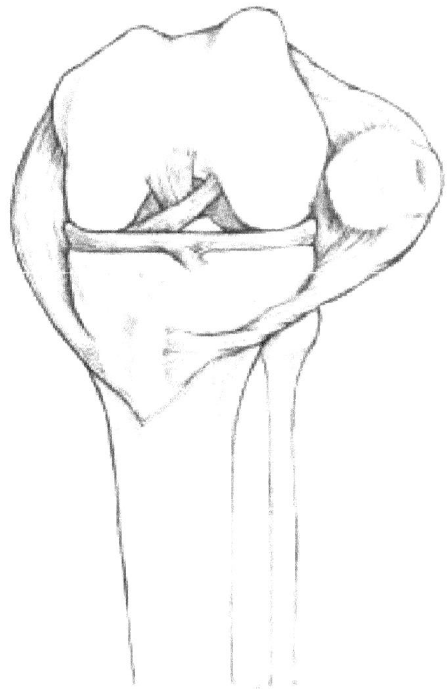

Figure 8. Patellar eversion and sufficient knee flexion.

Advantages	Precautions
- Very good exposure of the knee	- Risk of injuring the infrapatellar branch of saphenous nerve
- Very easy dislocation and eversion of the patella laterally	- Accidental avulsion of the patellar tendon from the tibial tubercle
	- Injuring the superior lateral geniculate artery

Table 1. Anteromedial parapatellar approach

4. Anterolateral parapatellar approach

Use a standard anterior midline incision of the skin (Figure 6) extending from a point 5 cm proximal to the apex on the patella until the tibial tubercle. Dissect the subcutaneous tissue and deepen the incision along its length through the subcutaneous fat and then the prepattelar bursa. Following the lateral side of the patella, perform a lateral parapatellar arthrotomy (Figure 9) extending from just superior to the patella, along the lateral side of the quadriceps tendon to the tibial tuberosity distally. Evert the patella medially with the knee still in extension. Keeping the patella everted medially, flex the knee to expose the knee joint (Figures 4 and 10).

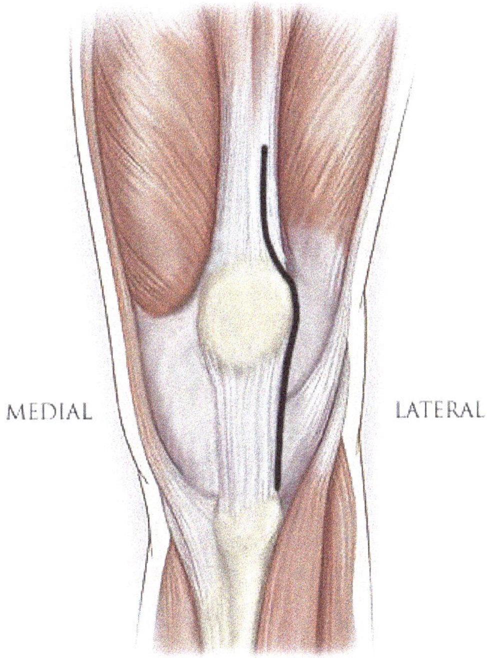

Figure 9. Lateral parapatellar approach.

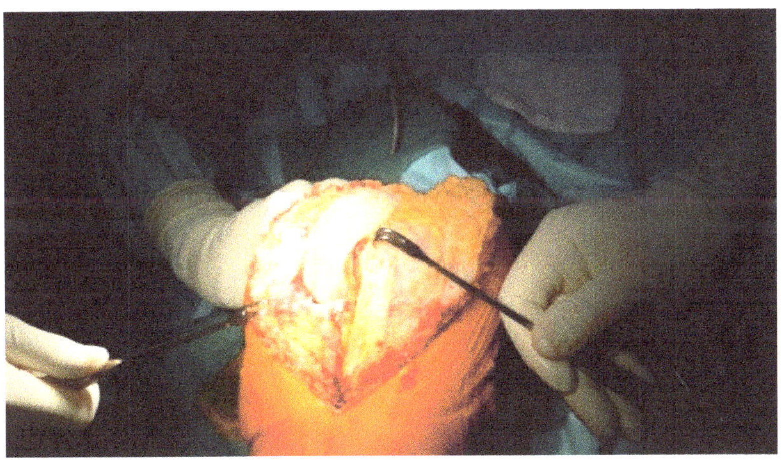

Figure 10. Evert the patella medially.

Advantages	Disadvantages
- Technically useful in valgus deformity cases	- Very rare
- Preserves the patellar blood supply	- Difficulty in everting the patella medially
- Prevents lateral patellar subluxation	- May require tibial tubercle osteotomy

Table 2. Lateral parapatellar approach

5. Subvastus approach [3]

Use a midline incision. Dissect the subcutaneous tissue but avoid incising the fascia covering the vastus medialis obliquus muscle. Identify the inferior border of the vastus medialis muscle and incise its overlying fascia medial to the patellar border. This should allow introducing the surgeon's finger or a retractor under the muscle's inferior border and pull the vastus medialis superiorly, separating it from the underlying synovial knee joint lining.

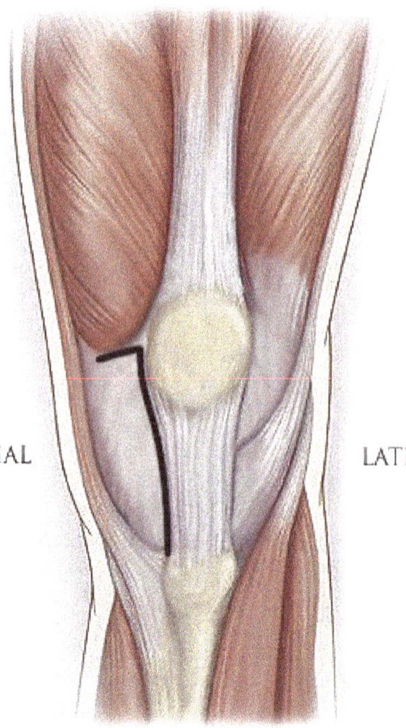

Figure 11. Subvastus approach

With the help of an electrocautery, the capsular incision is made under the vastus muscle's inferior border, starting posterolaterally, continuing laterally parallel to the border, and when the medial border of the patella is reached, the incision takes an L-shape, turning directly inferiorly at a 90° angle, parallel to the medial border of the patella (Figure 11). A small miofascial tissue cuff should be left attached to the medial border of the patella for closure. Tearing, splitting, or further damages to the muscle can be caused by incising along the inferior border of the vastus to the patellar superior pole and then inserting the retractors.

The arthrotomy consists in incising the underlying synovium incision that is performed across the joint line, in line with the patellar's tendon medial border.

Insert a bent Hohmann or a Z-retractor in the lateral flare in order to keep the patella and the extensor mechanism retracted with the quadriceps tendon and vastus medialis lying over the distal femur. The patella is either everted or subluxed. For additional exposure, the retropatellar bursa and fat pad can be excised or spared, depending on the surgeon's preference.

The knee is now flexed and extended in various degrees so as to vary the tension on the extensor mechanism and improve visualization.

Advantages	Disadvantages
- Claims of less intraoperative blood loss and more rapid rehabilitation	- Patella can be difficult to evert but it can be instead subluxated laterally
- Elevates the vastus medialis muscle instead of cutting into it	- Difficult to apply in muscular patients
- Preserving the quadriceps tendon intact	
- Preserving blood supply to the patella	

Table 3. Subvastus approach

6. Midvastus approach [4]

Similar to the subvastus approach, the dissection is carried out through the muscle of vastus medialis to facilitate exposure.

Use a longitudinal midline skin incision. Next, using electrocautery, the capsule should be incised parallel to the medial border of the patella and extended proximally and distally. The surgeon must leave a band of about 1 cm of capsule and peritenon that will later facilitate capsular closure.

The superficial fascia covering the quadriceps should be incised approximately 5 cm starting distally and extending proximally, so as to decrease the extensor mechanism's tension and permit mobilization of the quadriceps. In this manner, the quadriceps will be able to be translated laterally easier, facilitating the exposure of the knee joint.

The following step consists in dissecting through the muscular fibers of the vastus medialis itself, running oblique over a length of approximately 4–6 cm from proximal and lateral down to the medial border of the patella. From here, the dissection is continued proximally along the medial patellar border and ends around the tibial tuberosity (Figure 12). The knee is slightly flexed and the surgeon should decide whether to excise or preserve the retropatellar bursa and fat pad. The patella can be everted or subluxed. If the surgeon's choice is to evert the patella, then a release of the patella-femoral ligament should be made. Using a hook with two prongs, the patella is everted and dislocated laterally, or subluxed, exposing the articular surfaces.

Once the patella is everted, a bent Hohmann or a Z-retractor is introduced along the lateral gutter of the tibial metaphysis to maintain the dislocation of the patella and the extensor mechanism. For further flexing and exposing of the knee joint, the subperiosteal tissue should be dissected along the tibial insertion of the patellar tendon.

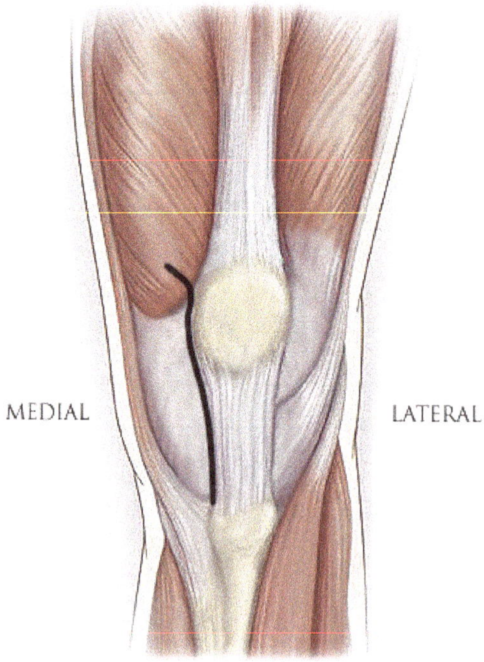

Figure 12. Midvastus approach.

Advantages	Disadvantages
- Better exposure than the subvastus	- Cutting and disrupting the vastus medialis muscular substance
- Allows rapid restoration of extensor mechanism	
- Advantage over the standard incision is that the vastus medialis insertion into the medial border of the quadriceps tendon is preserved	- Patella can be difficult to evert and can be instead subluxated laterally

Table 4. Midvastus approach

7. Lateral approach (Keblish)

Begin the incision laterally around the knee, following the femur line and curve the incision around the knee, keeping it parallel to the patella and then in line with the tibia (Figure 13). Deepen the incision down to the fascia. Divide the deep fascia between the biceps femoris and the iliotibial band, revealing the lateral collateral ligament. Perform an anterior arthrotomy parallel to the lateral side of the patella.

This approach was first described [5] in order to perform a release of lateral contracture structures in valgus knee. If a patellar maltracking is anticipated and further lateral release may be necessary, then this approach can be a start option in surgery. The approach needs experience and is more demanding. Anatomy is reversed, and the surgeon is not commonly used to work with the patella subluxed medially. The advantage is the direct approach to the concave side of the deformity, preserving patellar vascularization. Medial dissection is avoided, and the medial soft tissue, which is lax, is no longer jeopardized during surgery. Patellar everting is difficult in the original version of this approach. Tibial tubercle osteotomy may be necessary to overcome the patellar stiffness. After the lateral parapatellar approach itself, there are several tricks very important to avoid avulsion of the tibial tubercle. One is performing a lateral vastus snip about 2–3 cm long, and another is performing a minimal release of the patellar tendon from the tibial tuberosity. If it is not possible to slide the patella, then proceed with patellar osteotomy for patellar replacement. This can be done from the beginning, and then the bony surface can be protected with a metallic cap in order to avoid bony damage. At closure, the surgeon may confront with a problem, the remaining space between capsular incision sides. In order to avoid this, it is important to keep the Hoffa fat pad and damage it as little as possible. The Hoffa fat pad must be kept attached laterally, keeping the vascular pedicle and sutured between borders of capsular incision (Hoffa plasty). Generally, this approach is recommended in knees with more than 15° of valgus, with contracture of the lateral structures [6]. We could not find it especially useful even in valgus deformities with 30°.

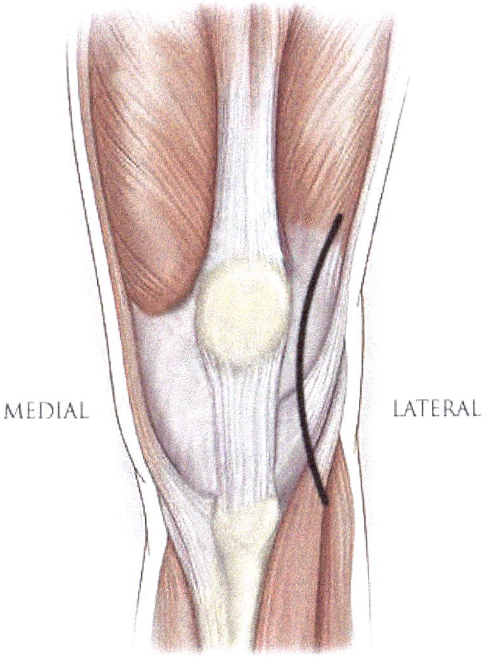

Figure 13. Lateral approach.

Advantages	Disadvantages
- Technically useful in valgus deformity cases	- Being rare becomes uncomfortable. Technically is more demanding and needs an experienced surgeon
- Preserves the patellar blood supply	- Difficulty in everting the patella medially
- Prevents lateral patellar subluxation	- May require tibial tubercle osteotomy

Table 5. Lateral approach

8. Tibial tubercle osteotomy technique (TTO)

This technique was introduced in 1983 [7]. The main indication is a stiff knee with shortening of the extensor mechanism and patella baja, but it must be left as one last alternative or avoided. Especially in revisions, it must be taken into consideration. This technique prevents the rupture of the patellar tendon but also allows lengthening of up to 2.5 cm of the extensor mechanism, enough to obtain good flexion in a stiff knee and avoid patella baja. Whiteside modified this technique and popularized it [8]. It is utilized with almost the same frequency as quad snip technique, especially in cases of high fibrosis stiff knees, knee arthroplasty revisions where median parapatellar approach rarely offers sufficient exposure. The tibial tubercle osteotomy should be as long as possible, 6–8 cm long and 1.5 times the width of tibial tubercule. Drilling holes can be useful to prepare the osteotomy, which is made with an osteotome or an oscillating saw. The proximal transverse cut is made oblique and upward in the methaphyseal area to create a ledge in order to prevent proximal migration. The distal transverse osteotomy is made at a 45° angle from the longitudinal cut. It is important to preserve lateral soft tissue attachments in order to prevent proximal displacement; a large tibial tubercle osteotomy will consolidate at least in few points to avoid nonunion (Figure 14). The tibial tubercle that has been osteotomized on the lateral side is everted to enlarge the exposure. At the end of the procedure, rigid fixation and good pattelar alignment are required to allow knee flexion in early postoperative interval and reduce further complications. Generally, two methods of fixation of the osteotomy fragment have been described: cerclage wire fixation and screw fixation. The fixation with cerclages is obtained with 3 or 4 loops of wire passed through drill holes in the tubercle and medial tibial cortex (Figure 15). The inclusion of the tibial prosthetic component into cerclage will increase the stability but it can create a bimetal reaction. The advantage of this type of fixation is that the wires are easier to place and provide a good fixation, but to avoid migration, a step cut on the proximal side of the segment needs to be made. On the other side, the proximal methaphiseal inclusion into cerclage could damage the popliteal artery. The complications might be as follows: anterior pain in the knee, migration of the tubercle, or soft tissue aggression caused by the tips of the wires. The fixation, with 2–4 bicortical screws, can provide a more reliable fixation (Figure 16), although it is more difficult to place the screws around a tibial revision stem for example. The subcutaneous prominence of the screw head can lead to knee pain, requiring screws removal. Other complication can be the tibial shaft fractures or the fracture of the tibial osteotomy fragment (Figure 14). Bleeding and skin healing problems may lead to infection in both cases. Passive range of motion of the knee must be intraoperatively tested till 90° and the fixation of must be rigid.

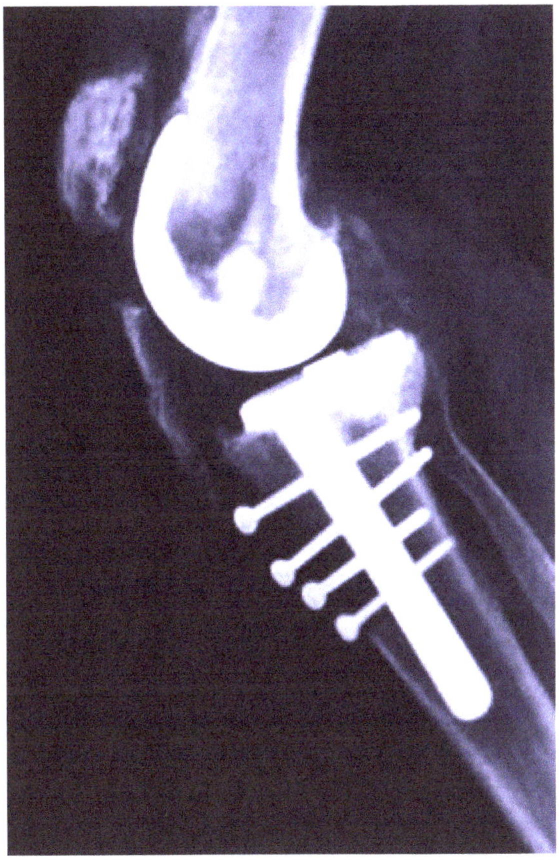

Figure 14. Migrated tibial tubercle

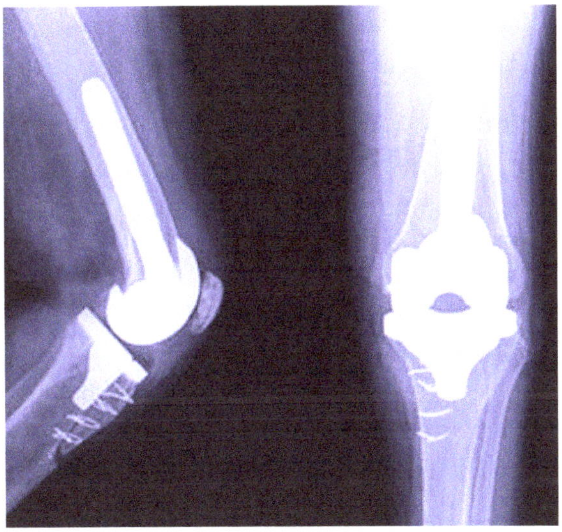

Figure 15. Tibial tubercle fixation with cerclages

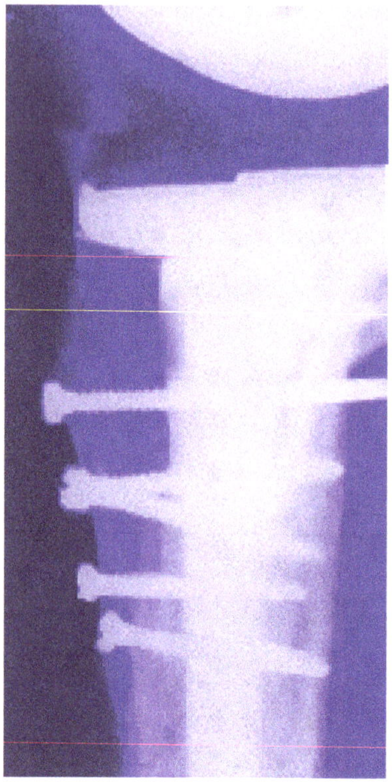

Figure 16. Tibial tubercle fixation with screws

9. Rectus snip technique

This is the main technique used in revision knee arthroplasty or in stiff knees. If the exposure is used in stiff knee, it is important that the stiffness is derived from proximal causes; otherwise, tibial tubercule osteotomy is a better solution.

The technique is easy and straightforward to perform, and good joint exposure is obtained in most of the revision cases or ankylosed knee, but it must be avoided.

The technique consists in cutting the rectus tendon at or near the musculotendinous junction in a 45° direction proximally and laterally, parallel with vastus lateralis' muscular fibers (Figure 17). As a general rule, the tendon must be divided completely and at the end of the procedure, all the muscular fibers should be reattached.

It is very important to remove all fibrotic tissue from the lateral gutter. Afterward, the knee must be flexed easily, and the patella must slide laterally. If this is not possible, a subperiosteal minimal lateral release can be performed around the medial patellar side. After this, if the patella cannot be everted, then the exposure must be extensive and the approach should continue with a rectus snip. John Insall[7] was the first to perform this technique in order to protect the extensor mechanism. The recovery period is a little bit longer, but no modification of postoperative rehabilitation protocol is necessary. Scott modified this technique [9] by dividing the quadriceps tendon not only obliquely but also downward and distally. This technique is known as V-Y quadricepsplasty (Figure 18). The main advantage of this exposure is that if the knee is very stiff and the joint cannot be exposed, this exposure can be converted in a full quadriceps turndown.

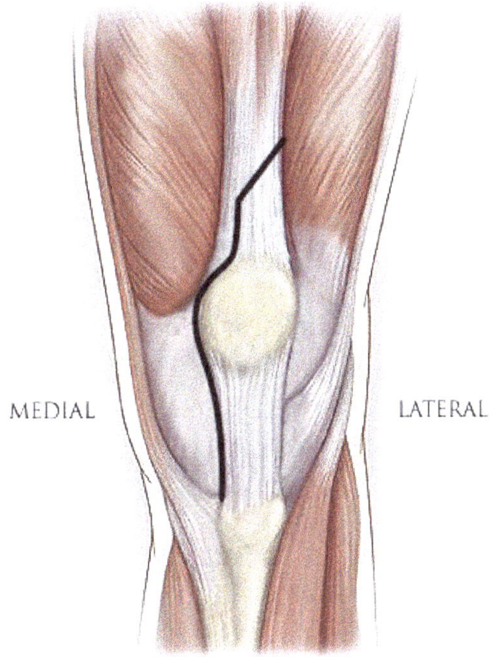

Figure 17. Rectus snip

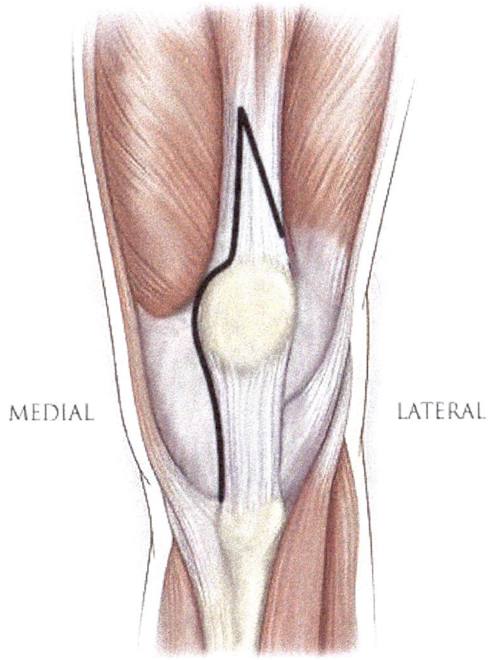

Figure 18. V-Y plasty.

10. Quadriceps turndown

This technique is rarely used. The main indication is severe ankylosed knee, where scaring is so impressive that bending of the knee is impossible. The decision of turndown should be taken after removing all the fibrotic tissue and osteophytes. If scarring of the extensor mechanism is major, then a turndown with lengthening is an option. Actually, there are 2 options for accessing the joint for such knees: one is quadriceps turndown and the other is tibial tubercle osteotomy. The decision is made according to the localization of the soft tissue contracture. If it is distal to the patellar pole, then a tibial osteotomy has to be done. If the contracture is more proximal and in the lateral gutter, then a quadriceps turndown is the solution. This was described by Coonse and Adams and modified by Insall in the patellar turndown approach.

The technique consists in a medial parapatellar approach, and then from the proximal pole of the incision, in a 45° angle, a second incision is made distally and laterally through vastus lateralis and the iliotibial tract. The base of the capsular incision must be broad and the vascularization of the patella through inferolateral genicular artery must be preserved. At the end of the procedure, the extensor mechanism can be lengthened by suturing in V-Y fashion(Figure 18).

Another possibility is the Japanese lamplike quadricepsplasty (Figure 19).

It is recommended to keep the knee in 30° of flexion when performing the lengthening. The recovery period is much longer; the knee must be kept in a brace with limiting knee flexion for the first 4–6 weeks. Sometimes an extension lag is present.

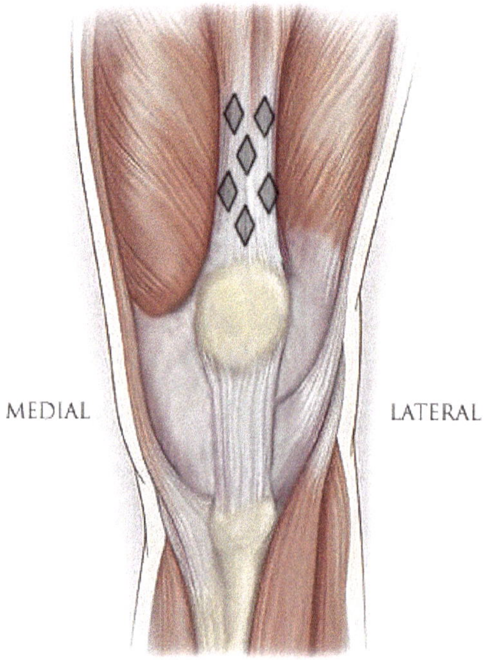

Figure 19. Japanese lamplike quadricepsplasty

11. Medial or lateral epicondylar osteotomy technique [10]

Medial epicondylar osteotomy is similar to the tibial tubercle osteotomy. Instead of releasing the medial soft tissue from the tibia, all the medial soft tissue is released from the femur, together with bony fragments. The technique is rarely used, for example, in cases where there is an important medial soft tissue contracture in flexion and extension. The procedure detaches the epicondyle with a bone fragment approximated 1 cm thick. After the final implant is cemented, the fragment is reattached with screws or sutures in order to have good medial stability. The secret is to keep the soft tissue's integrity between the medial collateral ligament, capsule, and adductor tendons. Sometimes the soft tissue is strong enough to stabilize the bone fragment even if this is not fixated to the femur (Figure 20). This kind of technique is also possible on the lateral side in difficult valgus knees where the lateral femoral epicondyle can be osteotomized and reattached in a new position. These techniques are demanding and can generally be avoided by using more conservative approaches. In our practice, they did not prove their utility.

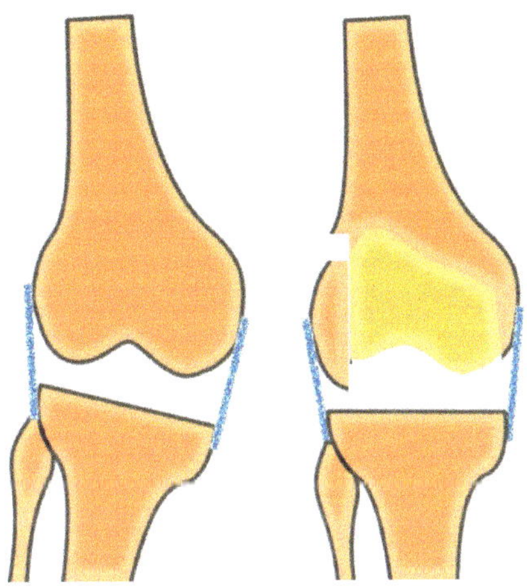

Figure 20. Lateral epicondylar osteotomy technique

Recovery after the knee arthroplasty is very important for a good surgical outcome, generally taking 4 weeks. To reduce the recovery period and the additional cost, many surgeons have developed new surgical techniques: minimal invasive approaches (MIS), new minimized specific instruments, navigation, and personalized surgical instruments (PSI).

After a long trial period of all these new trends, the classic approach remains the gold standard.

12. Minimal invasive surgery approaches (MIS approaches)

The needs to reduce surgery complications, hospital stay, and the need to accelerate functional postoperative recovery have lead surgeons to use smaller incisions that disrupt less tissue.

Additionally, blood loss is significantly lower than that in the classic incision cases; some patients may experience less postoperative pain, some may be able to resume their daily activities sooner, and some prefer the aesthetic aspect of the shorter scar (Figure 21).

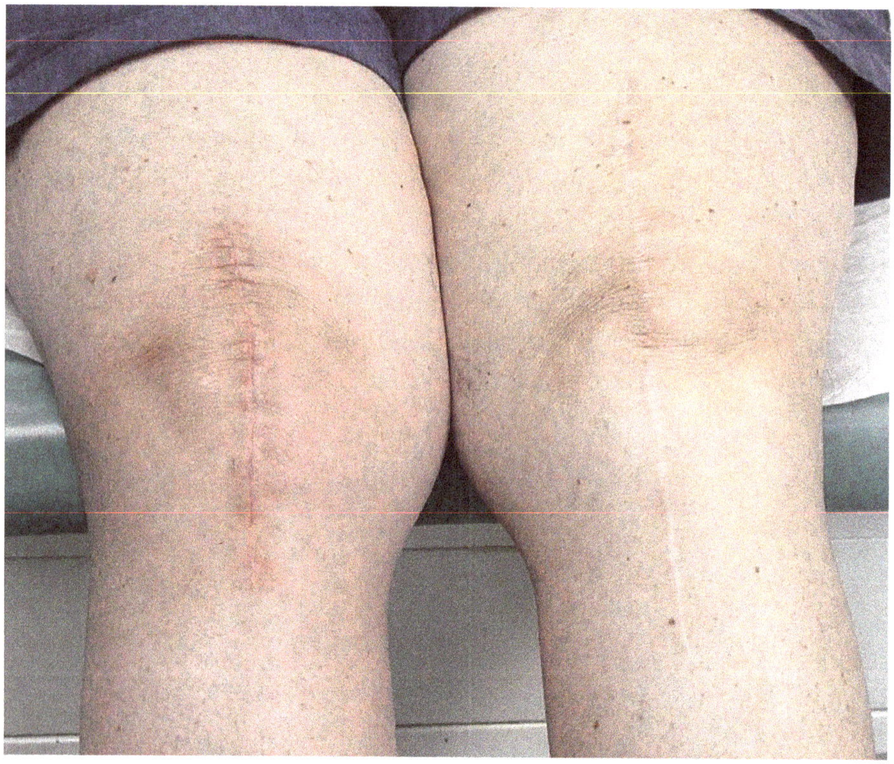

Figure 21. MIS incision versus classical in TKA.

The need for faster recovery time in total knee arthroplasty with less tissue disruption helped develop the mini-incision TKA technique in which the same surgical concepts are utilized, the same alignment goals are followed, but the original instruments have been minimized. A surgeon performing this technique should first have a good background in using the standard TKA procedure and should be familiar with the classical prosthesis components.

The mini-incision TKA is not indicated for all patients. Candidates for mini-incision arthroplasty must have preoperative flexion greater than 90% and must not be obese.

Extreme varus or valgus cases are contraindicated and also patients suffering from rheumatoid arthritis, for structural tissue reasons.

The incision may be made with the leg in extension or flexion depending on surgeon preference. First, the skin incision is made, being substantially smaller than the classical one (Figures 21 and 22). Then the surgeon can choose a mid-vastus approach, a subvastus approach, a mini-medial parapatellar arthrotomy (no quad), or a lateral approach (permits eversion of the patella) (Figure 23). Also, depending on the surgeon's preference, the patella can be either everted (if there is no tension on the patellar tendon) or subluxed (preferable in most cases).

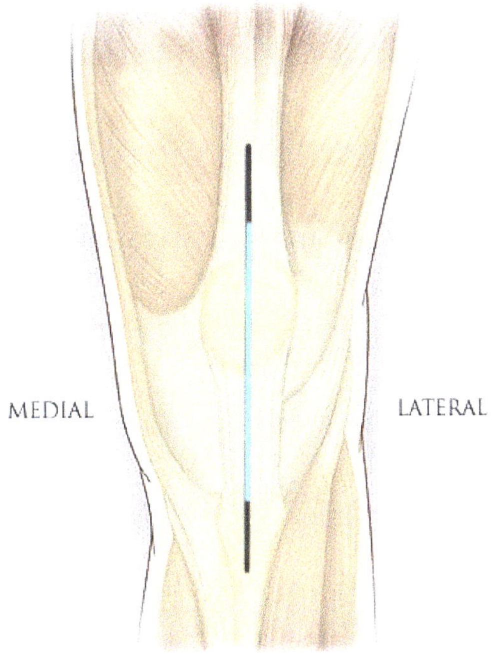

Figure 22. MIS skin incision vs classical.

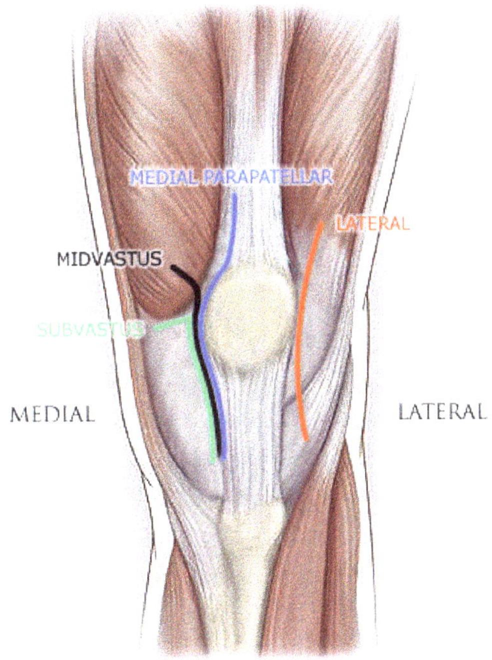

Figure 23. Different MIS incisions.

The length of the incision is dependent on the size of the femoral component needed. Although the goal of a mini-incision technique is to complete the surgery with an approximately 10 to

14 cm incision, extension of the incision is recommended if anatomical landmarks are not fully identified or patellar eversion is challenging, risking tibial tubercle avulsion. Maintaining extensor mechanism insertion is key in the mini-incision technique.

The first step in this procedure is the skin incision that is started at almost 2 cm proximal to the patellar superior pole and continued on the medial border of the patella. The subcutaneous tissue is carefully divided down to the retinaculum, facilitating access to the vastus medialis obliquus muscle. Following this step, the surgeon can choose his preferred type of arthrotomy. The incision's length should normally be about 50% above and 50% below the knee joint line. If it cannot be equally distributed, it is preferable that the longer portion be below the joint line. Electrocautery should be used during all steps of this exposure, minimizing bleeding after deflation of the tourniquet. Below are more detailed descriptions of each of the artrhrotomies used in MIS TKA.

13. MIS approaches – Mini-medial parapatellar arthrotomy [11, 12]

Minimally invasive total knee arthroplasty can be performed with a limited medial parapatellar arthrotomy. Begin by making a 10 to 14 cm midline skin incision from the superior aspect of the tibial tubercle to the superior border of the patella (Figure 22). Following subcutaneous dissection, develop medial and lateral flaps and dissect proximally and distally to expose the extensor mechanism. This permits mobilization of the skin and subcutaneous tissue as needed during the procedure. In addition, with the knee in flexion, the incision will stretch 2–4 cm due to the elasticity of the skin, allowing broader exposure.

The goal of minimally invasive surgery is to limit the surgical dissection without compromising the procedure. The medial parapatellar arthrotomy is used to expose the joint, but the proximal division of the quadriceps tendon should be limited to a length that permits only lateral subluxation. Candidates for mini-incision arthroplasty must have preoperative flexion greater than 90% and must not be obese.

The skin is first incised longitudinally around 10 cm starting from the superior patellar pole to the tibial tubercle. Medial and lateral flaps are now created, and with the flexion of the knee, even more exposure is obtained exposing the extensor mechanism. The dissection of the quadriceps tendon is carefully executed just to permit lateral subluxation of the patella without eversion. Incise the quadriceps tendon for a length of 2–4 cm initially. If is difficult to displace, the patella laterally or if the patellar tendon is at risk of tearing, extend the arthrotomy proximally along the quadriceps tendon until adequate exposure is achieved.

14. MIS approaches – Midvastus arthrotomy

The MIS-midvastus approach involves dividing 1–3 cm of the vastus medialis obliquus's (VMO) muscle fibers in full thickness starting from the superomedial patellar corner proximally (Figure 23). With the knee in flexion, the patella is subluxed laterally or everted. The incision may be extended if the surgeon needs more exposure of the joint.

15. MIS approaches – Subvastus arthrotomy

The MIS-subvastus approach necessitates specially modified instruments. It consists in entering the knee joint through the inferior border of the vastus medialis, making sure not to disturb the quadriceps mechanism (Figure 23). The patella is difficult to evert and is instead subluxed laterally. This approach limits the visibility of the lateral tibial condyle, so it requires a trained and experienced surgeon familiar with its requirements.

16. MIS approaches – Lateral arthrotomy

The MIS lateral approach has been recently described and used, having the advantages not to dislocate the knee joint, not to disturb the quadriceps mechanism, permitting the eversion of the patella but frequently requiring computer-assisted navigation. The approach consists in incising approximately 7–9 cm of the iliotibial band slightly below Gerdy's tubercle to the lateral epicondyle directly lateral to the patella (Figure 23). The distal femur is now exposed from the lateral side. A disadvantage of this lateral arthrotomy may be limited access to the tibia and to the posteromedial soft tissue attachments.

To reduce the recovery period and the additional cost, many surgeons have developed new surgical techniques: minimally invasive approaches, new minimized instruments, navigation, and personalized surgical instruments (PSI).

After a long period of testing of all these new trends, the classic anteromedial parapatellar approach is still the gold standard.

17. Posterior approach

This approach can be useful only in neurovascular complications, but also for repairing the posterior cruciate ligament avulsion fractures or excision of a cyst in the popliteal area.

Make a curvilinear incision 10 to 15 cm long over the popliteal space with the proximal limb following the tendon of the semitendinosus muscle distally to the level of the joint (Figure 24). Curve it laterally across the posterior aspect of the joint for about 5 cm and distally over the lateral head of the gastrocnemius muscle. Identify the posterior cutaneous nerve of the calf (the medial sural cutaneous nerve) lying beneath the fascia and between the two heads of the gastrocnemius muscle being the indicator in the dissection [13]. Expose the popliteal artery and vein, which lie directly anterior and medial to the tibial nerve.

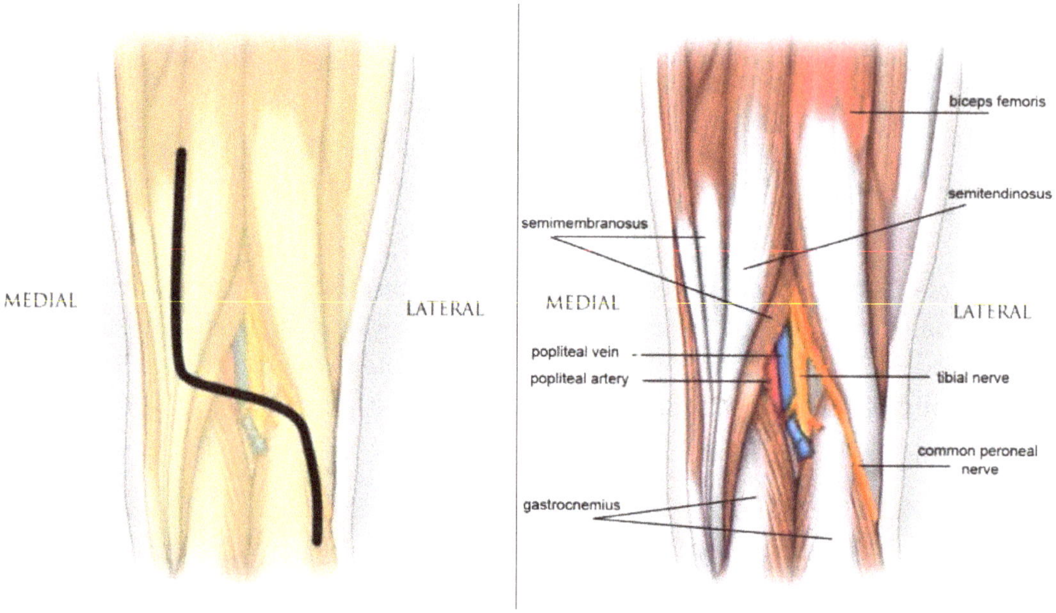

Figure 24. Posterior approach.

Author details

Stefan Cristea*, Vlad Predescu, Şerban Dragosloveanu, Ştefan Cuculici and Nicholas Mărăndici

*Address all correspondence to: drstefancristea@yahoo.com

Emergency Hospital of Saint Pantelimon, Carol Davila University of Medicine and Pharmacy, Bucharest, Romania

References

[1] Fehring TK, Odum S, Griffin WL Patella inversion method for exposure in total knee arthroplasty. J Arthroplasty. 2002:17(1): 101–104

[2] Insall JN. Surgical Approaches in the Knee. New York: Churcill-Livingstone 1984:41–54

[3] Jackson JD, Pagnano MW. The mini-subvastus approach for total knee arthroplasty. The Knee Joint. 2012, pp 775–781

[4] Vaughan LM. TKR through a mini incision. 17th Annual Vail Orthopaedic Symposium. State-of-the-art total hip and knee replacement controversies and solutions. January 19–24, 2003.

[5] Keblish PA. The lateral approach to the valgus knee. Surgical technique and analysis of 53 cases with over two-year follow-up evaluation. Clin Orthop Relat Res. 1991 Oct; (271):52–62.

[6] Barrack RE, Smith P, Munn B. Comparison of surgical approaches in total knee arthroplasty. Clin Orthop 1988; 356:16–21

[7] Dalin MG. Osteotomy the tibial tubercle in total knee replacement J Bone Joint Surg 1983;65-A:704–706

[8] Whiteside LA. Exposure in difficult total knee arthroplasty using tibial tubercle osteotomy. Clin Orthop 1995;321: 32–35

[9] Scott RD, Siliski JM. The use of a modified V-Y quadricepsplasty during total knee replacement to gain exposure and improve knee flexion in the ankylosed knee. Orthopedics 1985;8: 45–48

[10] Engh GA. Medial epicondylar osteotomy: a technique used with primary and revision arthroplasty to improve surgical exposure and correct varus deformity. Instr Course Lect 1999;48:153–156

[11] Scuderi GR, Tria, AJ, Jr., Berger RA (eds.). MIS Techniques in Orthopedics. Springer Science, 2006.

[12] Garvin KL, Scuderi G, Insall JN. Evolution of the quadriceps snip. Clin Orthop 1995;321:131–137.

[13] LaPrade et al. The anatomy of the posterior aspect of the knee, an anatomic study. JBJS 2007. 89 758–764.

4

Elbow Arthroscopy

Satish B. Sonar

Abstract

Introduction: Elbow joint is a complex articulation of three bones. It is a hinge joint with three types of motions; flexion-extension, varus-valgus and rotations. With advancement of instrumentations, our knowledge about surgical anatomy and surgical skills, elbow arthroscopy has become an excellent tool to treat a wide range of disorders with minimum risk and complications.

Pathologies such as tennis elbow, OCD, fracture radial head, fracture capitulum, stiff elbow, synovitis, loose bodies, etc, are now easily treated with arthroscopic technique.

Elbow arthroscopy has its role in the management of ligament injuries and instability.

There are three major neurovascular bundles in close proximity of elbow joint, the median nerve on posteromedial aspect, the radial nerve on posterolateral side and the ulnar nerve along with brachial vessels anteriorly.

Materials & Methods: Procedure can be performed either under general or regional anesthesia.

Usually, in young and cooperative patients, regional anesthesia in the form of interscalene, axillary, or Bier's block can be used.

In elderly and non-cooperative patients, general anesthesia with or without regional block for postoperative pain management can be used.

We usually prefer the lateral position with the elbow freely hanging on the support. But there are three positions described for elbow arthroscopy, supine position, prone position and lateral decubitus position.

Conclusion: Elbow arthroscopy is a minimally invasive procedure and provide good to excellent long term results. We can diagnose and treat concomitant intra-articular pathologies specially posterolateral plica, lateral gutter impingement, loose bodies and posterolateral rotator instability. We can fix fractures, treat tendinopathies, do chondroplasty and stiff elbow release. With the advancement of instrumentations, our knowledge about surgical anatomy and surgical skills, elbow arthroscopy has become an excellent tool to treat wide range of disorders with minimum risk and complications.

Keywords: Instability, Tennis Elbow, Fractures

1. Introduction

Elbow joint is a complex articulation of three bones. It is a hinge joint with three types of motions; flexion-extension, varus-valgus and rotations. With advancement of instrumentations, our knowledge about surgical anatomy and surgical skills, elbow arthroscopy has become an excellent tool to treat a wide range of disorders with minimum risk and complications.

Pathologies such as tennis elbow, OCD, fracture radial head, fracture capitulum, stiff elbow, synovitis, loose bodies, etc, are now easily treated with arthroscopic technique.

Elbow arthroscopy has its role in the management of ligament injuries and instability

There are three major neurovascular bundles in close proximity of elbow joint, the median nerve on posteromedial aspect, the radial nerve on posterolateral side and the ulnar nerve along with brachial vessels anteriorly

1.1. Materials and methods

Procedure can be performed either under general or regional anesthesia.

Usually, in young and cooperative patients, regional anesthesia in the form of interscalene, axillary, or Bier's block can be used.

In elderly and non-cooperative patients, general anesthesia with or without regional block for postoperative pain management can be used

We usually prefer the lateral position with the elbow freely hanging on the support. But there are three positions described for elbow arthroscopy, supine position, prone position and lateral decubitus position

1.2. Conclusion

Elbow arthroscopy is a minimally invasive procedure and provide good to excellent long term results. We can diagnose and treat concomitant intra-articular pathologies specially posterolateral plica, lateral gutter impingement, loose bodies and posterolateral rotator instability. We can fix fractures, treat tendinopathies, do chondroplasty and stiff elbow release. With the advancement of instrumentations, our knowledge about surgical anatomy and surgical skills, elbow arthroscopy has become an excellent tool to treat wide range of disorders with minimum risk and complications.

2. Elbow arthroscopy

2.1. Introduction

Elbow joint is a complex articulation of three bones. It is a hinge joint with three types of motions; flexion-extension, varus-valgus and rotations.

There are three major neurovascular bundles in close proximity of elbow joint, the median nerve on posteromedial aspect, the radial nerve on posterolateral side and the ulnar nerve along with brachial vessels anteriorly [5].

These things, along with a closely confined space, makes elbow arthroscopy a challenging procedure [4].

With the advancement of instrumentations, our knowledge about surgical anatomy and surgical skills, elbow arthroscopy has become an excellent tool to treat a wide range of disorders, with minimum risk and complications [1,4,5].

Pathologies such as tennis elbow, OCD, fracture radial head, fracture capitulum, stiff elbow, synovitis, loose bodies, etc, are now easily treated with arthroscopic technique [2].

Elbow arthroscopy has its role in the management of ligament injuries and instability [2].

Usually, a standard 4mm 30° arthroscope is sufficient for most of the procedures. In smaller joints, a 2.7mm scope can be used.

Procedure can be performed either under general or regional anesthesia [1].

Usually in young and cooperative patients, regional anesthesia in the form of interscalene, axillary, or Bier's block can be used.

In elderly and non-cooperative patients, general anesthesia with or without regional block for postoperative pain management can be used [1].

Position:-

We usually prefer the lateral position with the elbow freely hanging on the support.

There are three positions described for elbow arthroscopy.

1. Supine position: In 1985, Andrews and Carson first reported on supine positioning with a traction device for elbow arthroscopy. Morrey described supine positioning without a traction device in 1986 [1].

It is the most suitable position from the patient's and anesthetist's point of view.

But it requires special traction device to hold the limb in position. Though the position is best for anatomical orientation, it has certain disadvantages. An additional assistant is needed to support the elbow, elbow manipulation under traction is limited and access to posterior compartment is limited [1].

2. Prone position:- Poehling reported on elbow arthroscopy in the prone position in 1989.

This position greatly overcome the disadvantages of supine position, but is problematic from anesthesia point of view. With the patient in prone position, the elbow can be held on the bolster or arm holder in 90° flexion freely hanging on the side of the table. Accessing the posterior compartment, manipulation and conversion to open procedure is easier. Procedure in this position can be performed only under general anesthesia as maintaining the prone position under regional block will be difficult for the patient[1].

3. Lateral decubitus position: - O'Driscoll and Morrey described the lateral decubitus position for elbow arthroscopy in 1992. This is by far the most preferred position used for elbow arthroscopy [1]. It is easy to hold the arm on the support or bolster just like in the prone position. It has the same advantages as the prone position and avoids anesthesia problems also [1,2].

The procedure can be easily performed under regional anesthesia. With the distension of the joint the anterior neurovascular structures are pushed away making the procedure safer.

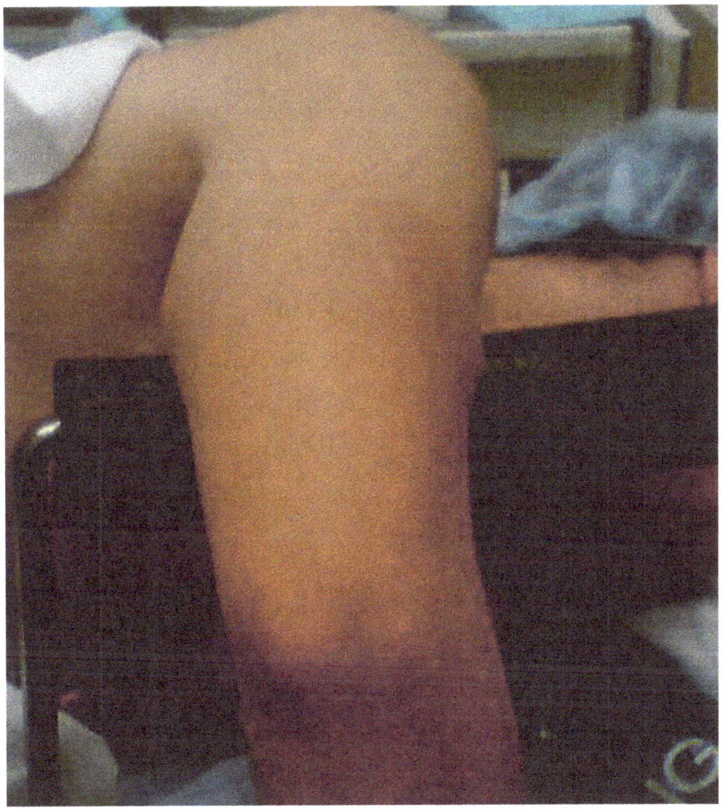

Figure 1. Lateral decubitus position

Portals:-

There are many portals described for elbow arthroscopy, but basically 5-6 portals are the most useful.

i. Basic portals

1. Anteromedial portal

2. Anterolateral portal

3. Midlateral portal

ii. Accessory portals

4. Proximal anterolateral portal

5. Proximal anteromedial portal

6. Posterolateral portal

7. Direct posterior portal

1. Anteromedial portal

This is the first portal made as a viewing portal.

It is 2 cm anterior to the medial epicondyle.

First, a small skin incision is made and a blunt trocar is advanced flush to the anteromedial surface of the humerus, directing toward the lateral epicondyle.

Since the anteromedial portal is anterior to the medial epicondyle, the ulnar nerve is at a minimal risk if the portal is placed properly [4, 5].

2. Anterolateral portal

This portal can be best made by the inside out technique from a anteromedial portal. It is situated about 1 cm anterior and 1cm distal to the lateral epicondyle. It coincides with the radiocapitular joint and is the safest lateral portal.

3. Midlateral portal

It is a direct soft spot portal situated in the anconeus triangle. Just like in knee arthroscopy, the trocar is introduced in the flexion and gently extending the elbow, it is directed towards the olecronon fossa. This portal is useful for viewing the inferior portions of the radial head, capitellum, ulnohumeral articulation, and olecronon fossa.

4. Proximal anterolateral portal

It is about 2 cm proximal and 1 cm anterior to the lateral epicondyle. A blunt trocar is directed toward the center of the joint flush to the anterior surface of the distal humerus.

This portal provides excellent visualization of the anterior compartment.

5. Proximal anteromedial portal (PAM)

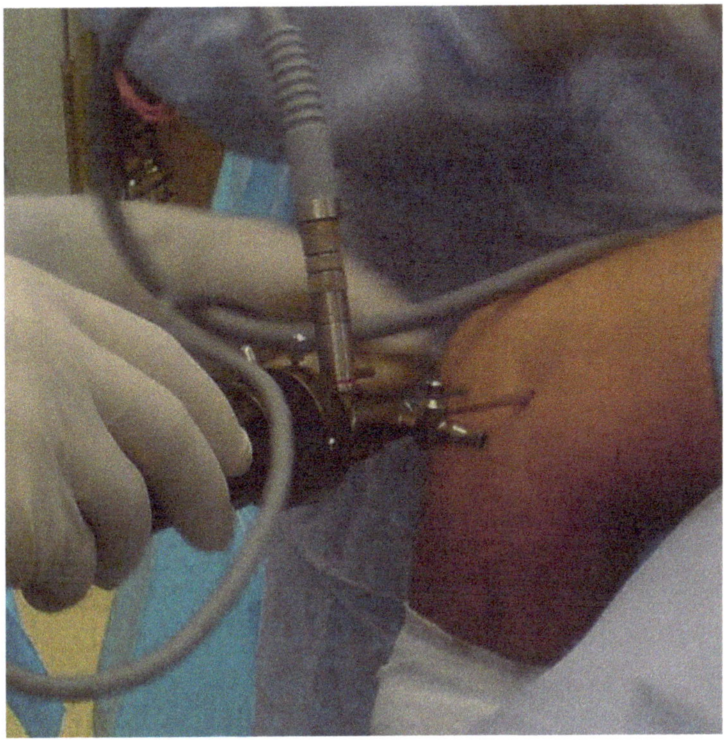

Figure 2. Anteromedial portal

The PAM portal is 2 cm anterior and proximal to the medial epicondyle. The medial intermuscular septum is palpated, and the portal is established anterior to the septum.

Just a skin incision is made and a blunt trocar is directed towards the radial head going flush to the anterior surface of distal humerus.

6. Posterolateral portal

It is just proximal to the olecranon and along the lateral border of the triceps tendon. After making a skin incision, a blunt trocar is directed toward the center of the olecranon fossa with the elbow in 45° flexion.

PLP is best for the visualization of the olecranon tip, olecranon fossa, and posterior trochlea, as well as the medial and lateral gutters.

7. Direct posterior portal (DPP)

The DPP is made in the midline posteriorly and 3 cm proximal to the olecranon tip. This portal is excellent for the visualization of the entire posterior compartment.

Examination:

- Inspection :-

The elbow joint is examined from the front, back and sides.

Lateral recess, medial epicondyle, antecubital fossa, and olecranon tip are inspected.

Prominence of the Olecranon tip may indicate posterior/posterolateral dislocation or triceps avulsion.

Ecchymosis anteriorly may indicate biceps tendon rupture.

Ecchymosis medially may indicate a fracture of the medial epicondyle or avulsion injury

Olecranon bursa should be inspected; if it is enlarged it may represent bursitis either aseptic or septic.

The ulnar nerve subluxation may be visible

- Palpation:-

Bony palpation is done in a step –wise manner:-

- Olecranon
    - Posteromedial tip (impingement)
    - Proximal shaft (stress fractures)
- Epicondyles:- Medial and lateral
    - Fractures
    - Epicondylitis

Medial Epicondylitis (golfer's elbow)

- Palpate medial muslce mass/epicondyle while resisting active pronation
- Pain either within muscle belly or directly over epicondyle

Lateral Epicondylitis (tennis elbow)

- Palpate mobile wad while resisting active supination (extensor carpi radialis brevis is the most common offender)
- Pain within muscle belly or over epicondyle
- Radial head
    - Fractures
    - Dislocations

Active followed by passive range of motion is checked.

Normal ROM in adult is 0 – 140 °(+/- 10°) in sagittal plane and 80-90°of forearm rotation in each direction.

With progressive flexion, the elbow moves into increasing valgus.

Impingement of the posteromedial tip of the olecranon in the olecranon fossa is examined by the vulgus extension and supination movement to diagnose vulgus extension overload (VEO) syndrome [2].

Soft tissues

- Antecubital fossa
  - Mobile wad, biceps tendon, brachial pulse
  - Median nerve not generally palpable
- Medial
  - Flexor-pronator mass
  - Ulnar nerve
  - UCL

Valgus stress test:-

With the patient in supine or prone position, abduct and maximally externally rotate the shoulder.

Elbow is flexed 25°and valgus stress applied.

Assess for end-feel and amount of opening and do not induce any pain in the normal elbow.

The radial collateral ligament and the lateral ulnar collateral ligament make up the lateral ligament complex [3].

Varus stress test;

Apply varus stress with the elbow flexed 15-20°and the arm is internally rotated to prevent shoulder rotation.

Assess any pain or increased varus laxity [3].

- Posterolateral rotator instability (PLRI):-
- Test for PLRI = "Pivot Shift"

Anesthetize supine patient and do forward flexion and external rotation of the shoulder.

Forearm supination and axial load with valgus stress as arm is gradually flexed.

Radial head subluxes posteriorly and "clunks" back into place.

- Stress x-ray

Graded stress x-rays in evaluation of the injury to the UCL of the elbow[3]

MRI:-

Diagnostic arthroscopy:-

After making the diagnosis and having decided for elbow surgery, the patient is prepared for the day care procedure. Preoperative intravenous antibiotics are given. After suitable anesthesia, we usually put the patient in the lateral decubitus position using an arm holder and a

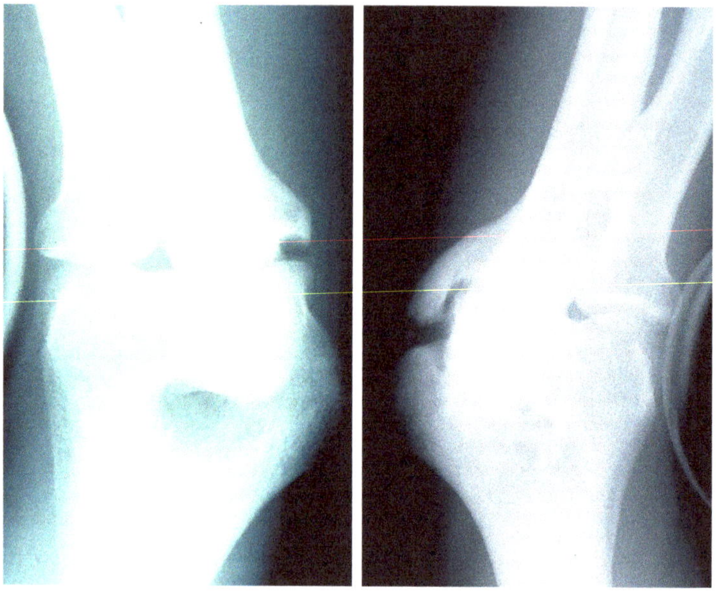

Figure 3. Medial joint opening-valgus stress

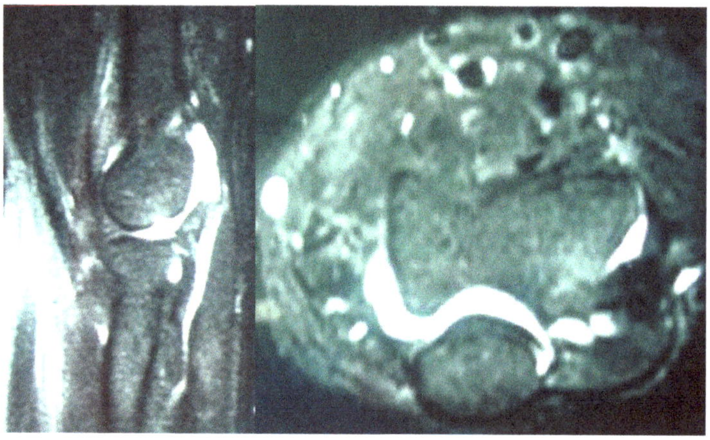

Figure 4. LUCL tear

bolster. The elbow should be positioned and draped so that the arm is supported by the holder at the proximal upper arm; the elbow rests at 90°. Care must be taken to keep the antecubital fossa free from contact with the bolster. The arthroscopy trolley is set on the opposite side of the patient. An examination under anesthesia is performed to determine elbow range of motion and stability. Prepping, draping and exsanguinations are done and the tourniquet is inflated. Surface landmarks of medial, lateral epicondyles, olecronon radial head, ligaments, and portals are marked with the sterile marker pen. The lateral soft-spot portal location is identified and 20 to 30 ml of saline is injected into the elbow joint space. A number 11 blade is used to incise the skin only to make an AM portal and blunt trocar -cannula for the 4-mm arthroscope are introduced toward the radial head maintaining contact with the anterior cortex of the distal Humerus. A 4-mm, 30°arthroscope attached to monitor via camera is then used to examine the capitellum, radial head, anterolateral capsule, coronoid process and fossa.

With pronation and in supination movements the radio-capitellar joint can be examined.

Now the anterolateral portal can be established by the inside out technique with Wisinger rod from the anteromedial portal directed towards the radial head. Or by the outside-in technique using a spinal needle introduced at about 1 cm anterior and 1cm distal to the lateral epicondyle. It coincides with radiocapitular joint and is the safest lateral portal. After this, using a Wisinger rod and sheath, a 4mm, 30°arthroscope is introduced through the anterolateral portal and medial capsule, trochlea, and coronoid can be examined.

The posterior compartment is examined by making a posterolateral portal just proximal to the olecranon and along the lateral border of the triceps tendon. After making a skin incision, blunt trocar is directed toward the center of the olecranon fossa with the elbow in 45° flexion. The olecronon process and fossa, medial and lateral gutters, and posterior radio-capitellar joint and capsule are examined.

Now through the soft spot midlateral portal, the posterior radial head, capitellum, and ulnohumeral articulation can be visualized. Direct posterior portal can be made for instrumentation if any pathology is found posteriorly.

Once the procedure is complete, portals are closed, compressive dressing applied, and the tourniquet is released.

Depending upon the procedure performed, a splint or brace is applied. An exercise program for the specific disorder is started on day two to be continued at home [1,2].

3. Medial elbow instability

The medial collateral ligament (UCL/MCL) is the only primary static stabilizer on the medial side in 30-90° flexions [6]. Though the common flexor muscles, radio-capitellar articulation, and ulnohumeral articulation provide secondary restrains, UCL is the main medial support in throwing, backhand tennis or badminton serve, golf, and activities of daily living requiring flexion-valgus movements of the elbow [6]. Repetitive valgus stresses to the elbow occurring during the throwing can lead to MCL incompetence, ulnar neuritis, and vulgus extension overload [7].

Acute injury to the MCL (UCL) can occur with a fall of an outstretched hand with the elbow in valgus and supination [6].

MCL consists of the anterior bundle, posterior bundle, and transverse segment.

The anterior bundle is the primary restraint to valgus stress at the elbow.

In cases of MCL insufficiency due to repeated micro trauma, pain is localized to the medial elbow generally in throwing, backhand serve, underarm throw in cricket, etc. Since it's a cumulative injury over time, the patient does not remember the injury [7]. Associated ulnar neuritis causing paresthesias in the posteromedial elbow to the ring and small fingers may be the first complaint [7].

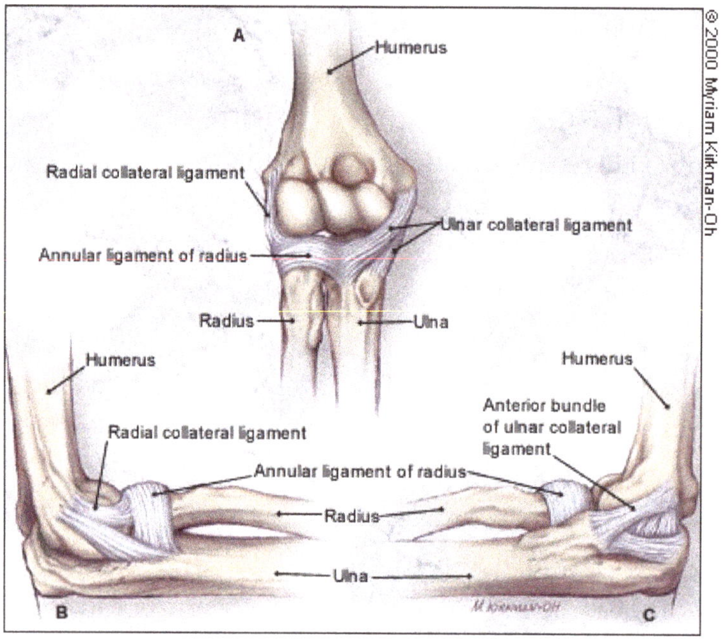

Figure 5. Medial collateral ligament-anatomy

But in acute traumatic injury, there is an event followed by a "pop" sensation, pain, swelling and inability use the elbow with without bruising [6,10].

Complications of chronic instability:-

Ulnar neuritis, posteromedial olecranon impingement (VEO), and ulnohumeral arthritis [7].

Examination:-

Inspection:- Swelling and bruising along the medial aspect.

Palpation: - Tenderness along the MCL course; may feel gapping, restricted and painful ROM.

Valgus stress test: valgus load applied to the elbow with the elbow flexed 20°. Positive results means the reproduction of medial elbow pain and valgus laxity greater on the injured side as compared to contra lateral side.

Moving valgus stress test: Rrapid extension from full flexion while maintaining a constant valgus stress. Positive result means the reproduction of medial elbow pain.

Milking maneuver: Patient or examiner pulls on the patient's thumb creating a valgus stress, with the patient's forearm supinated and elbow flexed 90°. Medial elbow pain indicates medial elbow instability.

Xray / MRI

X-rays are generally normal, but may show MCL calcification, medial humeral osteophytes, ulnar osteophytes, posterior olecranon spurring, or loose bodies [8].

Valgus stress x-rays: > 3 mm medial opening on side-to-side comparisons is diagnostic of valgus instability [8].

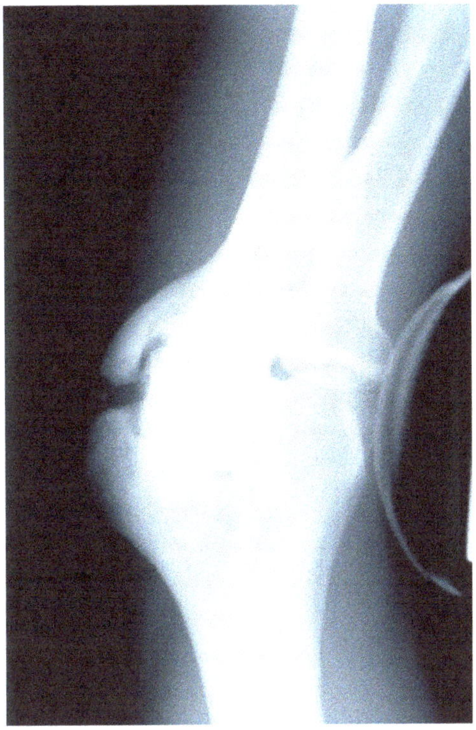

Figure 6. Valgus stress X-ray- medial opening.

MRI: 3 Tesla MRI will accurately show the MCL tear; T- sign of ulnar avulsion, humeral MCL avulsion or midsubstance tearing [8].

CT arthrography: Rarely needed in todays world with the availability of high resolution MRI [8].

Treatment

Primary treatment for the player is rest from throwing and for others to avoid repetitive elbow valgus extension movement. Taping and physical therapy with lateral stretching, flexor-pronator strengthening and modalities are also applied. Gradual arm and forearm muscle strengthening and sports specific rehabilitation are done after 10-12 weeks [6, 7].

If after the above schedule the patient fails to improve through conservative treatment, he/she will need MCL repair, MCL reconstruction +/-capsular placation.

Arthroscopy: Elbow arthroscopy is performed as a surgical adjunct performed in concert with open surgical procedures and arthroscopic elbow instability assessment can provide valuable information [4]. Medial joint opening and ligament laxity can be demonstrated and documented [9]. It is indicated for those patients who maintain symptoms of posteromedial impingement despite non-operative management.

Reconstruction:- A palmaris longus or semitendinosus tendon is harvested and prepared.

Medial approach:- The approach to the elbow is a muscle-splitting technique described by Thompson. Medial skin is incised from the medial epicondyle to 5 cm distally along the medial

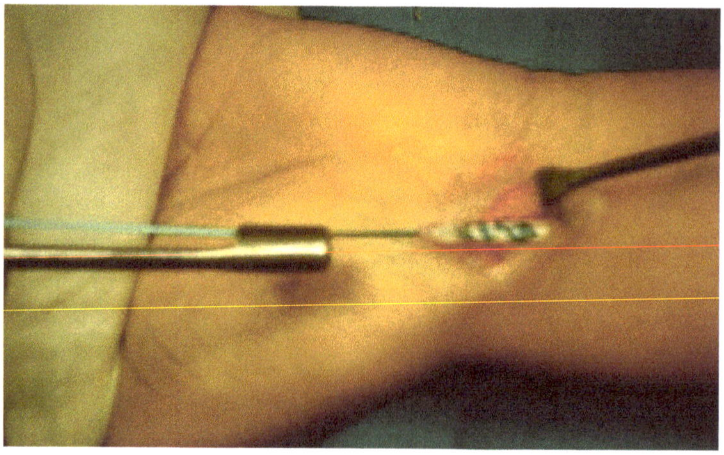

Figure 7. Palmaris longus tendon harvest.

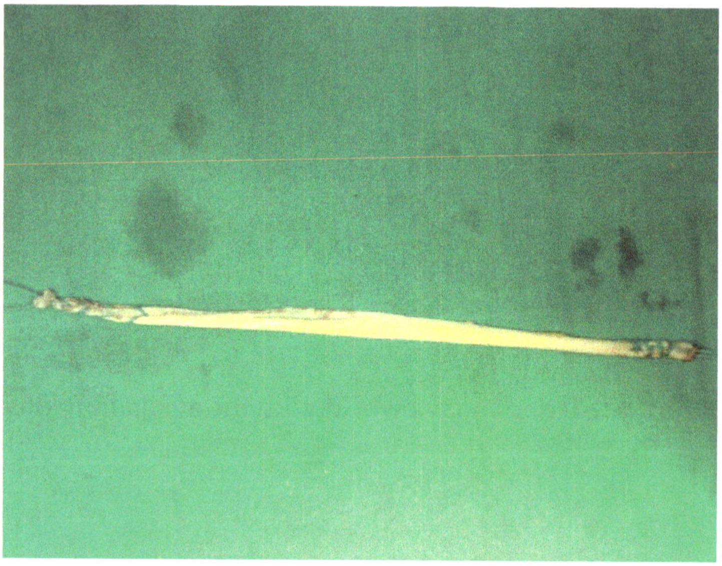

Figure 8. Graft preperation

border of ulna is made. Blunt dissection is used to develop a plane in line with the fibers of the flexor Carpi ulnaris, beginning at the medial epicondyle down to the sublime tubercle of the ulna [7, 10]. The muscle is retracted to expose the native UCL and care is taken not to injure the ulnar nerve. The UCL is incised in line with the muscle fibers and the fascial incision. Anterior and posterior leaflets are created by sharply dissecting the ligament off of the ulna, exposing the sublime tubercle. A safe zone has been described as 1 cm distal to the insertion of the UCL two, 4.5 mm tunnels are made around, unicorticaly, and then connected to each other using large towel clip [11].

After making the ulnar tunnes, humeral tunnels are made. The anterior band of the UCL originates at the anterior and inferior portion of the medial epicondyle and the posterior band from the posteroinferior portion. The tunnel is made at the isometric point between these two bundles. To expose the anterior surface of the medial epicondyle, a separate fascial incision is made proximal to the medial epicondyle. The muscle fibers are gently elevated off the bone. A total of three tunnels are made in the medial condyle; first at the isometric point at the base of medial epicondyle, second anterosuperiorly, and third posterosuperiorly by a 4.5mm drill bit [11]. The inferior tunnel is enlarged and all three tunnels then interlinked using a towel clip.

Graft is passed in the ulnar tunnels using No. 5 Ethibond as a relay and then through the humeral tunnels and exiting one anterosuperiorly, and another posterosuperiorly. The sutures are pulled, and the graft tensioned and tied at the desired flexion angle of the elbow about 60°–70° of flexion [7, 11].

The wound is closed in layers and a splint is applied at 70° flexion [11].

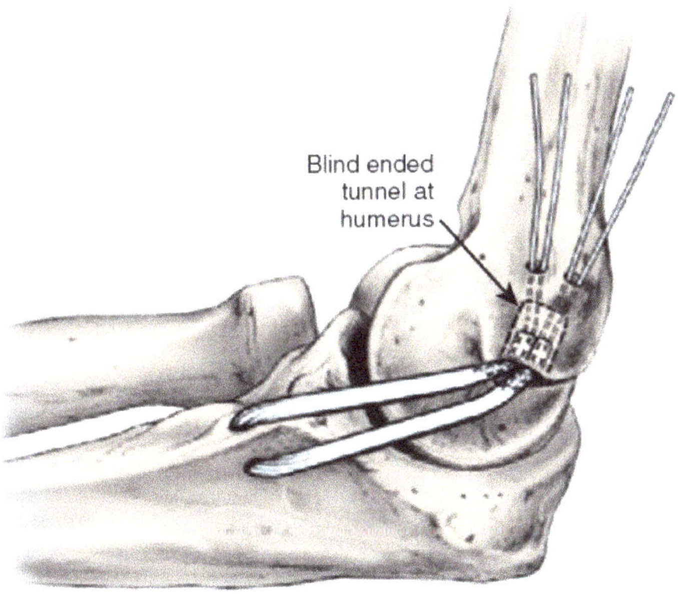

Figure 9. Two ulnar and three humeral tunnels.

Postoperative Rehabilitation :-

A splint is applied in 60°-70° of flexion for 3 weeks. Initially, 0°-30°of movement is restricted for 4 weeks.

The range of 60°-90° of movement is started from 1st two weeks, 40°-100° of movement from 3- 5weeks and 20°-110° from 6-8 weeks.

After about two months, full range of movement is started along with isotonic strengthening, concentric flexor-pronator and eccentric elbow flexor exercises.

After 3 months, sports specific training, arm and forearm muscles strengthening and proprioceptive exercises are started.

The athlete can return to sports after 6- 8 months, depending upon elbow strength and overall fitness status.

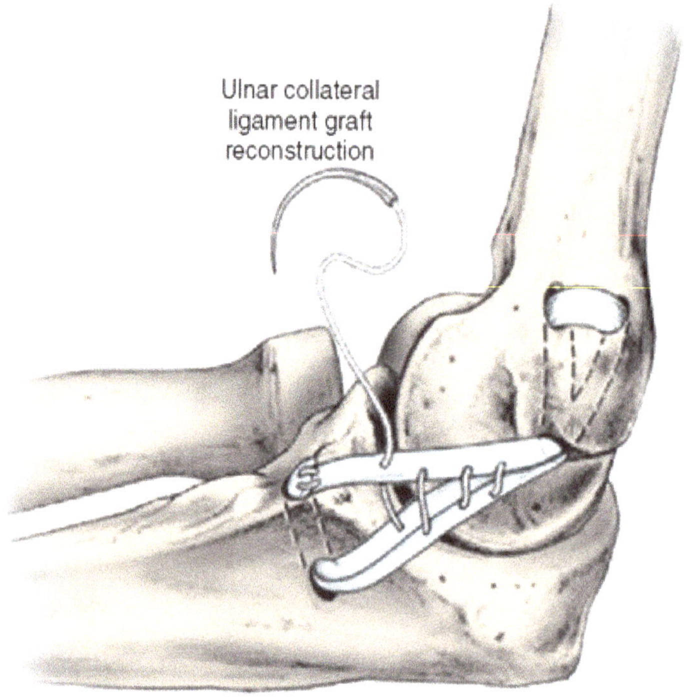

Figure 10. Docking technique.

Full speed pitching, strong backhand serve, and powerful golf swing is not recommended for 12 months after reconstruction [7, 11].

Medial elbow instability is most often a chronic attenuation and insufficiency of UCL due to repeated micro trauma in throwing athletes, baseball players, and workers involved in repeated throwing activities [7].

Valgus stress test and milking maneuver can clinch the diagnosis, but MRI is the investigation of choice to diagnose the tear. Arthroscopy helps in treating concomitant pathologies [9].

UCL reconstruction using Palmaris longus or semitendinosus tendon graft, provide good medial stability and with proper rehab, a player can return to sports in 6- 8 months [6].

4. Lateral instability and Posterolateral Rotatory Instability (PLRI)

Posterolateral rotatory instability is the most common pattern of elbow instability, particularly that which is recurrent.

Posterolateral rotatory instability can be considered a spectrum consisting of three stages according to the degree of soft tissue disruption [12].

Patients typically present with a history of recurrent painful clicking, snapping, clunking, or locking of the elbow and careful examination reveals that this occurs in the extension portion of the arc of motion with the forearm in supination [12, 13].

Deficiency of LUCL and laxity/tear of the posterolateral capsule leads to the abnormal rotation of the ulna posteriorly taking the radius along with it. It is an initial stage in the pathology of unstable elbow. Radial head excision or any lateral bony loss further aggravates the instability [12, 13, 15].

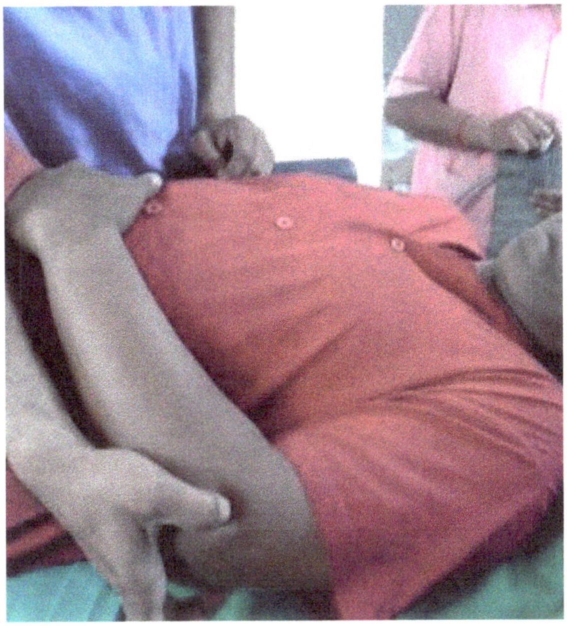

Figure 11. Tenderness over LUCL

Pain along the posterolateral aspect of the elbow is the main symptom. The patient usualy has pain in standing from the sitting position with hand resting on chair arms, in lifting weight, and in throwing. In severe cases, patients also complain about instability [12, 13].

Examination:-

Patients had varus instability in 30° flexion, tenderness over PL elbow, and chair test and push-up test were positive in most of the patients.

Chair test:

Ask the patient to stand up from the armed chair with both elbows taking the upper body weight.

At about 20°- 30°extension, patient feels pain and sudden click or instability due to postero-lateral subluxation of the ulna.

Push up test:

Similar symptoms can be produced by asking the patient to do push ups. At about 20°-30°extension, patient feels pain and sudden click or instability due to posterolateral subluxation of the ulna.

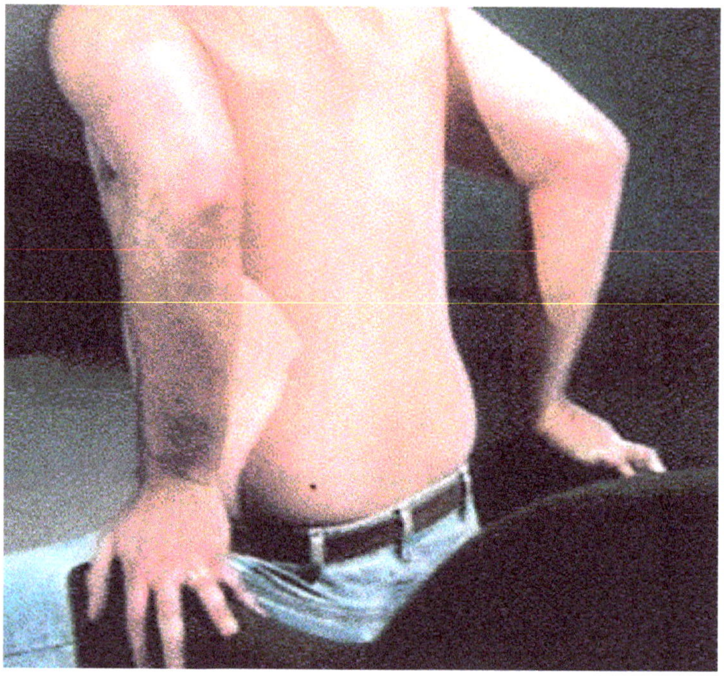

Figure 12. Chair test

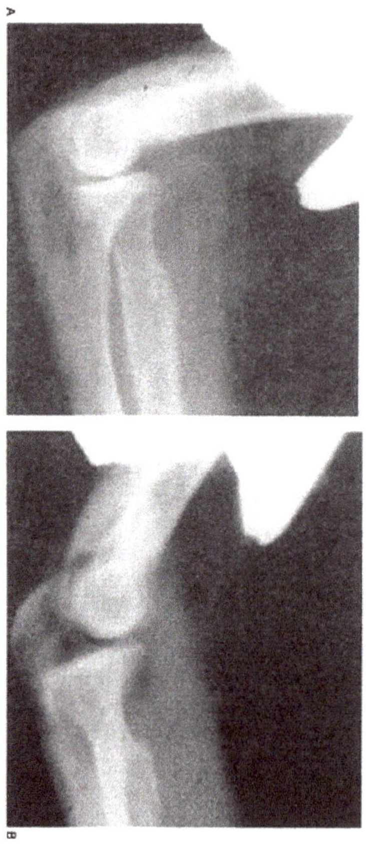

Figure 13. Varus stress x-ray

5. Surgical details

The pivot shift test which was negative in all on OPD examination was positive under anesthesia in all. Stress x-ray showed significant lateral opening. MRI is an effective tool in the preoperative, noninvasive diagnosis of posterolateral rotatory instability [12, 16].

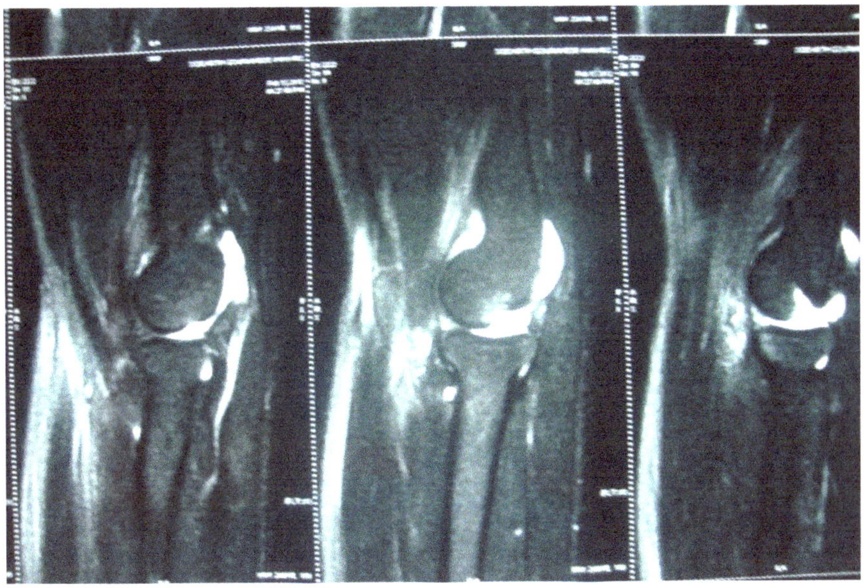

Figure 14. Sagital T2 MRI-showing LUCL and posterior capsular tear

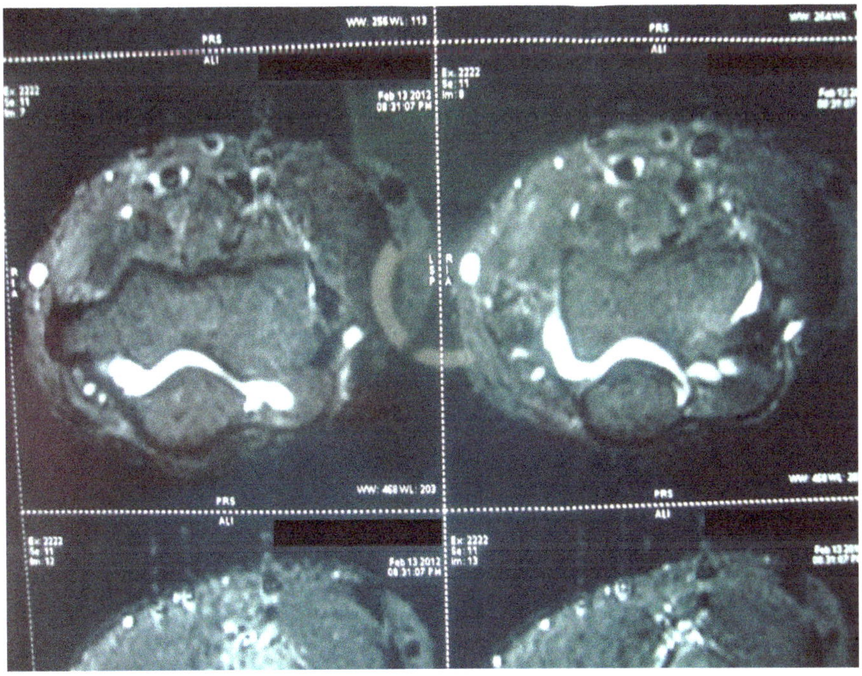

Figure 15. Axial section T2 MRI- showing LUCL tear

6. Arthroscopy

The patient is placed in lateral decubitus position with the elbow free and arm supported on a bar. Tourniquet is applied well proximally for free access [15]. Anteromedial and anterolateral portals are used with special attention to the median and the radial nerves. Anteromedial was used as a viewing portal and the anterolateral as the working portal. Cartilage flakes are removed, debridement done using a shaver through anterolateral portal and chondroplasty is done. You will see the torn or stretched capsule posterosuperior to radial head. Lateral ulnar collateral ligament tear or attenuation will be seen and the area around its origin can be debrided and marked for open reconstruction [13, 14]. Arthroscopy is helpful in not only diagnosing the condition but also treating other pathologies that coexist with PLRI [14].

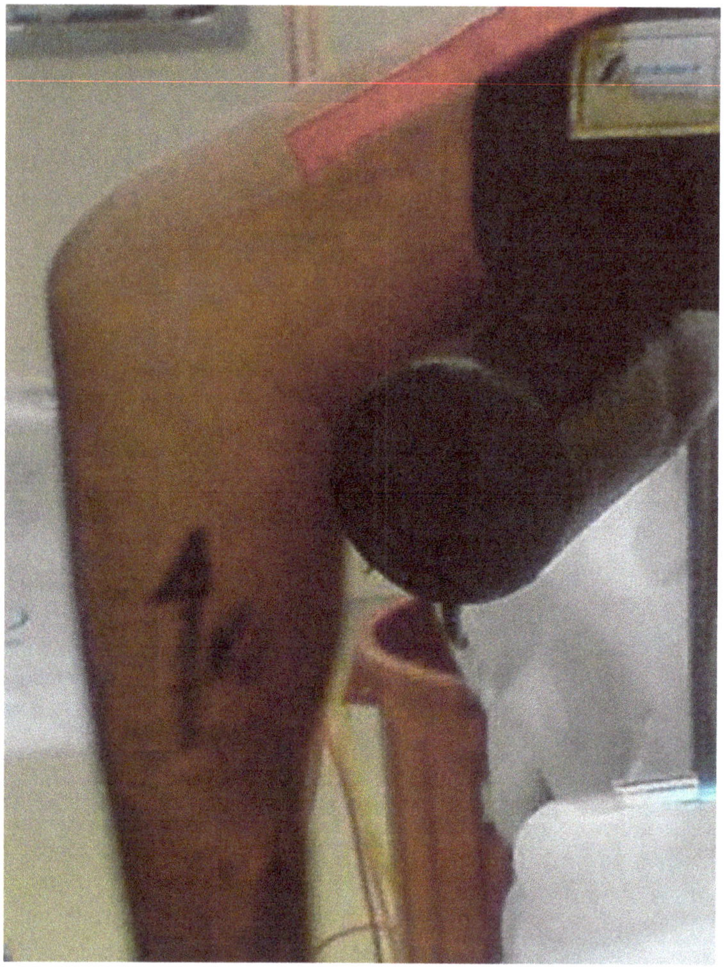

Figure 16. Lateral position

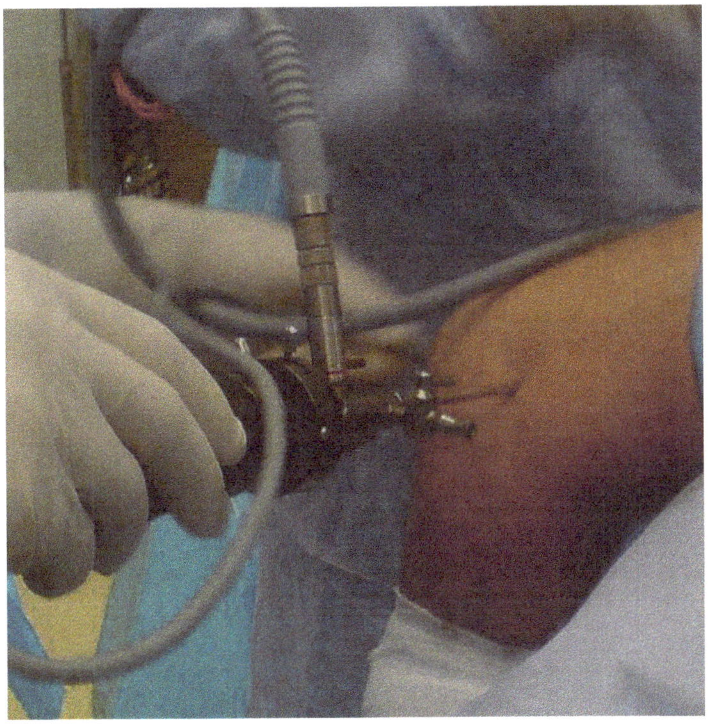

Figure 17. Anteromedial viewing portal

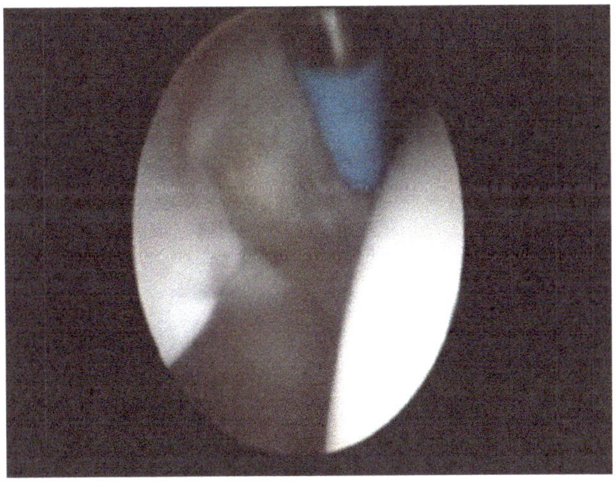

Figure 18. Arthroscopic view of humeral attachment of LUCL

7. Open procedure

7.1. Graft harvest

Patient made supine and painting and redrapping is done. Reconstructive procedure started with harvesting palmaris longus graft from the same side [15, 16]. A 1 cm incision is made in the palmer wrist crease. The palmaris longus graft is identified, released gently, and harvested using a tendon stripper. In one patient, it was absent so gracilis tendon was harvested instead. The graft was prepared using No.2 Ethibond. The graft is wrapped in wet gauze with amikacin, and kept in a bowl.

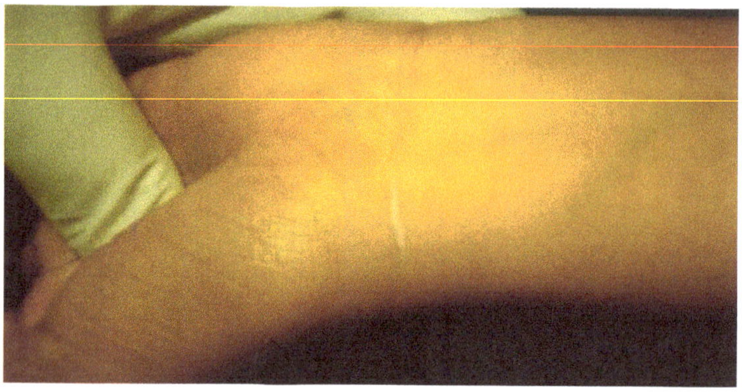

Figure 19. Palmaris longus tendon harvest- incision.

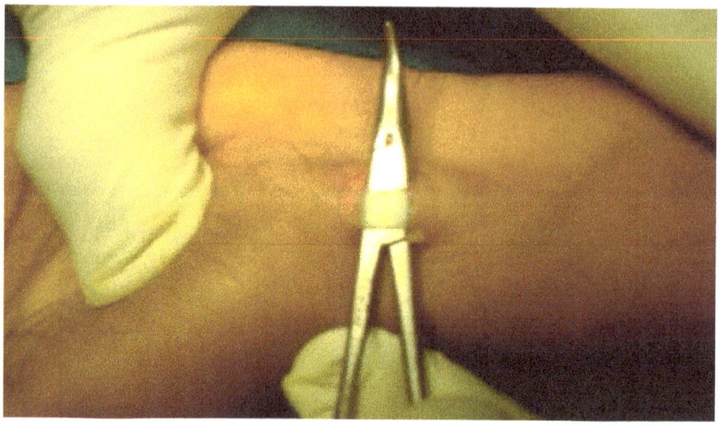

Figure 20. Palmaris longus tendon- isolated.

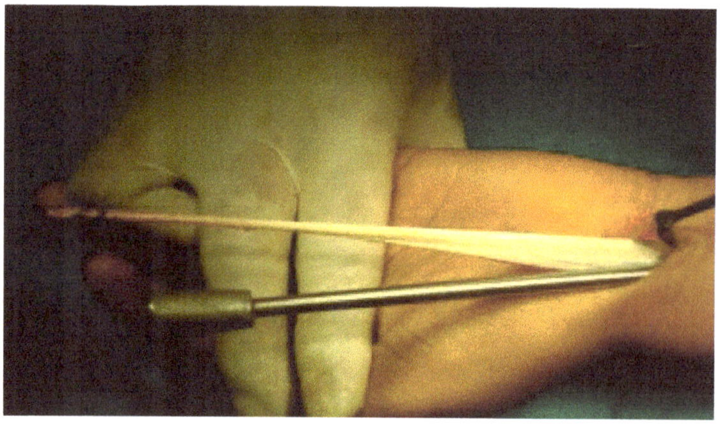

Figure 21. Palmaris longus tendon- harvested.

7.2. Kocher's approach

7.2.1. Reconstruction of LUCL

Kocher's approach was used to do ligament reconstruction and capsular surgery. Begin skin incision over the lateral epicondyle (or proximal to it) and continue it distally and obliquely directly over lateral epicondyle to end at the proximal ulna. Incise through the fascia overlying the anconeus and the extensor carpi ulnaris. Keep this dissection in line with the fibers of the extensor carpi ulnaris (not the axis of the arm) in order to preserve the fascial contributions of the extensor carpi ulnaris to the posterolateral ligamentous complex [12, 16].

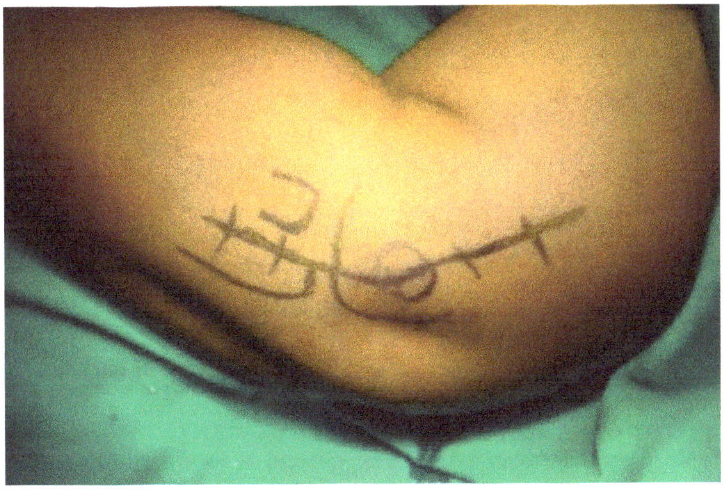

Figure 22. Lateral approach

Keep the arm pronated during this dissection in order to avoid injury to the posterior interosseus nerve (PIN); bluntly dissect through this interval and dissect down to the joint capsule. The interval between these muscles is more easily found distally, since these muscles share a common proximal fascial origin. The extensor carpi ulnaris and a portion of the supinator are elevated off capsule and are elevated anteriorly. PIN is protected at this point by the ECU and EDC. Sub-periosteally dissect the aconeus off its humeral origin in order to expose joint capsule.

8. Lateral collateral ligament complex

At this point the LCL should be exposed [13,16, 18]. Visualization of the LCL, is achieved through anterior retraction of the extensor digitorum communis and extensor carpi ulnaris. LCL complex will be seen torn or attenuated. Capsular incision should be made anterior to radial humeral ligamentous complex. Incision over the radial head in line with the radius should avoid the LCL remnants. Two 4.5 mm tunnels are made at the insertion point of LUCL over the ulnar crest in line just distal to the radial head [17, 18].

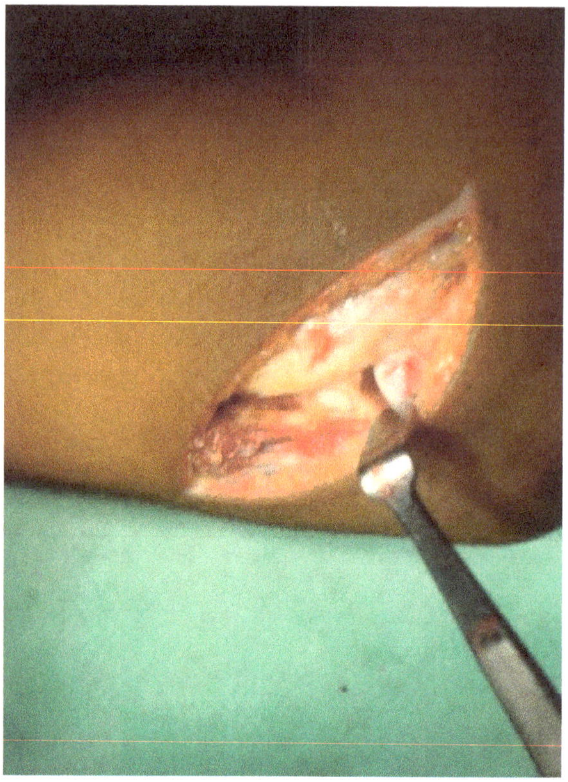

Figure 23. LUCL and posterior capsular tear

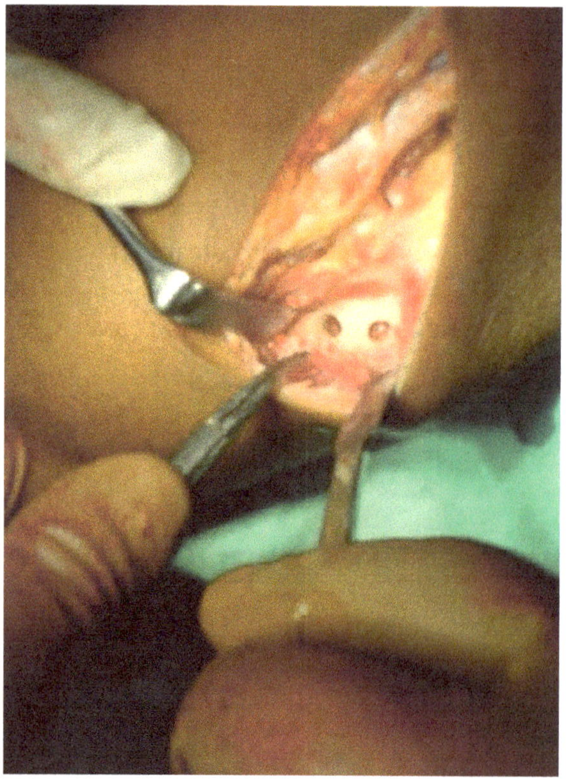

Figure 24. Two ulnar tunnels

Three tunnels are made in the lateral epicondyle in a triangle fashion [14,17, 18]. Lower one at the isometric point at the base of epicondyle and other two anterosuperior and posterosuperior part of the epicondyle. The graft is passed through the ulnar tunnels and then through the humeral tunnels.

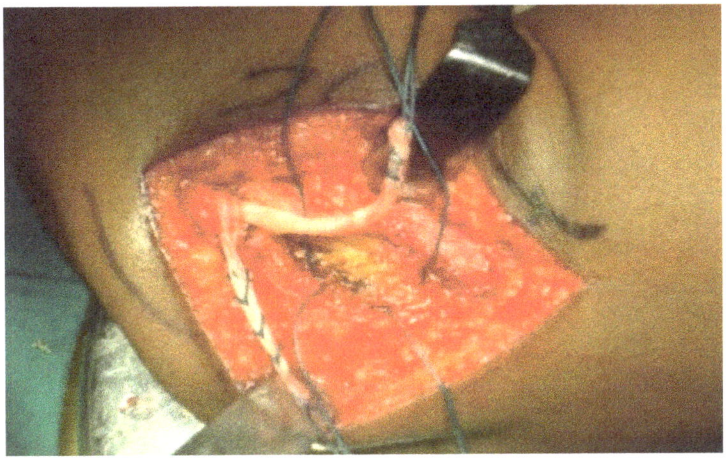

Figure 25. Graft being passed.

The lateral ulnar collateral ligament was reconstructed using the docking technique and graft was tied with the elbow in 30° flexion, valgus and internal rotation.

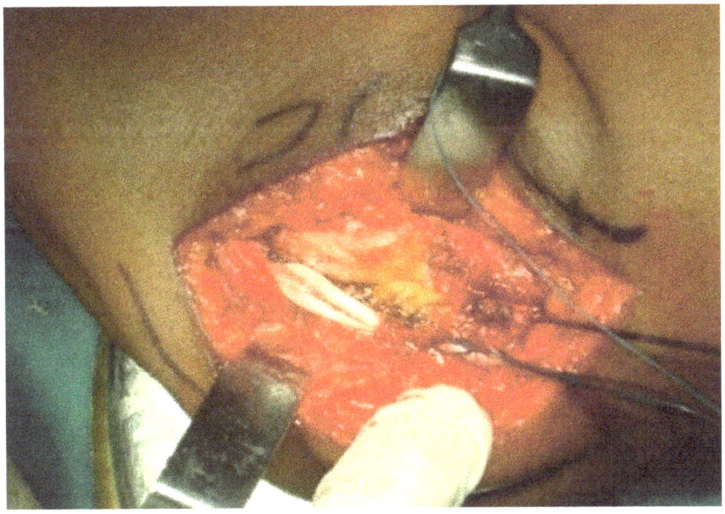

Figure 26. Graft passed through 3 humeral tunnels

Capsular repair was done, [13, 15, 16] and wound closed in anatomical layers.

Postoperatively all patients were applied with a hinge elbow brace for 6 weeks [16].

Initially restricted range of movements were allowed from 30°- 100° for 2 weeks, and then 15°- 110 ° for another 2 weeks.

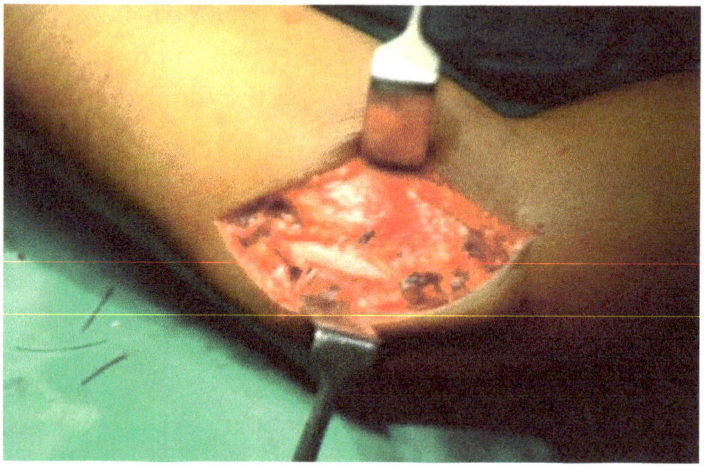

Figure 27. Graft tied with elbow in 20-30° flexion, valgus and pronation.

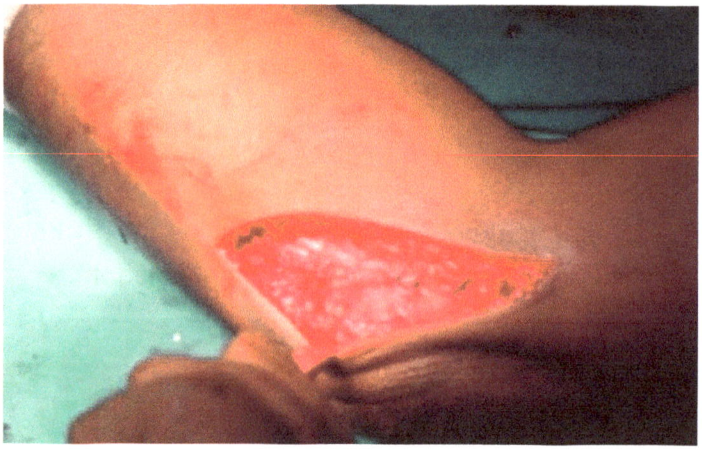

Figure 28. Final repair

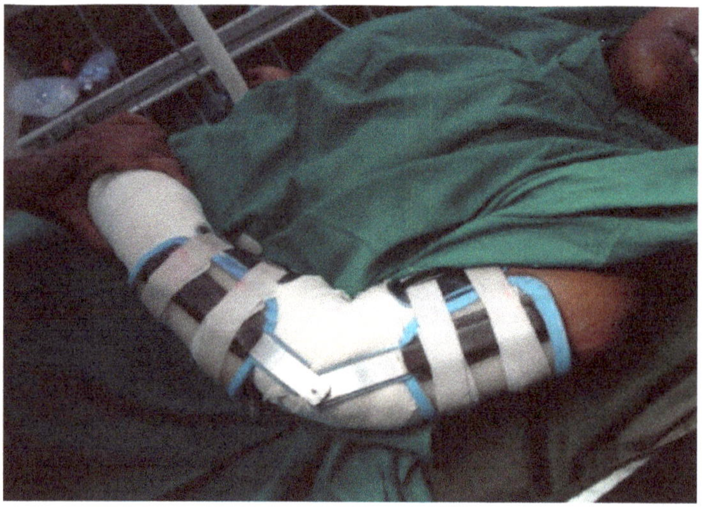

Figure 29. Brace with elbow in 60°- 70° flexion

Full range of movement to be achieved by 6 weeks, followed by strengthening exercises [12, 13]

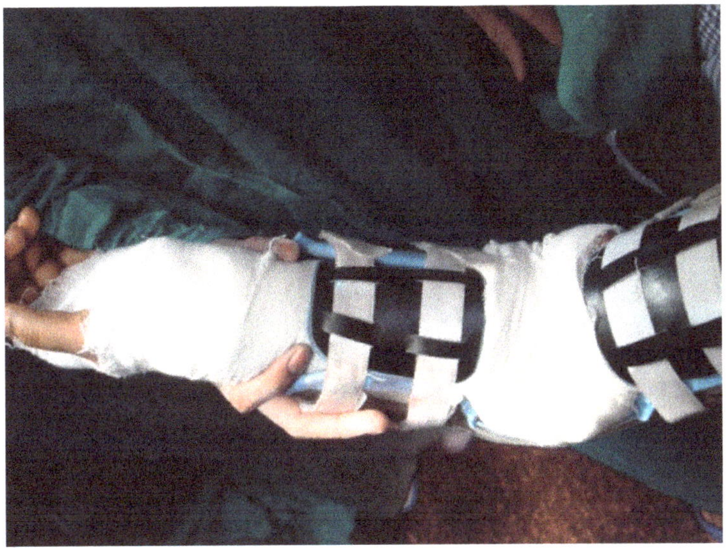

Figure 30. Hinge elbow brace

Routine activities such as lifting, pulling, pressing, etc were allowed after 3 months and sports activities after 5- 6 months after assessing muscle strength and agility [12, 15, 17].

Stability was obtained as the patient had good functional result as per Mayo elbow performance scores [16].

There is no difference in results as per age, sex or sidedness [13, 17].

Capsular repair and plication provides excellent rotational and varus stability in addition to LUCL reconstruction as seen by Mayo performance scores with a mean of 88.

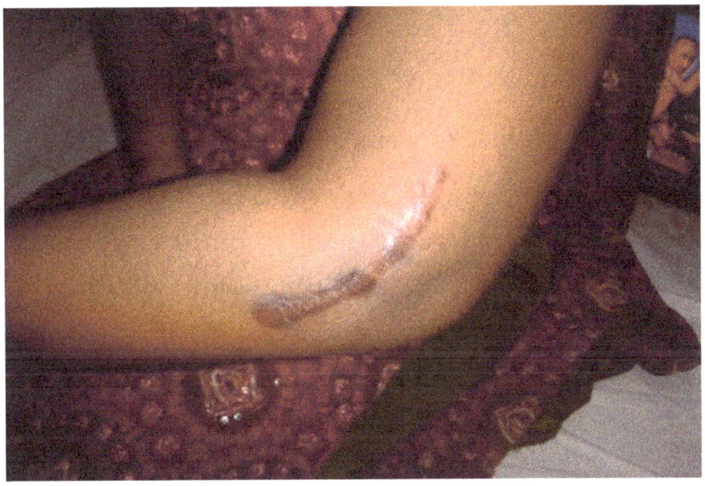

Figure 31. Postop hypertrophic scar in one of the patient.

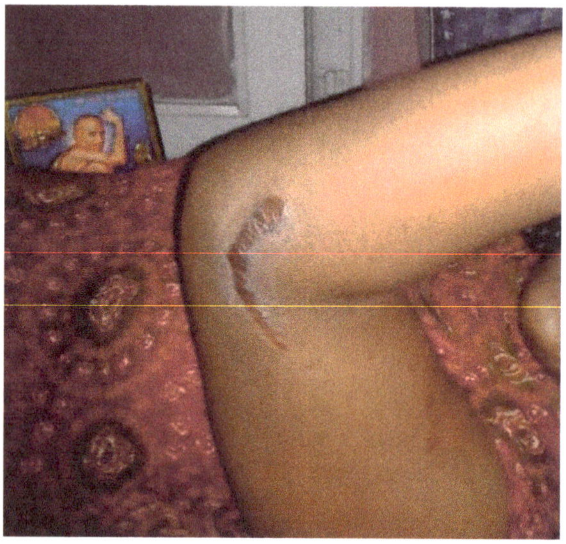

Figure 32. ROM

Capsular surgery is important in PLRI, as it is an important posterolateral structure assisting LUCL [12, 15, 17].

Surgical treatment of PLRI was mainly ligament repair or augmentation. In our technique after complete evaluation, we performed elbow arthroscopy that helps in diagnosing the instability and treat additional pathologies such as chondral injury, loose bodies, gutter impingement, and marking correct humeral attachment [14, 17]. Taking palmaris longus graft from the same side, decreases the morbidity. Only when it is absent, we use semitendinosus graft. This type of reconsruction with capsular repair gives excellent stability and we can start early rehabilitation. Most of the patients can return to normal work in 3- 4 months. For a sports person, it takes 7- 8 months to return to competitive sports [16].

9. Lateral epicondylitis

It is one of the common elbow disorders we encounter in daily orthopaedic clinics.

Females are more commonly involved, specifically those doing household chores.

It is most famously known as tennis elbow because of its early association with lawn tennis. It is usually due to chronic repetitive trauma to the common extensor muscle origin near the lateral epicondyle. Involvement of the extensor carpi radialis bravis is the main source of pain and disability [18, 21].

Symptoms:-

Patients usually have pain in supination extension movements. Passive wrist extension recreates symptoms.

Treatment:-

Conservative treatment usually involve avoiding provocative activities such as sweeping, chapatti making, squeezing clothes, tennis forehand serve, heavy cricket/ baseball bat etc.

Anti-inflammatory drugs, tennis elbow support and physical therapy usually, give relief to 90% of the patients [19].

Even after this about 5% - 10% of patients develop chronic symptoms [19, 22]. These patients will need some form of intervention in the form of percutaneous, open, radiofrequency, or arthroscopic procedures. Combining ESWT with eccentric loading appears to show superior results. Low-dose thermal ablation-RF- devices helps in angiogenesis and growth factor stimulation [21, 22].

PIN entrapment, radiocapitellar degenerative, C7 radiculitis, anconeus muscle compartment syndrome, posterolateral plica, and posterolateral rotatory instability has to be ruled out before embarking on an intervention [20, 23].

Intervention:

10. Percutaneous needling technique

- Followed by platelet rich plasma (PRP) injection is associated with less morbidity and fairly good results in term of pain and functional improvement on American shoulder elbow society(ASES) scale [1]. Growth factors are stored in the alpha granules of the platelets. Platelets are the first to arrive at the injury site and they mediate the healing response. Platelet-rich therapies allow for an opportunity to utilize the body's own healing (growth) factors to improve the quality and speed of recovery from injury. Even with the limited published scientific data, PRP appears to be the most attractive option available, with minimal side effects; the relative ease of preparation, cost effectiveness and the ability to complete the procedure as a day care procedure goes in favor of PRP. Leukocyte-reduced PRP may be the optimum preparation to stimulate superior healing without scar tissue formation.
- But inadequate resection and the inability to address intra-articular pathology are the main causes of failures in some patients and in 11% to 19% of cases there is intra-articular involvement.

11. Extracorporeal Shock Wave Therapy(ESWT)

Combining ESWT with eccentric loading appears to show superior results. It acts by inducing trauma to degenerated tendon through shock waves and 5- 8 settings for 15 minutes at weekly intervals show encouraging results. It induces the inflammatory response to aid natural healing of the lesion.

12. Radiofrequency probes

These can be used through a small incision to induce the inflammatory response to aid natural healing of the lesion. It acts by inducing trauma to degenerated tendon through Radiofrequency waves. It is in its early stages and long-term results are still awaited.

13. Open procedure

With debridement of ECRB origin and in severe cases anconeus transfer provide long-term relief from the symptoms [23]. With gradual physical therapy, and rehab, the patient can return to sports.

14. Arthroscopic release of ECRB

This is a minimally invasive procedure and provide good to excellent long term results. We can diagnose and treat concomitant intra-articular pathologies specially posterolateral plica, lateral gutter impingement, loose bodies, and posterolateral rotator instability. In two recent series, we found that at 2-year follow-up, patients treated with arthroscopic ECRB release subjectively reported feeling "much better" to "better" in 83% to 95% of cases [21, 22].

15. Other elbow pathologies

- Osteochondritis dissecans (OCD) is a disease whose cause is unknown, although overuse, microtrauma, and ischemia caused by repetitive valgus movements can be considered as causes [24, 25]. In OCD there is a separation of a portion of articular cartilage and is a source of loose bodies that ultimately can cause painful mechanical symptoms in the elbow. The most common site of OCD in the elbow is the capitellum [24].

In earlier stages, treatment consists of conservative management with avoidance of activities, bracing, and physical therapy.

In later stages, treatment options include arthroscopic joint debridement, abrasion chondroplasty, removal of loose bodies, drilling of lesions, and fixation of large OCD fragments [24].

- Elbow synovitis can occur as a localized disease, such as an inflamed lateral synovial plica or commonly, as proliferative and generalized disease, such as rheumatoid arthritis, synovial chondromatosis, pigmented villonodular synovitis, and hemophilic synovitis [26, 27].

Initially it causes pain and gradual restriction of movements. Later on there is articular cartilage involvement, periarticular soft tissue injury, and in the end subchondral bone erosion and loss. Articular and subchondral bony loss result in severe pain and instability [26].

Disease is can be treated with conservative nonoperative treatment such as medications, splinting, physiotherapy, and steroid injections.

Arthroscopic synovectomy is needed in chronic cases not responding to conservative medical line of treatment. It reduces disease load, improve ROM, and provide pain relief.

Arthroscopic synovectomy has many advantages over open procedure: it is minimally invasive, thorough debridement in all compartments is possible, other pathologies can be addressed, decreased postoperative pain, and earlier rehabilitation [26, 27].

- Elbow impingement:

Synovial plica can cause elbow impingement adjacent to the radiocapitellar joint. The patient usually complains about painful locking or catching of the elbow relieved by gentle manipulation. It is most commonly misdiagnosed as lateral epicondylitis or tennis elbow.

Another cause of elbow impingement is valgus extension overload [29].

In this condition, excessive valgus force applied to the thrower's elbow can cause impingement of the posteromedial olecranon into the olecranon fossa during extension. Gradual chronic medial elbow instability due to UCL insufficiency can lead to chondromalacia, osteophyte formation and loose bodies to develop [29].

There is pain in the terminal extension and gradual restriction of extension.

A thorough clinical history, specific tests, and investigations are needed to differentiate isolated valgus extension overload from MCL insufficiency.

Elbow arthroscopy is a boon in these conditions [29]. Arthroscopic excision of olecronon osteophytes, olecronon tip, clearing the fossa and debridement gives good results if followed by medial stabilization, if present [29].

- Stiff elbow

Restricted movements of the elbow can be traumatic, non traumatic, inflammatory, or non inflammatory. It can be extra-articular or intra-articular. Even in intra-articular pathologies, there is some element of extra-articular involvement [30].

In most of the cases, some form of modalities, such as ultrasonic heat and physiotherapy along with anti-inflammatory medications improves the ROM. But in severe elbow stiffness surgery is generally needed [31].

Manipulation under anesthesia after inflating the joint with saline can be done in a controlled manner in less severe contractures. But it is a risky procedure with complications such as muscle tear, fractures, neurovascular, and ligament injury [30, 31].

Arthroscopic capsular release and intraarticular debridement improves ROM in refractory cases provided there is no bony pathology causing a block in the elbow motion. Arthroscopic release is a technically demanding procedure in a stiff joint with neurovascular structures nearby [31, 32].

Open contracture release is a morbid procedure and causes further trauma to soft tissues. But in severe contractures where entry into the joint is difficult, in bony involvement, and inexperienced surgeons, open release is a treatment of choice [30]. Extensive lateral approach can provide access to both posterior and anterior compartments. Occasionally, medial approach needed.

- Fractures

Elbow arthroscopy is expanding its horizon to newer indications. Smaller, delicate instrumentations, improved clinico-anatomical knowledge, and surgical skills are making it possible to treat various intra-articular fractures [34].

Fractures of radial head, coronoid, trochlea, capitulum,, and olecronon can be treated with elbow arthroscopy [33, 34].

Radial head and capitellum fractures are the most common intra-articular fractures treated arthroscopicaly [33].

16. Conclusion

Elbow arthroscopy is a minimally invasive procedure and provide good to excellent long-term results. We can diagnose and treat concomitant intra-articular pathologies specially posterolateral plica, lateral gutter impingement, loose bodies, and posterolateral rotator instability. We can fix fractures, treat tendinopathies, do chondroplasty, and stiff elbow release. With the advancement of instrumentations, our knowledge about surgical anatomy, and surgical skills, elbow arthroscopy has become an excellent tool to treat a wide range of disorders with minimum risk and complications.

Author details

Satish B. Sonar

Address all correspondence to: stshsonar@yahoo.com

Sports Med-Joint Care Centre, Nagpur, India

References

[1] Bennett JM. Elbow arthroscopy-the basics. Journal of Hand Surgery Am. 2013 Jan; 38(1):164-7.

[2] Yeoh KM, King GJ, Faber KJ, Glazebrook MA, Athwal GS. Evidence-based indications for elbow arthroscopy. Journal of Arthroscopy and Related Research. 2012 Feb; 28(2):272-82.

[3] Van Tongel A, Macdonald P, Van Riet R, Dubberley J. Elbow arthroscopy in acute injuries. Journal of Knee Surgeries, Sports Traumatology and Arthroscopy. 2012 Dec; 20(12):2542-8.

[4] Elfeddali R, Schreuder MH, Eygendaal D. Arthroscopic elbow surgery, is it safe? Journal of Shoulder and Elbow Surgery; 2013 May; 22(5):647-52.

[5] Nelson GN, Wu T, Galatz LM, Yamaguchi K, Keener JD. Elbow arthroscopy-Early complications and associated risk factors. Journal of Shoulder and Elbow Surgery; 2014 Feb; 23(2):273-8.

[6] Floris S, Olsen BS, Dalstra M, Søjbjerg JO, Sneppen O. The medial collateral ligament of the elbow joint: Anatomy and kinematics. Journal of Shoulder Elbow Surgery. 1998 Jul-Aug; 7(4):345-51.112.

[7] Grace SP, Field LD. Chronic medial elbow instability. Orthopedic Clinics of North America. 2008 Apr; 39(2):213-9, VI. D

[8] Beltran LS, Bencardino JT, Beltran J. Imaging of sports ligamentous injuries of the elbow. Seminars of Musculoskeletal Radiology. 2013 Nov; 17(5):455-65.

[9] Field LD, Altchek DW. Evaluation of the arthroscopic valgus instability test of the elbow. American Journal of Sports Medicine. 1996 Mar-Apr; 24(2):177-81.

[10] Richard MJ, Aldridge JM 3rd, Wiesler ER, Ruch DS. Traumatic valgus instability of the elbow: Pathoanatomy and results of direct repair. Journal of Bone Joint Surgery Am. 2008 Nov; 90(11):2416-22.

[11] Rohrbough JT, Altchek DW, Hyman J, Williams RJ 3rd, Botts JD. Medial collateral ligament reconstruction of the elbow using the docking technique..American Journal of Sports Medicine. 2002 Jul-Aug; 30(4):541-8.

[12] Anakwenze OA, Kancherla VK, Iyengar J, Ahmad CS, Levine WN. Posterolateral rotatory instability of the elbow. American Journal of Sports Medicine. 2014 Feb.

[13] O'Brien MJ, Savoie FH 3rd. Arthroscopic and open management of posterolateral rotatory instability of the elbow. Journal of Sports Medicine and Arthroscopy. 2014 Sep.

[14] Anakwenze OA, Kwon D, O'Donnell E, Levine WN, Ahmad CS. Surgical treatment of posterolateral rotatory instability of the elbow. Journal of Arthroscopy and Related Research. 2014 Jul.

[15] Kim BS, Park KH, Song HS, Park SY. Ligamentous repair of acute lateral collateral ligament rupture of the elbow. Journal of Shoulder and Elbow Surgery. 2013 Nov.

[16] Lin KY, Shen PH, Lee CH, Pan RY, Lin LC, Shen HC. Functional outcomes of surgical reconstruction for posterolateral rotatory instability of the elbow. Injury Journal. 2012 Oct.

[17] Jones KJ, Dodson CC, Osbahr DC, Parisien RL, Weiland AJ, Altchek DW, Allen AA. The docking technique for lateral ulnar collateral ligament reconstruction: surgical technique and clinical outcomes. Journal of Shoulder Elbow Surg. 2012 Mar.

[18] Shiple BJ. How effective are injection treatments for lateral epicondylitis? Clinical Journal of Sport Medicine. 2013 Nov; 23(6):502-3.

[19] HO, Kose O, Guler F. Injection of autologous blood versus corticosteroid for lateral epicondylitis: A randomised controlled study. Journal of Orthopaedic Surgery (Hong Kong). 2014 Dec; 22(3):333-7.

[20] Raeissadat SA, Sedighipour L. Effect of platelet-rich plasma (PRP) versus autologous whole wlood on pain and function Improvement in tennis elbow: A randomized clinical Trial. Journal of Pain Research and Treatment. 2014; 2014:191525.

[21] Sauvage A, Nedellec G. Arthroscopic treatment of lateral epicondylitis: A prospective study on 14 cases. Chirurgae Main. 2013 Apr.

[22] 22].Adams JE, King GJ. Elbow arthroscopy: Indications, techniques, outcomes, and complications. Journal of American Academy of Orthopedic Surgery. 2014 Dec; 22(12).

[23] Ruch DS, Orr SB. A comparison of débridement with and without anconeus muscle flap for treatment of refractory lateral epicondylitis. Journal of Shoulder and Elbow Surgery. 2015 Feb;24(2):236-41.

[24] De Graaff F, Krijnen MR. Arthroscopic surgery in athletes with osteochondritis dissecans of the elbow. Journal of Arthroscopy. 2011 Jul; 27(7):986-93.

[25] Marshall KW, Marshall DL, Busch MT. Osteochondral lesions of the humeral trochlea in the young athlete. Journal of Skeletal Radiology. 2009 May; 38(5):479-91.

[26] Kang HJ, Park MJ, Ahn JH, Lee SH. Arthroscopic synovectomy for the rheumatoid elbow. Journal of Arthroscopy. 2010 Sep; 26(9):1195-202.

[27] Ekman EF, Cory JW, Poehling GG. Pigmented villonodular synovitis and synovial chondromatosis arthroscopically diagnosed and treated in the same elbow. Journal of Arthroscopy. 1997 Feb.

[28] 28].Cohen SB, Valko C, Zoga A. Posteromedial elbow impingement: Magnetic resonance imaging findings in overhead throwing athletes and results of arthroscopic treatment. Journal of Arthroscopy. 2011 Oct; 27(10):1364-70.

[29] Ahmad CS, Conway JE. Elbow arthroscopy: Valgus extension overload. Instruction Course Lecture. 2011; 60:191-7.

[30] Pederzini LA, Nicoletta F, Tosi M. Elbow arthroscopy in stiff elbow. Journal of Knee Surgery Sports Traumatology and Arthroscopy. 2014 Feb; 22(2):467-73.

[31] Singh H, Nam KY, Moon YL. Arthroscopic management of stiff elbow. Journal of Orthopedics. 2011 Jun 14;34(6):167.

[32] Koh KH, Lim TK, Lee HI, Park MJ. Surgical release of elbow stiffness after internal fixation of intercondylar fracture of the distal humerus. Journal of Shoulder Elbow Surgery. 2013 Feb; 22(2):268-74.

[33] Wijeratna M, Bailey KA, Pace A, Arthroscopic radial head excision in managing elbow trauma. International Journal of Orthopaedics. 2012 Dec; 36(12):2507-12.

[34] Van Tongel A, Macdonald P, Van Riet R, Dubberley J. Elbow arthroscopy in acute injuries. Journal of Knee Surgery Sports Traumatology and Arthroscopy. 2012 Dec; 20(12):2542-8.

5

Cervical Disc Arthroplasty

Christopher Paul O'Boynick and Bruce V. Darden II

Abstract

Anterior cervical discectomy and fusion (ACDF) has long been considered the gold standard for treating myelopathy and radiculopathy due to disk degeneration. One major complication of this procedure is adjacent segment degeneration. Cervical disc arthroplasty (CDA) has been proposed as an alternative to ACDF and as a means to reduce ASD. This chapter briefly recounts the advent of CDA. Additionally, it describes the most common implants and biomechanical properties associated with those designs. Critical to CDA is meticulous operative technique including implant positioning and hemostasis. Data in the form of FDA IDE studies and more recent meta-analyses of existing studies have demonstrated non-inferiority of CDA when compared to ACDF. This chapter also reviews the most common complications associated with CDA including heterotopic ossification and ankylosis of the involved segment. While more technically demanding than ACDF, CDA does represent a viable alternative in the proper patient.

Keywords: Cervical disc, disc arthroplasty, spine surgery

1. Introduction

Anterior cervical discectomy and fusion (ACDF) has long been considered the gold standard for treating myelopathy and radiculopathy due to disk degeneration [1]. Secondary to this success it has become the archetype by which all subsequent techniques are judged. The clinical success of ACDF is evident across the literature, reaching as far back as the middle of the last century [1-4].

As with any surgical intervention, ACDF is not without its complications. The most notable of these complications is adjacent segment degeneration (ASD). Described as the radiographic appearance of degenerative changes above or below a fused segment, this anomaly has a reported incidence of up to 92% in some studies [5]. Instrumental in its management is understanding the difference between adjacent segment degeneration and adjacent segment disease. The latter being degeneration severe enough to cause clinical symptoms and/or require surgical intervention [6]. Keeping this distinction in mind, Hilibrand et al. [6] described a 3% chance of symptomatic ASD per year following ACDF. In the symptomatic group approximately two thirds required a repeat surgery. Taking the group as a whole, 25% demonstrated new symptoms within 10 years of the index procedure. Goffin et al. [7] demonstrated similar rates of ASD between older patients treated for degeneration and younger patients treated in the traumatic setting. Combining this data with the biomechanical studies demonstrating increased motion and intradiscal pressures at juxtafusional levels, it stands to reason that altered biomechanics following ACDF may play a role in ASD.

Complications related to graft materials have also come under scrutiny. In addition to increased operative time, iliac crest harvest has been linked to numerous complications including donor site pain, infection, nerve injury, and pelvic fracture [8, 9]. While allograft options do eliminate the risks listed above it does carry the risk of disease transmission [10].

Nonunion is also a risk associated with ACDF. Rates of 3%-11% have been reported in the literature for single-level fusions with rates increasing to over 25% in multi-level cases [1, 11].

It is with these complications in mind, that alternatives to fusion have come to the forefront in treating cervical degenerative disease.

Cervical disk arthroplasty (CDA) has come of age over the last two decades. From its crude beginnings in the 1950's, through its re-emergence in the late 80's and 90's, CDA has evolved to include multiple devices and bearing options. The following chapter will work to describe the most clinically relevant implants, outline the current state of the art, and highlight the results of landmark studies for this emerging procedure.

2. Implants

The implants described in the following section were chosen based on relevant data that will be described in the clinical outcomes section. It is not meant to be a representation of all available devices.

2.1. The Porous-Coated Motion Cervical arthroplasty (PCM) (Figure 1)

The PCM made by Nuvasive (San Diego, California) consists of a cobalt-chrome-molybdenum (CrCoMo) alloy with an ultra-high molecular weight polyethylene (UHMWPE) insert. The concave surface of the superior endplate articulates with the convex superior surface of the polyethylene over a large radius of curvature. The endplates have a coating of titanium/ calcium phosphate in addition to serrated edges to promote ingrowth. The disk is designed to match the natural contour of the uncovertebral joint. This design allows for minimal limitations of range of motion and minimal constraint.

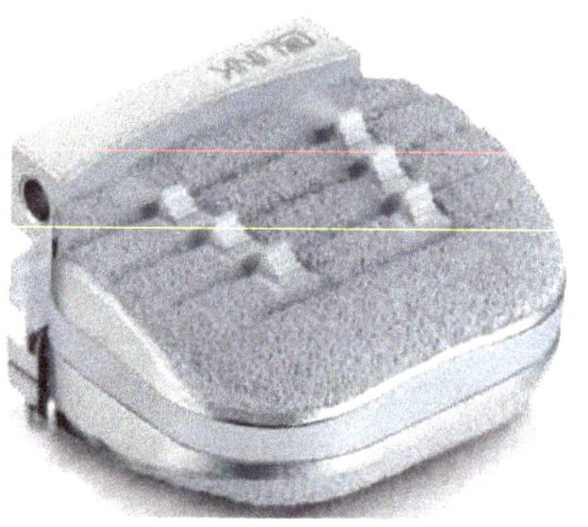

Figure 1. PCM (Courtesy of Nuvasive, San Diego, California)

2.2. ProDisc-C (Figure 2)

ProDisc-C made by Synthes (West Chester, Pennsylvania) has a ball and socket design, with endplates made of a cobalt-chrome alloy. Initial fixation comes from keels on each endplate combined with titanium plasma spray to promote bony in-growth. The bearing surface has an articulating dome of UHMWPE secured to the inferior endplate and a concave socket integral to the superior endplate. The implant allows for motion only in a specific range.

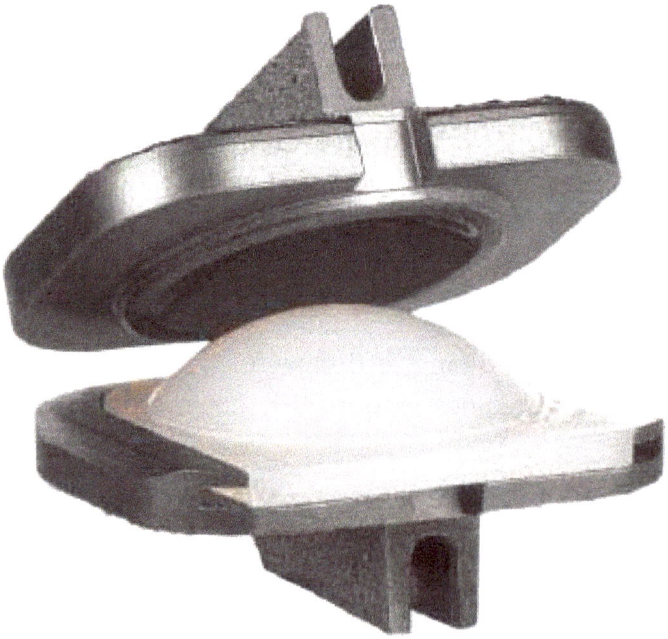

Figure 2. ProDisc-C (Courtesy of Synthes Spine, West Chester, Pennsylvania)

2.3. Bryan cervical disc prosthesis (Figure 3)

Bryan Cervical Disc Prosthesis made by Medtronic Sofamor Danek (Memphis, Tennessee) consists of a nucleus made of polyurethane between two titanium alloy endplates in a clamshell configuration. The two bearing surfaces in the arthroplasty at the interfaces between the nucleus and the endplates are contained by a polyurethane sheath that attaches to the endplates. Sterile saline is injected between the outer sheath and the nucleus as lubricant as part of the implantation. Ideally, this sheath contains any wear debris and prevents soft tissue in-growth. The endplates have a titanium porous coating and a flange to prevent migration. This implant is unconstrained.

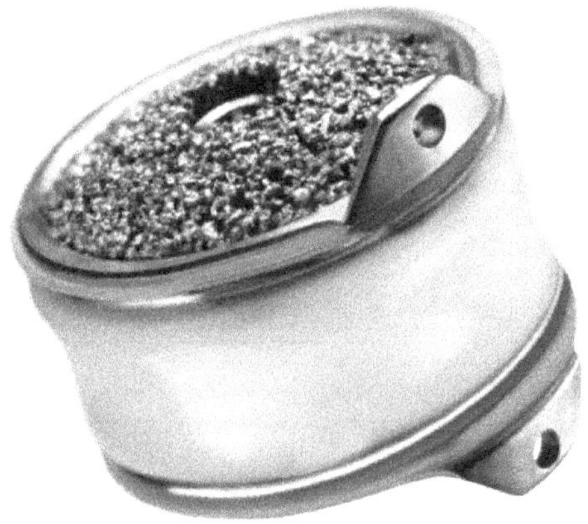

Figure 3. Bryan Cervical Disc (Courtesy of Medtronic Sofamor Danek, Memphis, Tennessee)

2.4. Prestige (Figure 4)

The current prestige disc replacement has a long history. Its initial design was taken from the technology developed by Cummins et al. and acquired by Medtronic Sofamor Danek (Memphis, Tennessee). Over many derivations the implant has morphed from a stainless steel ball and socket articulation into a cobalt chrome alloy with a ball and groove design. This allows for coupled motion. The implant uses locking screws as well as grit blasted implant surfaces for fixation. In its most recent design change the Prestige LP moved to titanium ceramic composition and traded the flange and locking screw construct for a titanium plasma spray with rails for immediate fixation.

2.5. Mobi-C (Figure 5)

The Mobi-C LDR spine (Austin, Texas) is a metal on the UHMWPE device. It has mobile bearing technology allowing both the superior and inferior endplates to articulate with the polyethylene for an increased range of motion. The articulation between the insert and the inferior endplate is limited by two lateral stops on the inferior endplate. The endplates, made

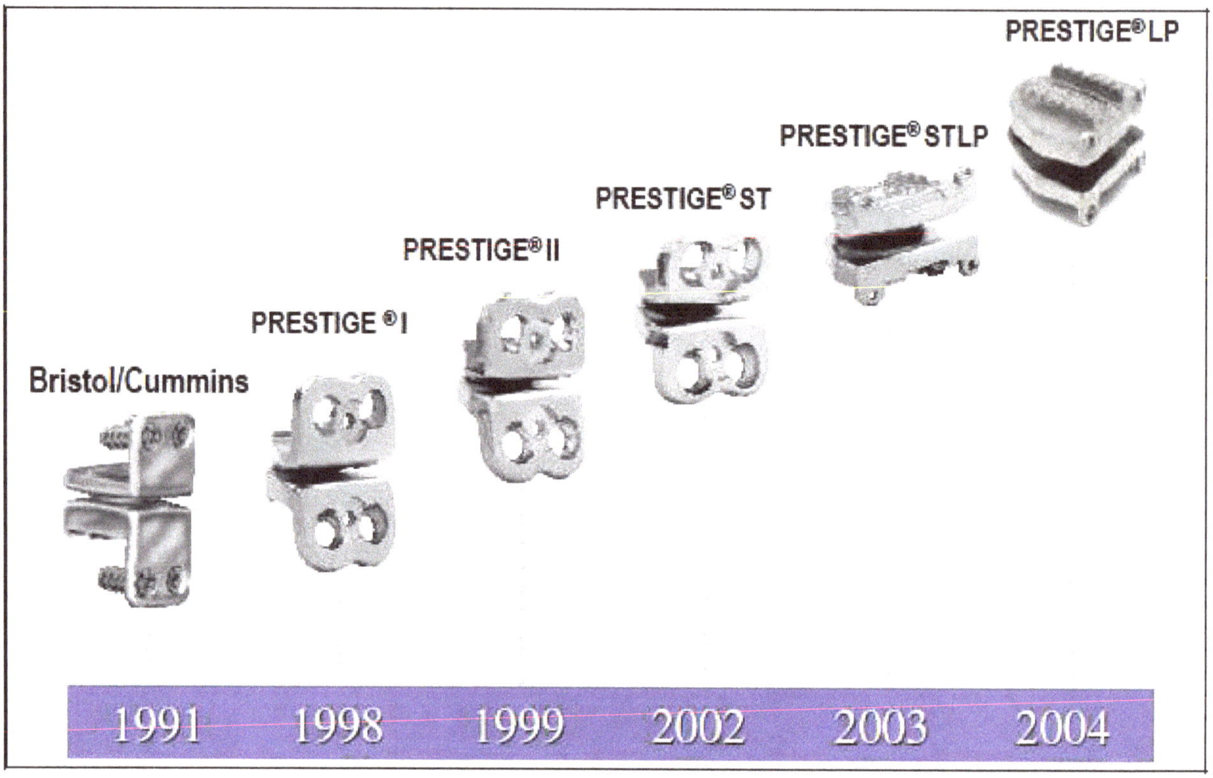

Figure 4. Evolution of the Prestige Cervical Disc (Courtesy of Medtronic Sofamor Danek, Memphis, Tennessee)

of cobalt chromium alloy, are coated with plasma sprayed titanium and a hydroxyapatite coating to promote ingrowth.

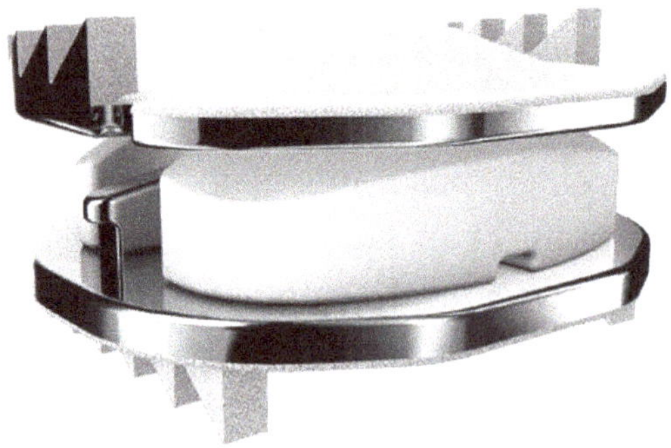

Figure 5. Mobi-C (Courtesy of LDR, Austin, Texas)

3. Biomechanics

Critical to understanding the biomechanics of cervical disk replacement is a knowledge of normal cervical spine kinematics. Normal motion in the subaxial cervical spine requires coupled motions at the disc space. There is anterior-posterior translation during flexion and extension as well as lateral translation during bending and axial rotation. Secondary to this complex motion is the concept of varying constraint through normal cervical spine range of motion. During flexion the facet joints unshingle and provide less constraint across the involved disc. During extension the opposite occurs and the motion segment becomes more constrained. Understanding the varying amounts of constraint in the native disc is vital when considering the concept of constraint within an implant. Huang et al. [12] defines constraint in the cervical spine as a limitation of anterior-posterior translation typically found during normal flexion and extension activity. An unconstrained or semi-constrained device theoretically allows for more natural motion across a given segment. On the other hand, a constrained implant dictates all motion at that segment and could result in decreased motion and more stress across the segments as the implant and facet joints work against each other. Additionally, the complex nature of each motion segment results in varying centers of rotation. Building on the work of Penning and Amevo [13, 14], the normalized instantaneous centers of rotation were identified and can be seen in Figure 6 [15]. These centers of rotation become increasingly important with respect to implant positioning particularly for devices with a more constrained design. Failure to position the implant appropriately could result in increasing strain on the facets. Figure 7 demonstrates ideal placement on the lateral view with slightly asymmetric insertion on the AP. Ideal placement can be seen in figures 13 and 14.

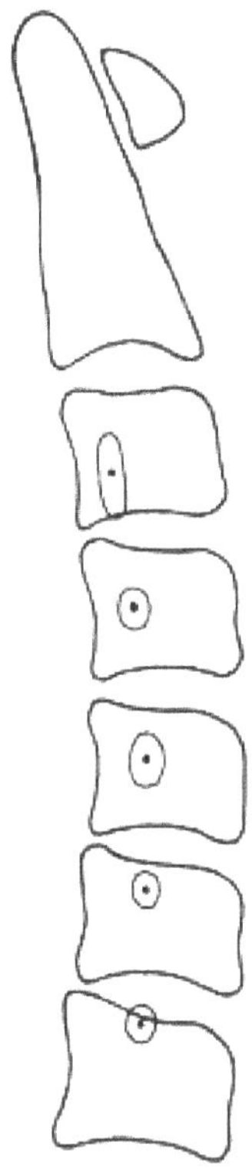

Figure 6. Mean instantaneous axes of rotation for each level of the cervical spine. Circles represent a two standard deviation range of distribution. Knowledge of their location is instrumental for proper placement of CSA implants. (Image reprinted from Bogduk N, Mercer S. Clin Biomechanics, 2000 [15])

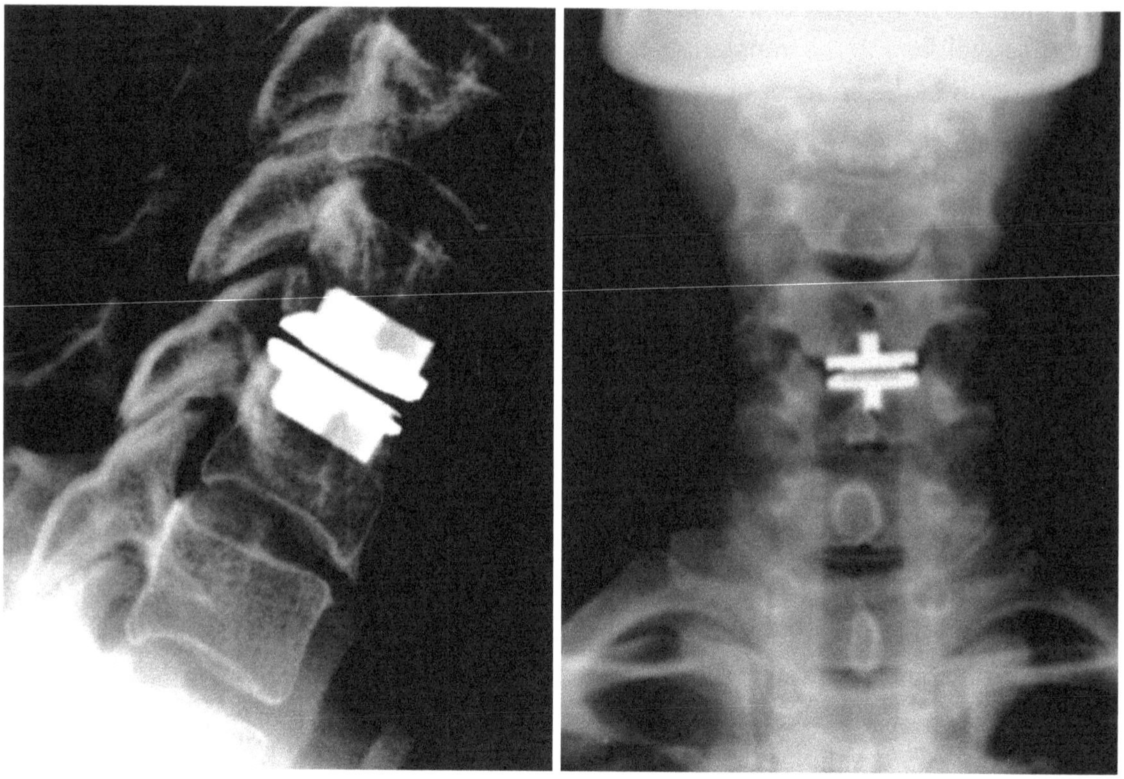

Figure 7. AP and lateral radiographs of a ProDisc-C

4. Surgical technique

- Patient positioning: Proper positioning is key to proper orientation and alignment of the prosthesis. Obtaining anatomic lordosis is critical prior to procedure commencement. This can be achieved with a rolled towel or similar placed behind the neck. Additionally, AP and lateral fluoroscopic imaging is necessary to ensure proper placement of the implant. The head should be secured to prevent rotation. The shoulders may be taped with caudal retraction as necessary for visualization. Figures 8 and 9 demonstrate proper positioning.
- Approach and discectomy: A standard Smith-Robinson approach may be utilized and the index level exposed. The center of the vertebral body must be identified for proper implant placement (Figure 10). Aggressive hemostasis will help to prevent blood loss and reduce risk of heterotopic ossification. Additionally, the surgeon must obtain parallel distraction of the disc space (Figure 11), release the foramen bilaterally, and re-establish normal disc height prior to implant placement.
- Device insertion: Implant placement and fixation should be done under fluoroscopic guidance utilizing implant specific devices as outlined in each respective technique guide (Figure 12). The surgical site should be thoroughly irrigated and closed in a standard fashion.

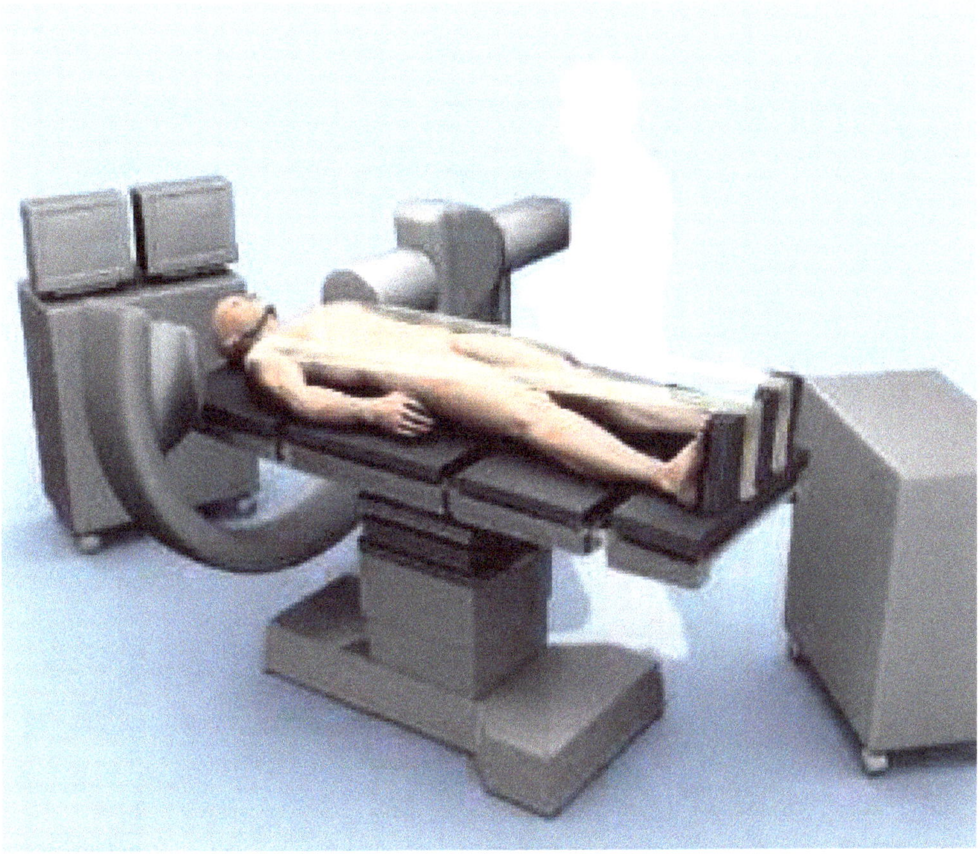

Figure 8. Illustrations of proper positioning for cervical disc replacement (Courtesy of Synthes Spine, West Chester, Pennsylvania)

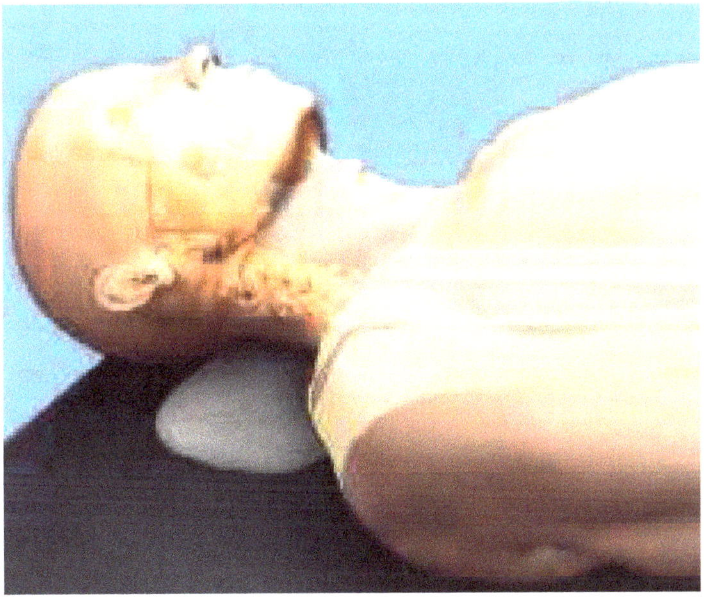

Figure 9. Illustrations of proper positioning for cervical disc replacement (Courtesy of Synthes Spine, West Chester, Pennsylvania)

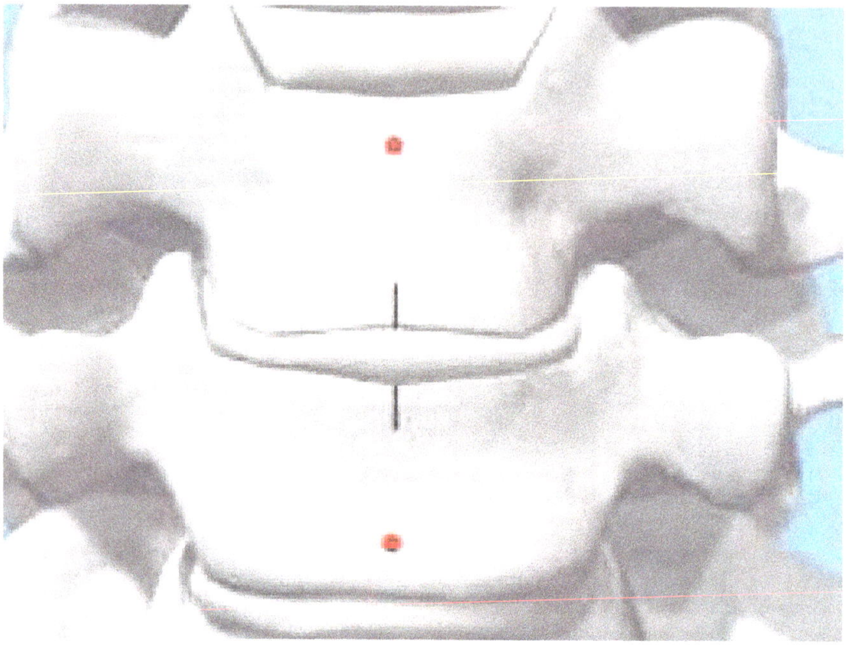

Figure 10. Illustrations of midline identification of the vertebral body and parallel distraction of the disc space for optimal implant placement (Courtesy of Synthes Spine, West Chester, Pennsylvania)

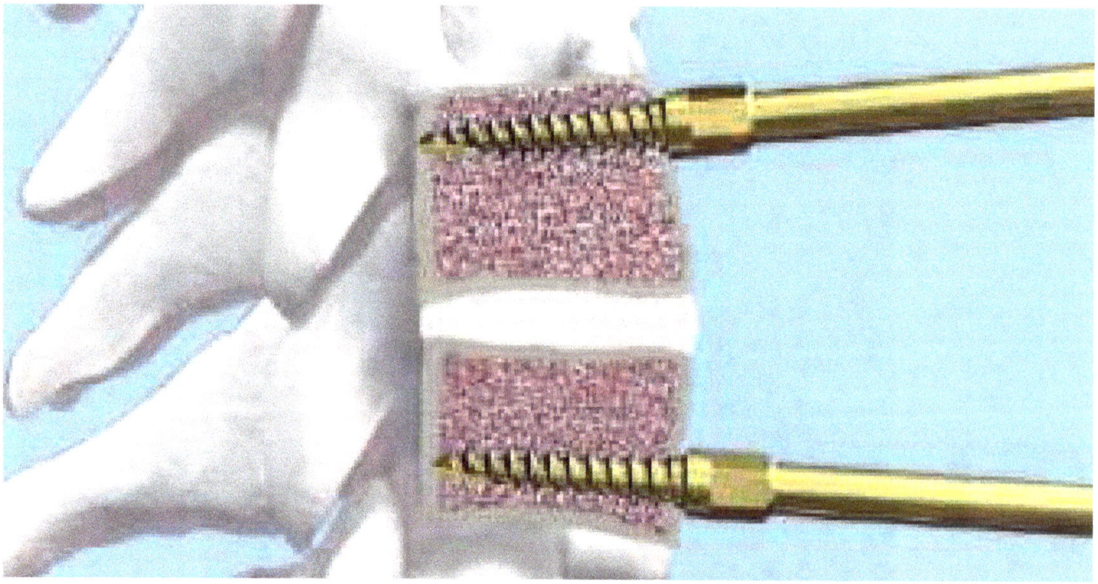

Figure 11. Illustrations of midline identification of the vertebral body and parallel distraction of the disc space for optimal implant placement (Courtesy of Synthes Spine, West Chester, Pennsylvania)

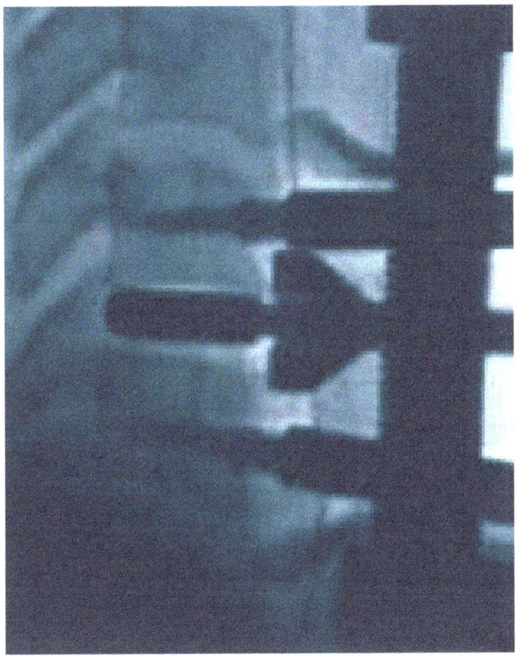

Figure 12. Lateral fluoroscopic view demonstrating optimal trial placement along the posterior margin of the vertebral bodies. Note the parallel distraction of the endplates and placement of the distraction pins. (Courtesy of Synthes Spine, West Chester, Pennsylvania)

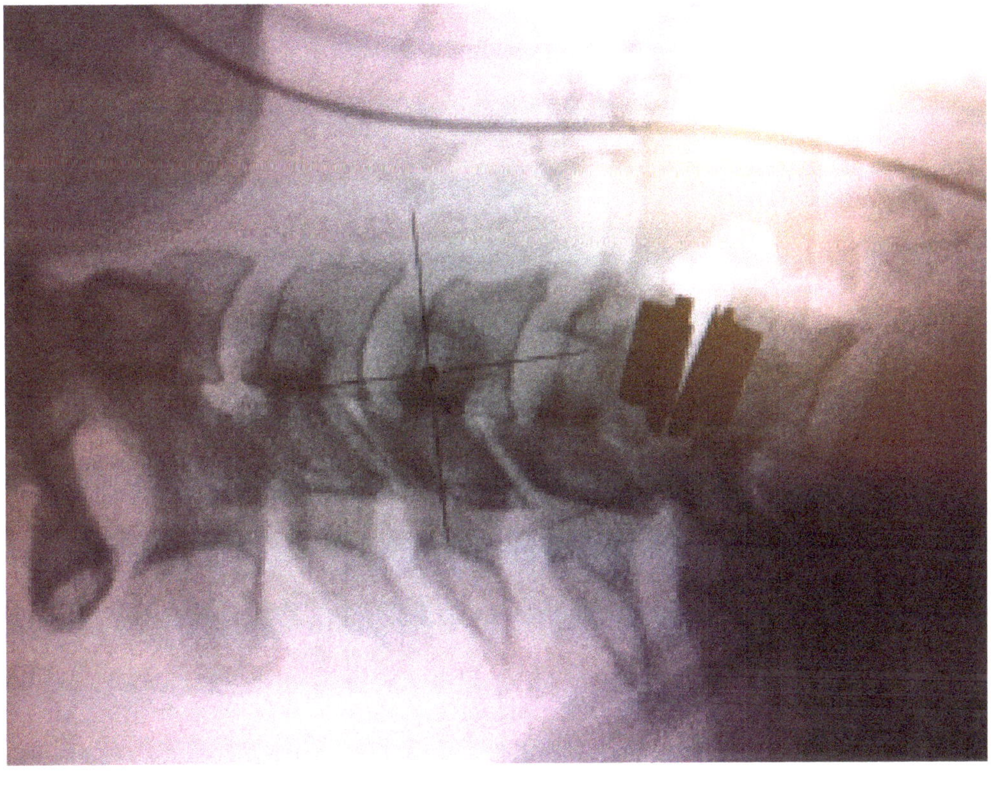

Figure 13. Intra-operative views showing optimal placement of cervical disc arthroplasty in the AP and lateral views (Courtesy of Synthes Spine, West Chester, Pennsylvania)

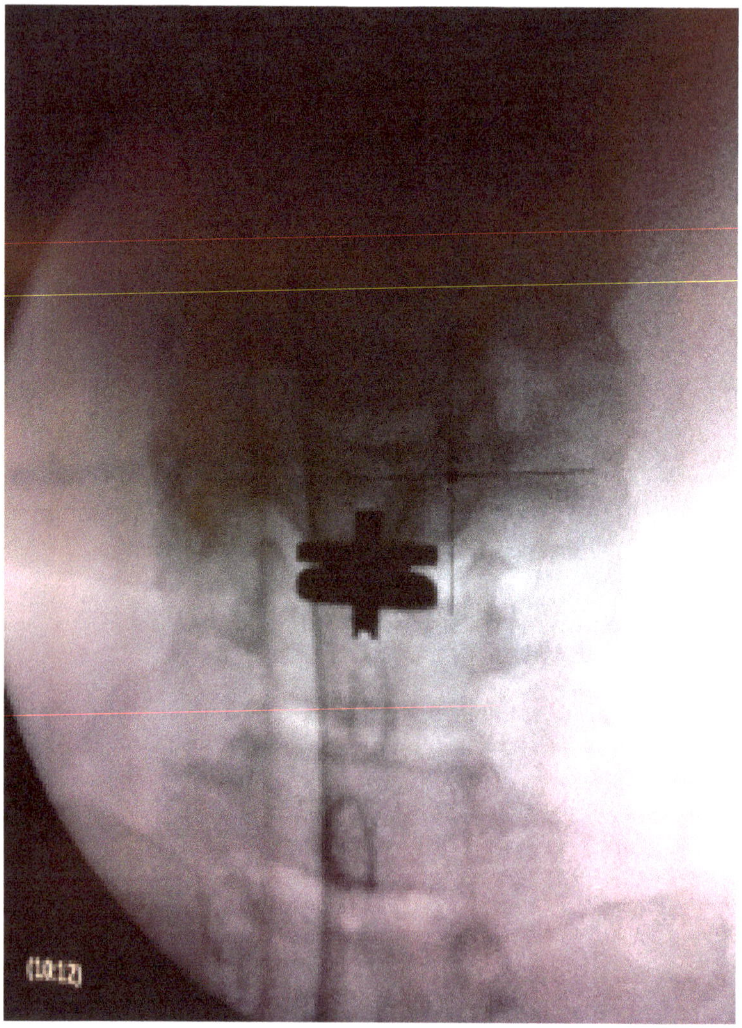

Figure 14. Intra-operative views showing optimal placement of cervical disc arthroplasty in the AP and lateral views (Courtesy of Synthes Spine, West Chester, Pennsylvania)

5. Clinical outcomes

Most of the data available surrounding CDA, at least in the US, is the result of numerous clinical evaluations as part of the US FDA IDE studies. This data from these individual studies has been summarized previously by many authors and will be touched on later in this section. Some of the most recent data comes in the form of meta-analyses of these existing studies as well as retrospective review of large clinical databases.

McAfee et al. [16] performed a meta-analysis of four FDA IDE studies examining four separate CDA devices. At 24 months, over 1200 patients were available across all studies for evaluation. Pooling all this data, a significant treatment effect favoring arthroplasty was demonstrated with an overall success rate of 78% for CDA compared to 71% for ACDF. This significance was also borne out in the subcomponent analysis for neurological status and survivorship. Their overall conclusions suggest superiority of CDA compared to ACDF.

Gao et al. [17] reviewed 27 randomized clinical trials. Twelve of these demonstrated level 1 evidence with the remaining studies identified as level 2. The arthroplasty group had lower VAS neck and arm pain scores, better neurological success, and fewer secondary procedures. The remaining variables including duration of hospital stay, NDI, and rates of adverse events demonstrated no significant difference across the groups.

Davis et al. [18] reported a four year follow up on 2-level disc replacement versus ACDF. This study is part of the US FDA IDE study evaluating the Mobi-C device. Of the 225 patients receiving CDA, 202 were available for follow up along with 89 of the original 105 patients receiving ACDF. ASD was found in 86% of ACDF cases compared with 42% of CDA cases. Rates of subsequent surgeries were also elevated in the ACDF group at 15% compared to 4% with CDA. From the baseline, CDA patients improved more in NDI, SF-12, patient satisfaction, and overall success when compared to ACDF. Another study, again looking at the Mobi-C device in single-level constructs over the course of four years identified significantly higher rates of subsequent surgery and adjacent segment disease is the ACDF group when compared to CDA [19]. At no point during this study were CDA scores significantly worse than ACDF scores with respect to NDI, VAS, or SF-12.

Heller et al. [20] published two-year results on the Bryan FDA IDE study. They had over 200 in each group available at follow up. At two years, the Bryan patients had improved NDI scores, VAS scores, and higher overall success when compared to ACDF. The longest follow-up study of the Bryan disc comes from the work of Goffin and his colleagues out of Europe [21]. This was a multicenter, prospective, non-randomized study, which included both multi-level and single-level constructs. At their 4-6-year follow up, there were 89 single-level patients and nine two-level patients available for examination. All patients remained clinically improved compared to preoperatively. Nearly 90% had good or excellent results based on Odum's criteria. Kaplan-Meier analysis showed and estimated success rate over 90% at the seven-year mark.

The Prestige disc (ST or LP) does not have the long-term data yet to match the longer but non-randomized study of the Bryan disc. Mummaneni et al. [22] presented the results of the Prestige ST at two years. Again, this data was from a prospective, randomized, multicenter trial between ACDF and CDA. With better than 75% follow up, the rate of adjacent level surgery was statistically greater for the ACDF patients versus the CDA group. This trend continued with respect to neurological success favoring CDA in 93% of patients compared to 84% of ACDF patients. Overall success including improved NDI, maintained neurological improvement, and the absence of implant related adverse events again favored CDA 79% vs. ACDF 68%. SF-36, VAS, and NDI showed no differences at the two-year time point. A two-year prospective trial out of Japan showed no difference between ACDF and CDA with the Prestige LP when evaluating VAS, NDI, SF-36, or Japanese Orthopedic Association scores [23].

Data on the ProDisc-C IDE study comes from Murrey et al. [24]. Similar to previous studies the 1:1 randomized, controlled, multicenter trial had over 100 patients available in each arm at two-year follow up. Each group had improvement in the clinical parameters measured but no significant difference was elucidated between groups. Rates of revision surgery, however, did favor the CDA group (2%) compared to ACDF (8.5%). Delamarter in 2010, re-examined the ProDisc-C IDE data in addition to 136 patients that received CDA in the continued access arm of the study [25]. Again, clinical parameters improved significantly from baseline in both groups. Mirroring the work of Murrey et al., the rates of secondary surgical procedures were higher in those patients receiving ACDF (11%) vs. CDA (3%). Half of these ACDF patients required adjacent segment surgery while the other half required revision ACDF for pseudarthrosis at the index level. While three CDA patients required conversion to fusion for axial pain, none required surgical intervention at adjacent segments.

Phillips et al. [26] most recently published on the two-year results of the PCM US FDA IDE clinical trial. At two years the follow-up rate was nearly 90% (195) for the PCM group and 82% (151) for the ACDF group. Similar to data presented previously, all patients had significant improvement from baseline in clinical scores. The mean NDI was significantly lower in the CDA group compared to ACDF (p=0.029). Reported dysphagia scores were also lower in the CDA group. Overall success rates determined by combined NDI scores, lack of complications, no need for revision surgery, and radiographic evidence of motion (PCM) and fusion (ACDF) favored PCM (75%) over ACDF (65%) with a p=0.02. Overall findings from this study suggest at minimum an equivalency between ACDF and CDA with the PCM device.

In 2008, Riew et al. examined the effectiveness of CDA in the setting of myelopathy due to single level disc herniation [27]. This study combined subset data from both the Bryan trial and the Prestige trials. Myelopathy was diagnosed based on hyperreflexia, presence of clonus, or a Nurick grade of greater than or equal to 1. Radiographic diagnosis was limited to single-level disc disease and patients with multi-level lesions were excluded. In comparing myelopathic patients that underwent CDA vs. ACDF, there was no significant difference between groups with respect to clinical improvement. This data suggests that CDA is a viable treatment option for patients with cervical myelopathy resulting from single level pathology.

6. Heterotopic ossification

Heterotopic ossification (HO) is frequently associated with CDA and has a reported prevalence approaching nearly 70% by some authors [28-34]. Similar to the previously described clinical results some of the most recent data comes from meta-analysis, which demonstrated an average prevalence of 45% at one year and 58% at two years [35]. HO is not unique to a single device. The rates associated with Bryan Disc, Mobi-C, and ProDisc-C are 21%, 53%, and 71% respectively [33]. Not surprisingly, the risk of HO formation increases with multi-level instrumentation from 41% to 75% in one reported study [36]. To date, no other causal relationship has been elucidated between HO rates and diagnosis, alcohol, tobacco, operative level, operative time, or pre-existing ossified lesions [29, 34]. Secondary to its increasing prevalence a classification scheme was proposed by McAfee et al. [37] adapted from systems previously used to describe hip and lumbar spine HO. This simple system attempts to quantify the amount of HO while qualifying the remaining motion at the involved segment [Table 1].

Briefly, grade 0 shows no HO, while grade IV represents complete ankylosis across the segment [37]. Incidentally, there is some evidence that post-operative NSAID use may reduce the rates of HO formation. Review of the continued access arm of Delamarter et al. [25] in which NSAIDS were more frequently prescribed demonstrated no ankylosis at the treated level compared with five grade IV lesions in the initial IDE study at four years. Mehren et al. [28] showed a two-fold decrease in the rate of grade IV HO between two centers in their multicenter trial in which NSAIDS were routinely prescribed postoperatively at one site but not at the other. Currently, there is no published data suggesting a correlation between HO and a negative clinical outcome following CDA. Barbagallo et al. [38] found HO in over 40% of CDA patients but no difference in reported functional scoring between groups. Some segmental motion was preserved in 94% with some grade of HO. It should be noted that current follow-up data on HO is still short term and the long-term natural history as well as its implications for index level and adjacent level motion remains to be seen.

Class		Description
0	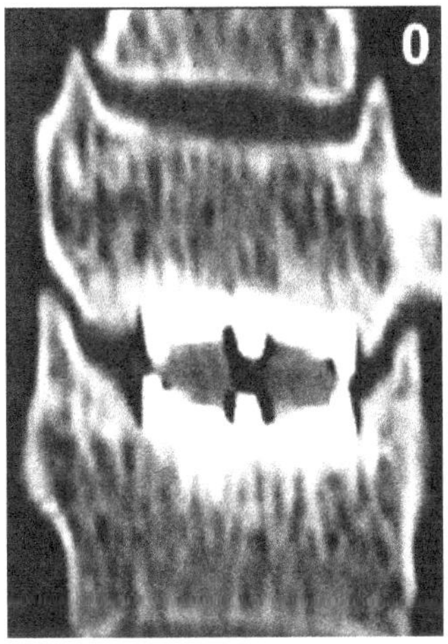	No HO present
I	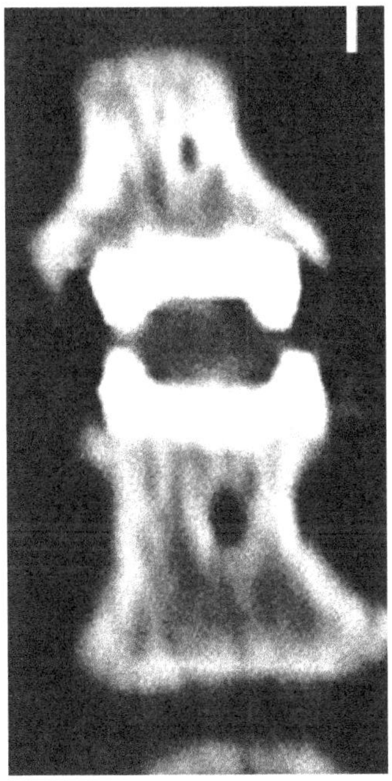	HO present but is not in the disc space and does not appear to interfere with motion

Class		Description
II	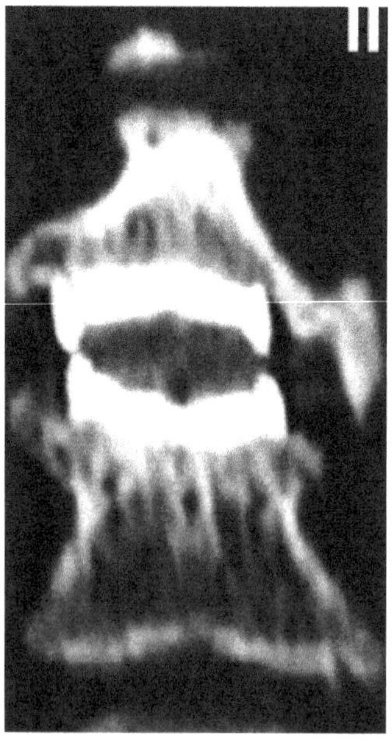	HO has violated the disc space and may be affecting the normal function of the prosthesis
III	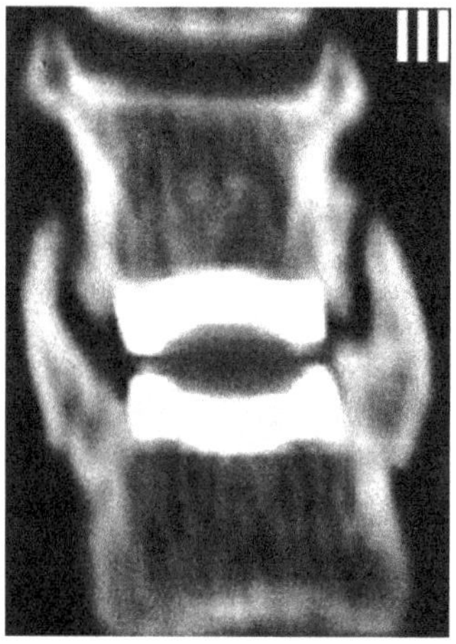	Bridging ossifications may limit function of the implant, but motion remains
IV	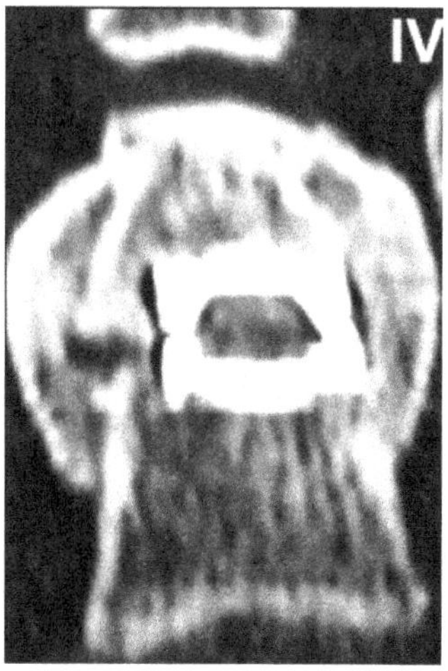	Bridging HO resulting in complete fusion of the segment

Table 1. Classification of HO Scale with computed tomography images (Adapted from [37])

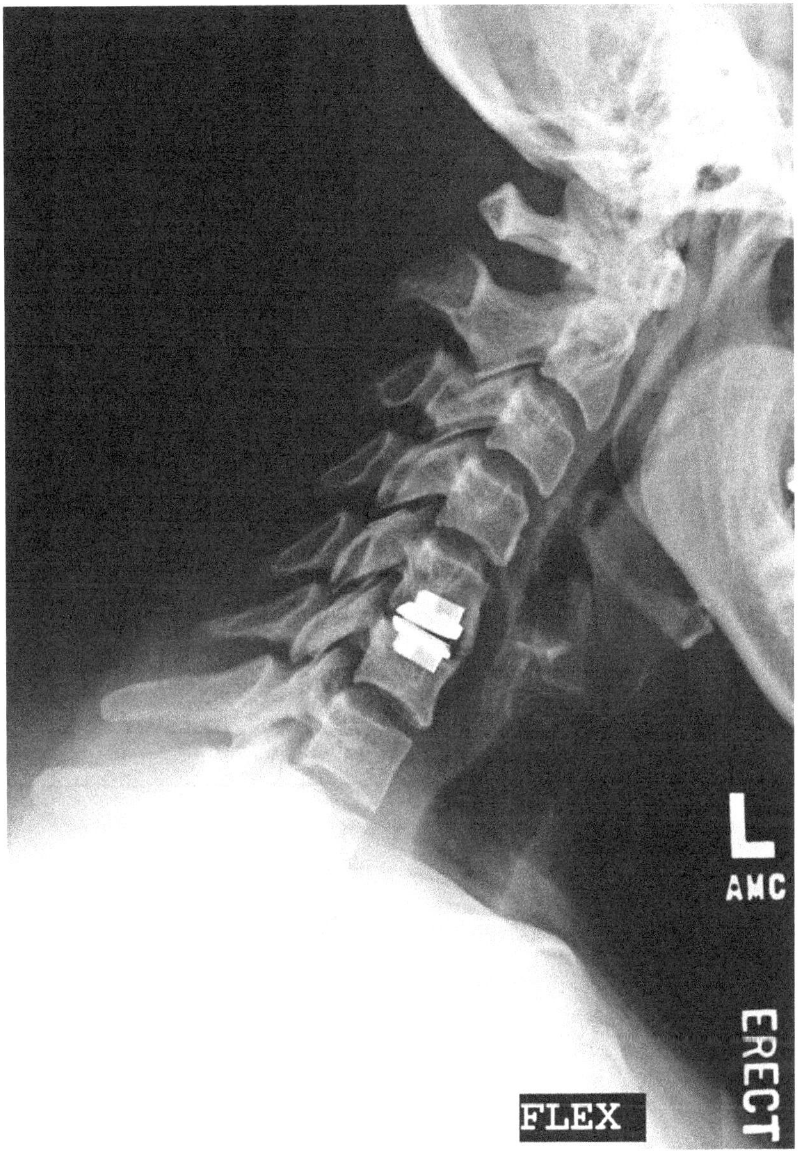

Figure 15. Lateral radiograph of ProDisc-C with HO formation and preserved motion

7. Complications, infection, and wear

To date, none of the large clinical series have reported catastrophic neurological complications. As described above, the rates of revision surgery at the index level have been on par or better when compared with ACDF in a non-inferiority study design. The authors are unaware of any published reports of CDA revision secondary to infection.

No chapter on arthoplasty would be complete without a discussion on wear and osteolysis. According to work done on the Bryan disc by Anderson et al., [39] the particles generated were larger than those associated with hip and knee arthroplasty and occurred in a much smaller volume. In a mouse model there was no evidence of local or systemic inflammatory response.

A brief search of the literature identified two case reports of local inflammatory response in the setting of CDA. The first [40] involved return of radicular symptoms following a metal-on-metal CDA. Repeat MRI revealed a posterior soft tissue mass encroaching on the spinal canal. Surgical exploration revealed hypertrophic cartilaginous material and chronic inflammatory debris. The patient was treated with explantation and conversion to ACDF. After revision surgery, the patient had complete resolution of symptoms. The second case reported by Tumialan and Gluf [41] recounts a 30-year-old male that developed axial neck pain nine months postoperatively. Repeat imaging studies revealed progressive osteolysis on the superior endplate. Infection workup was negative and revision to ACDF was completed without complication. Examination of the implant showed no abnormal wear characteristics and the authors hypothesized that the process was related to a local immune response.

Table 2 highlights the most common complications associated with CDA.

Approach	Infections, hollow viscera injury, vascular injury, dysphagia
Technique	Malposition, improper sizing, migration, end plate fracture, subsidence, heterotopic ossification (Figure 14), ankylosis (Figure 15)
Implant	Heterotopic ossification, implant failure, wear debris (inflammatory response)

Table 2. Complications of Cervical Spinal Arthoplasty

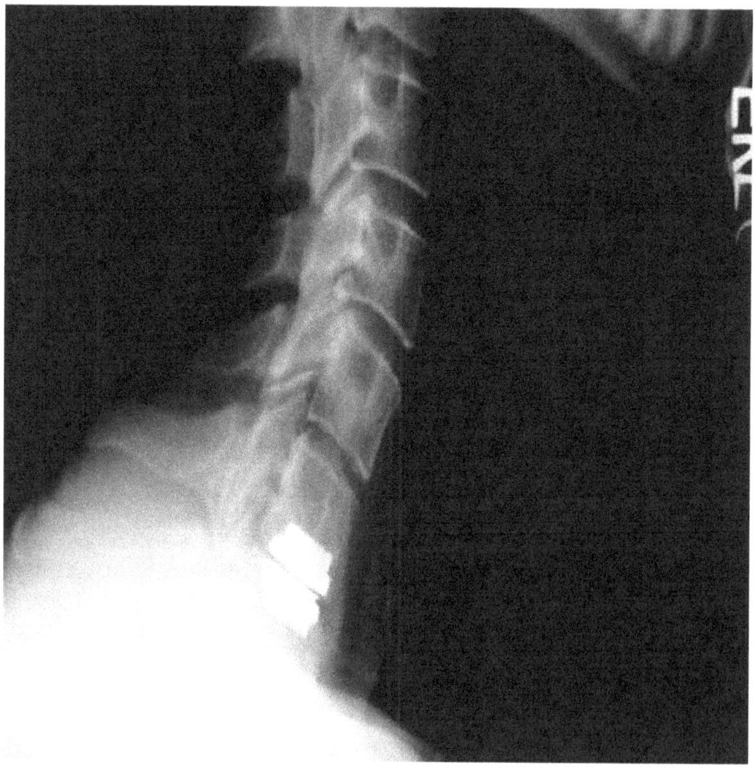

Figure 16. Ankylosis of a cervical disc arthroplasty

8. Conclusions

Cervical disc arthroplasty has evolved significantly since its introduction over 60 years ago. Multiple randomized, controlled, multicenter trials have been performed to assess its validity compared to the gold standard of ACDF. Unfortunately, despite the large trials the numbers are still small and the long-term follow up remains to be seen. Recent meta-analyses of existing data have attempted to extrapolate this data and do show promise for CDA but again only time will tell.

Author details

Christopher Paul O'Boynick* and Bruce V. Darden II

*Address all correspondence to: coboynic@gmail.com

OrthoCarolina Spine Center, Charlotte, USA

References

[1] Bohlman HH, Emery SE, Goodfellow DB, et al. Robinson anterior cervical discectomy and arthrodesis for cervical radiculopathy: Long-term follow-up of one hundred and twenty-two patients. J Bone Joint Surg Am 1993;75 1298-1307.

[2] Bailey R, Badgely C. Stabilization of the cervical spine by anterior fusion. Journal of Bone and Joint Surgery Am 1960;42(4) 565-594.

[3] Robinson R, Smith G. Anterolateral cervical disc removal and interbody fusion for cervical disc syndrome. Bull. John Hopkins Hospital 1955;96 223-224.

[4] Gore DR, Sepic SB. Anterior cervical fusion for degenerated or protruded discs: A review of one hundred forty-six patients. Spine 1984;(9) 667-71.

[5] Goffin J, Geusens E, Vantomme N, et al. Long-term follow-up after interbody fusion of the cervical spine. Journal of Spinal Disorders and Techniques 2004;17(2) 79-85.

[6] Hilibrand AS, Carlson GD, Palumbo MA, et al. Radiculopathy and myelopathy at segments adjacent to the site of a previous anterior cervical arthrodesis. Journal of Bone and Joint Surgery Am 1999;(81) 519-528.

[7] Goffin J, Van Loon J, VanCalenbergh F, et al. Long-term results after anterior cervical fusion and osteosynthetic stabilization for fractures and/or dislocation of the cervical spine. Journal of Spinal Disorders and Techniques 1995;(8) 500-508.

[8] Brown CA, Eismont FJ. Complications in spinal fusion. Orthop Clin North Am 1998;(29) 679-699.

[9] Summers BN, Einstein SM. Donor site pain from the ilium: A complication of lumbar spine fusion. J Bone Joint Surg Br 1989;(71) 677-680.

[10] Mroz TE, Joyce MJ, Lieberman IH, et al. The use of allograft bone in spine surgery: Is it safe? Spine J 2009;(9) 303-308.

[11] Brodke DS, Zdeblick TA. Modified Smith-Robinson procedure for anterior cervical discectomy and fusion. Spine1992;(17) S427-430.

[12] Huang RC, Girardi FP, Cammisa FP et al. The implications of constraint in lumbar total disc replacement. Journal of Spinal Disorders and Techniques 2003;(16) 412-417.

[13] Penning L. Normal movements of the cervical spine. Am J Roentgenol 1978;(130) 317-326.

[14] Amevo B, Worth D, Bogduk N. Instantaneous axis of rotation of the typical cervical motion segments: A study in normal volunteers. Clinical Biomechanics 1991;(6) 111-117.

[15] Bogduk N, Mercer S. Biomechanics of the cervical spine. I: Normal kinematics. Clinical Biomechanics 2000;(15) 633-648.

[16] McAfee P, Reah C, Gilder K, et al. A meta-analysis of comparative outcomes following cervical arthroplasty or anterior cervical fusion. Spine 2012;(37) 943-952.

[17] Gao Y, Ming L, Tao L, Fuguo H, et al. A meta-analysis comparing the results of cervical disc arthroplasty with anterior cervical discectomy and fusion (ACDF) for the treatment of symptomatic cervical disease. J Bone Joint Surg Am 2013;(95) 555-561.

[18] Davis RJ, Nunley PD, Kim KD, et al. Two-level total disc replacement with Mobi-C cervical artificial disc versus anterior discectomy and fusion: A prospective, randomized, controlled multicenter clinical trial with 4-year follow results. J Neurosurg Spine 2015;(22) 15-25.

[19] Hisey MS, Bae HW, Davis R, et al. Prospective, randomized comparison of cervical total disc replacement versus anterior cervical fusion: Results at 48 months follow-up. J Spinal Disord Tech 2014; Epub ahead of print.

[20] Heller JG, Sasso RC, Papadopoulos SM, Anderson PA, Fessler RG et al. Comparison of Bryan Cervical Disc Arthroplasty with anterior cervical decompression and fusion. Spine 2009;(34) 101-107.

[21] Goffin J, VanLoo J, VanCalenbergh F et al. A clinical analysis of 4-6 year follow-up results after cervical disc replacement using the Bryan Cervical Disc Prosthesis. J Neurosurg Spine 2010;(12) 261-9.

[22] Mummaneni et al. Clinical and radiographic analysis of cervical disc arthroplasty compared with allograft fusion: A randomized controlled trial. J Neurosurg Spine 2007;(6) 198-209.

[23] Peng CW, Yue WM, Abdul B et al. Intermediate results of the Prestige LP cervical disc replacement: Clinical and radiological analysis with minimum two-year follow-up. Spine 2011;(36) 105-111.

[24] Murrey et al. Results of the prospective, randomized, controlled Food and Drug Administration Investigational Device Exemption Study of the ProDisc-C total disc replacement versus anterior discectomy and fusion for the treatment of one level symptomatic cervical disc disease. Spine Journal 2009;(9) 275-286.

[25] Delamarter RB, Murrey D, Janssen MI et al. Results of 24 months from the prospective, randomized, multicenter investigation device exemption trial of ProDisc-C versus anterior cervical discectomy and fusion with 4-year follow-up and continued access patients. SAS Journal 2010;(4) 122-128.

[26] Phillips FM, Lee JY, Geiser FH, et al. A prospective, randomized, controlled clinical investigation comparing PCM cervical disc arthroplasty with anterior cervical discectomy and fusion. 2-year results from the US FDA IDE clinical trial. Spine 2013;(38) E907-918.

[27] Riew KD, Buchowski JM, Sasso R, Zdeblick T, Metcalf NH, Anderson PA. Cervical disc arthroplasty compared with arthrodesis for the treatment of myelopathy. J Bone Joint Surg Am 2008;(90) 2354-2364.

[28] Mehren C, Suchomel P, Grochulla F, et al. Heterotopic ossification in total cervical artificial disc replacement. Spine 2006;31(24):2802-6.

[29] Leung C, Casey AT, Goffin J, et al. Clinical significance of heterotopic ossification in cervical disc replacement: A prospective multicenter clinical trial. Neurosurgery. 2005;57(4):759-63; discussion 63.

[30] Heidecke V, Burkert W, Brucke M, et al. Intervertebral disc replacement for cervical degenerative disease--clinical results and functional outcome at two years in patients implanted with the Bryan cervical disc prosthesis. Acta neurochirurgica 2008;150(5): 453-9; discussion 9.

[31] Beaurain J, Bernard P, Dufour T, et al. Intermediate clinical and radiological results of cervical TDR (Mobi-C) with up to 2 years of follow-up. European spine journal: Official publication of the European Spine Society, the European Spinal Deformity Society, and the European Section of the Cervical Spine Research Society. 2009;18(6): 841-50.

[32] Suchomel P, Jurak L, Benes V, 3rd, et al. Clinical results and development of heterotopic ossification in total cervical disc replacement during a 4-year follow-up. European spine journal: Official publication of the European Spine Society, the European

Spinal Deformity Society, and the European Section of the Cervical Spine Research Society 2010;19(2):307-15.

[33] Yi S, Kim KN, Yang MS, et al. Difference in occurrence of heterotopic ossification according to prosthesis type in the cervical artificial disc replacement. Spine 2010;35(16):1556-61.

[34] Lee JH, Jung TG, Kim HS, et al. Analysis of the incidence and clinical effect of the heterotopic ossification in a single-level cervical artificial disc replacement. The spine journal: Official journal of the North American Spine Society 2010;10(8):676-82.

[35] Chen J, Wang X, Bai W, et al. Prevalence of heterotopic ossification after cervical total disc arthroplasty: a meta-analysis. European spine journal: Official publication of the European Spine Society, the European Spinal Deformity Society, and the European Section of the Cervical Spine Research Society 2012;21(4):674-80.

[36] Wu JC, Huang WC, Tsai HW, et al. Differences between 1- and 2-level cervical arthroplasty: More heterotopic ossification in 2-level disc replacement: Clinical article. Journal of neurosurgery Spine. 2012;16(6):594-600.

[37] McAfee PC, Cunningham BW, Devine J, et al. Classification of heterotopic ossification (HO) in artificial disk replacement. Journal of spinal disorders & techniques 2003;16(4):384-9.

[38] Barbagallo GM, Corbino LA, Olindo G, et al. Heterotopic ossification in cervical disc arthroplasty: Is it clinically relevant? Evidence-based spine-care journal 2010;1(1): 15-20.

[39] Anderson PA, Sasso RC, Rouleau JP, et al. The Bryan Cervical Disc: wear properties and early clinical results. Spine Journal 2004;(4) 5303-5309.

[40] Cavanaugh DA, Nunley PD, Kerr EJ, et al. Delayed hyper-reactivty to metal ions after cervical disc arthroplasty: A case report and literature review. Spine 2009;34(7) E262-265.

[41] Tumialan LM and Gluf, Wm. Progressive vertebral body osteolysis after cervical arthroplasty. Spine 2011;36(14) 973-8.

6

Failure Mechanisms in Hip Resurfacing Arthroplasty

Hiran Wimal Amarasekera

Abstract

Hip resurfacing arthroplasty has been a popular alternative for total hip replacement in young active patients since the early 1990s.

Early results have been promising and a large number of arthroplasties were performed in the United Kingdom, North America, and Western Europe during the last decade. However, due to a series of complications, such as pseudo-tumours, femoral neck fractures avascular necrosis and aseptic loosening, the long-term results were poor and failure rate has been high.

This chapter attempts to identify the different biological and biomechanical mechanisms that may contribute to these failures. It also discusses some considerations to be noted when designing resurfacing implants in the future.

This is a research study based on the author's primary research work carried out with retrieval specimens taken from failed hip arthroplasties.

Keywords: Hip Resurfacing, pseudo-tumours, retrieval specimens, metal-on-metal designs, surgical approaches, avascular necrosis, aseptic lymphocyte-dominated vasculitis-associated lesions (ALVAL)

1. Introduction

1.1. History

The concept of hip resurfacing arthroplasty or surface replacement of the hip was originally introduced by John Charnley in the 1950s [1] but had to abandon the idea due to high wear rate [2]. Since then, many surgeons, such as *Wagner et al* [3], have been using hip resurfacing arthroplasty as an alternative to total hip replacements (THR). [4, 5]

Due to high wear rate and metal plastic debris giving rise to a number of complications, this procedure did not gain popularity among orthopaedic surgeons until the early 1990s.

1.2. Modern hip resurfacing

In the early 1990s, there was resurgence in hip resurfacing arthroplasties when *McMinn et al.* introduced metal-on-metal-resurfacing. [6] Instead of metal-on-plastic, the design was changed to metal-on-metal. Since then, there has been a rapid increase in hip resurfacing throughout the world mainly in Europe, the United Kingdom [7], and North America peaking in late the 90s and the early part of this decade. [8]

The main reasons for this popularity among surgeons were the advantages of hip resurfacing as compared to the conventional hip replacements such as minimal bone loss, less dislocation rates, and easier conversion to a revision. Due to these factors resurfacing was introduced mainly as an alternative to THR in young active adults. [9] Modern hip resurfacing also addressed the problems associated with previous designs. The new design was built using better materials (metal-on-metal), modified surgical techniques including new surgical approaches, and better instrumentation for implant positioning. [10]

1.2.1. Indications for modern hip resurfacing

Indications were broad-based, but the ideal candidate is described as young, active adult males in their late forties to early sixties [9] with good bone stock having primary or secondary osteoarthritis.

Hip resurfacings have been done in young females [11], including patients with dysplasia and avascular necrosis (AVN) of the femoral head. [12]

1.2.2. Complications of hip resurfacing

There are many complications associated with hip resurfacing some are common for any orthopaedic procedure such as infection, nerve palsy, deep vein thrombosis, and dislocation. Even though the complications are similar the complication rates differ between hip resurfacing and total hip arthroplasty.

These complications can be classified in many ways:

1. Based on common and specific: Common to all hip arthroplasties and specific to hip resurfacing
2. Based on timing: Early and late
3. Based mainly on site of failure; femoral or acetabular components: Femoral, acetabular, both, or none

Common complications to all hip arthroplasty procedures include bleeding, nerve damage, deep vein thrombosis, malpositioning of implants, and dislocations. Out of these, dislocation is relatively rare in hip resurfacing compared to THR due to the larger size head in the femoral component. However, the large head increase the surface area and can lead to high wear rates leading to eventual failure. Malpositioning is a contributory factor for the high wear rates. [13]

The complications that are more specific to hip resurfacing arthroplasty can be further divided into early and late complications.

The early complications are usually seen within the first weeks to the early years. These are loosening of implants, femoral neck fractures, femoral head notching [14] and AVN. [15]

The late complications are set of complications recognized recently, following the long-term outcome of patients. [16] Among these are osteolysis, pseudo-tumours, bone resorption, ALVAL, loosening of components, high metal ion levels in blood, and tissue metallosis. These complications can eventually lead to failure of the hip resurfacing implant. [17, 18]

2. Causes of failure/complications in hip resurfacing

1. AVN of the femoral head
2. Loosening of implants
3. Femoral neck fractures
4. Impingement
5. High metal ion levels in blood
6. Metallosis
7. Pseudo-tumours formation
8. ALVAL
9. Resorbtion of head

2.1. Pathogenesis of early complications

It is widely believed that early complications such as AVN, femoral neck fractures, and loosening of implants, are mainly associated with the decrease in the blood flow to the femoral head. Understanding the basic mechanisms of failure in each complication will help us to prevent these at present and design better implants in the future.

2.1.1. Reducing blood flow to the femoral head possibly leading to AVN and implant failure

This has been mainly attributed to the posterior surgical approach that reduces the femoral head blood flow by damaging the branches of the medial circumflex femoral artery. Unlike in THR where the femoral head and neck is removed in resurfacing the neck and part of the head is preserved, the blood flow to this area appear to play a crucial role in the long-term outcome. This is the main reason why many surgeons have challenged the posterior approach. Alternatively many surgical approaches have been tried. Many studies have attempted to demonstrate this by comparing the blood flow between posterior and other approaches [19 - 22].

Ganz et al has described trochanteric flip approach as an alternative surgical approach to the posterior approach to be used during hip resurfacing to preserve the blood flow. [23]

Even though many studies show a clear drop in blood flow intra-operatively during posterior approach, post-operatively some studies fail to establish a clinical significance and a direct link to this fall as a cause of AVN; other studies show this as a transient drop that recovers during the post-operative period [24]. Some have argued that AVN is not caused by the procedure. [25] Some have even used hip resurfacing as a treatment option for patients having established AVN and Perthes disease. [12, 26, 27, 28]

Due to these reasons, many studies have been conducted comparing different surgical approaches when hip resurfacing is performed. This has also led to many different surgical approaches being tried by many surgeons in the past decade. [29] The posterior, poster-lateral [30], direct lateral, Ganz trochanteric flip [31], direct anterior [32], and antero-lateral [33] approaches. [34] Some complications of resurfacings shown in Fig 1A-1C.

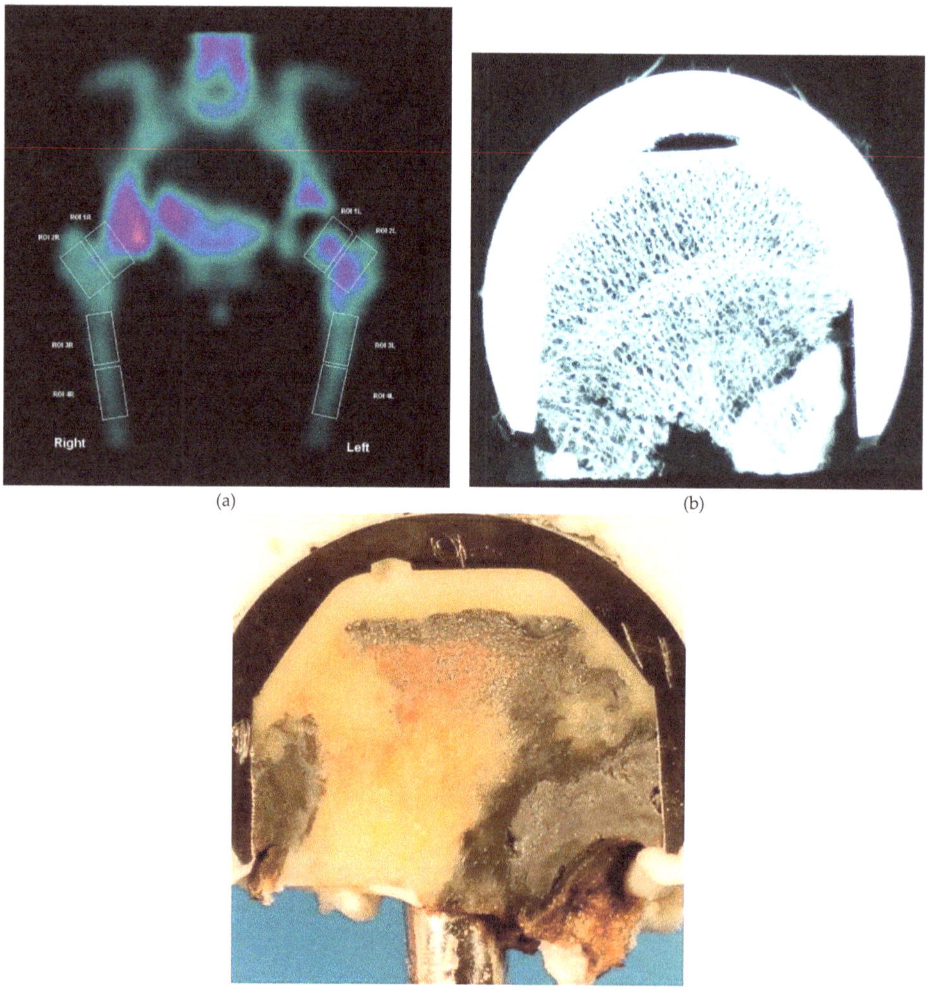

(a) (b) (c)

Figure 1. (a). Single cut section of a Single Positron emission Computed Tomography (SPECT) image. The most likely areas to develop AVN and fractures are ROI L (L: Operated, R: Normal). (b). Mocroradiograph shows bone thinning under the metal implant with a fracture at the lower margin. (c). The cut section of a retrieval head with metallosis and early pseudo-tumour formation

2.1.2. *Femoral neck fractures following hip resurfacing*

Femoral neck fractures is a common and specific complication of hip resurfacing (Fig. 1B and 2). There are many factors attributed to this including AVN, poor patient selection (patients with osteoporosis such as older age groups, post menopausal female patients), and poor implant positioning that may cause notching. [15] Some also believe that notching may affect the blood flow. [14] Proper patient selection and careful surgical technique is important to minimise neck fractures. [35 - 37]

The ideal patient for hip resurfacing is the young active adult male. [38] Hip resurfacing in post-menopausal females is not recommended. Hip resurfacing in younger females is a debatable issue among many surgeons as revision rates and femoral neck fractures appear to be higher in females than in males. [39] Bone density and good bone stock appear as an important feature to prevent complications. [40] Obesity is another risk factor for neck fractures. [35]

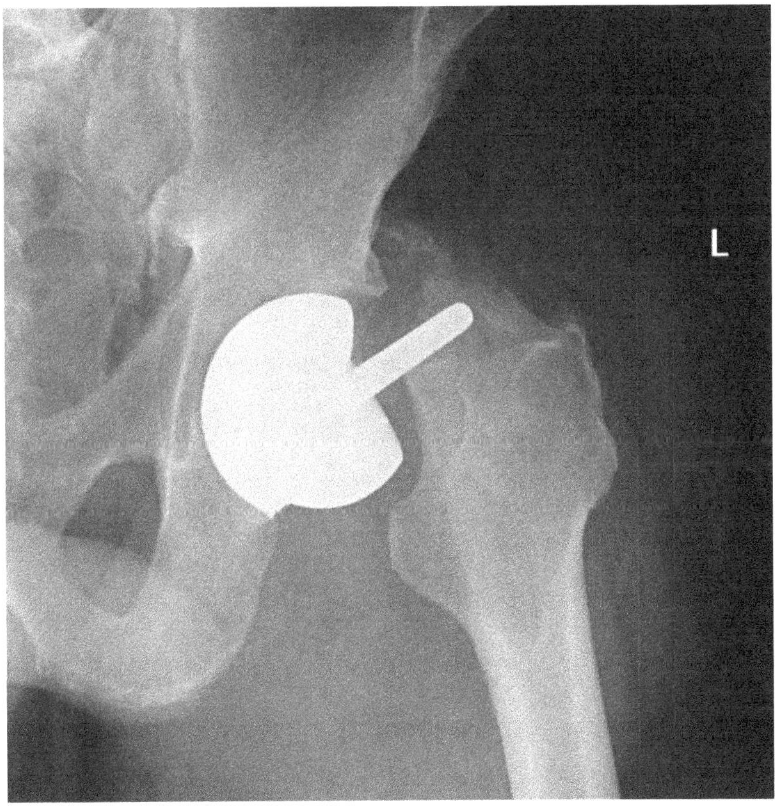

Figure 2. X-ray of a femoral neck fracture following hip resurfacing arthroplasty

2.1.3. *Loosening of components*

Loosening of components is another cause for early and late failure of resurfacing, mainly acetabular failure, in young adults. [41] Loosening can be further divided to acetabular, femoral or both. Loosening of components can be due to many reasons. Poor positioning, poor cementing, poor surgical technique, and infection can all cause loosening. Even though cementing of both components are common, some prefer cementing the femoral head with un-cemented acetabular component, while some do not use cement at all. [42, 43] Initial failure rates for cemented acetabular component were high and led to the re-introduction of the cementless components. [44] If cement is used, the cementing technique becomes a key factor in improving long and short-term results. [45] Another complication associated with cementing is the possibility of thermal necrosis (Fig. 3) that can lead to loosening and this needs to be minimised for better outcomes. [46]

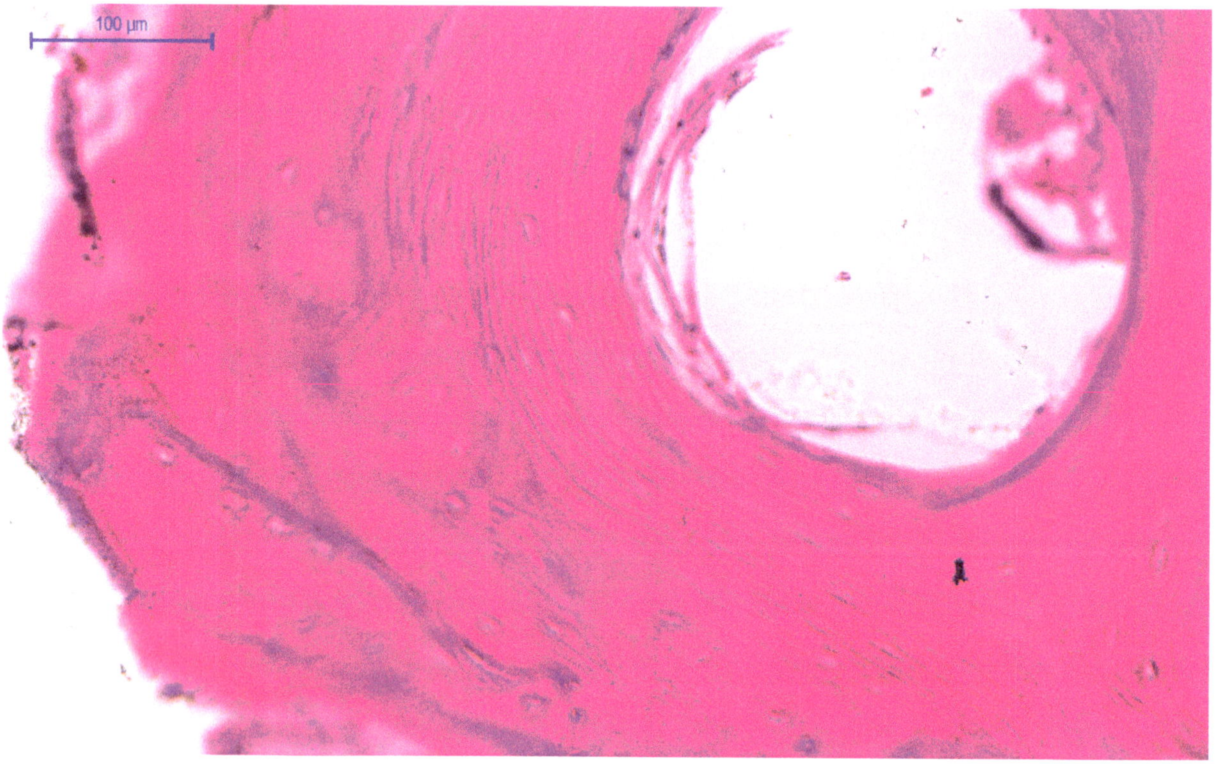

Figure 3. Features of necrosis at the margin of cemented implant with empty lacunae, most likely due to thermal necrosis (Cement metal interface) (H & E 20X)

2.2. Pathogenesis and possible mechanisms of failure in late complications

Most late complications that lead to eventual failure of the implants seem to be associated with high wear rates leading to increased metal ion released to soft tissues and blood leading to the following changes:

1. High metal ions in the blood
2. Metal sensitivity
3. Metallosis in tissues
4. ALVAL
5. Development of pseudo tumours (Fig. 4)

6. Osteolysis
7. Bone resorption

Pseudo-tumours have been reported [47] following resurfacing arthroplasty (Fig. 1C and 4). In a Canadian study of around 3,400 hips, pseudo-tumours were reported in four, giving a prevalence of 0.10%. [48].

The commonest hypothesis suggested for pseudo-tumour formation is the release of metal ions due to the increased surface area and malpositioning of implants. [49] This triggers a delayed Type IV hypersensitivity reaction leading to osteolysis and ALVAL presenting as pseudo tumours. [50 - 53]

Acetabular component malpositioning appear to cause more ALVAL formation due to high wear. [50, 54, 55] Blood metal ion levels, mainly Cobalt and chromium (Co and Cr), have been found to be high following resurfacing arthroplasty but the link between high blood ion levels and the formation of pseudo-tumours is not well established. [56] Some studies suggest the presence of asymptomatic pseudo-tumours with high blood ion levels among patients after resurfacing arthroplasty (RA). [57]

Blood metal ion levels may be high following both THR and RA, as many studies suggest [58 - 61], but the local effect on the hip may differ between the two.

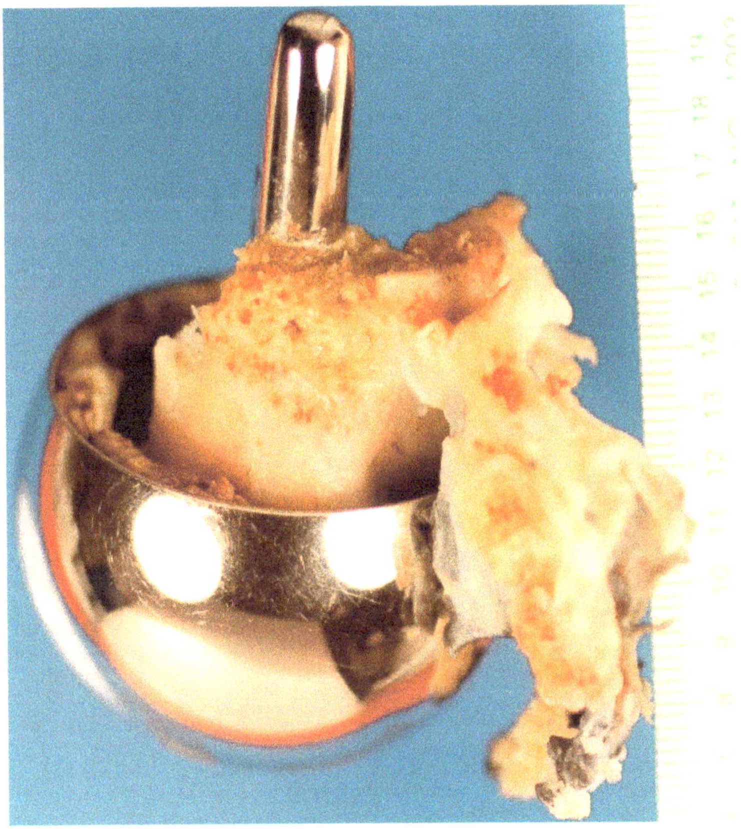

Figure 4. Retrieved head with extensive resorption of head osteolysis and growth of a pseudo-tumour

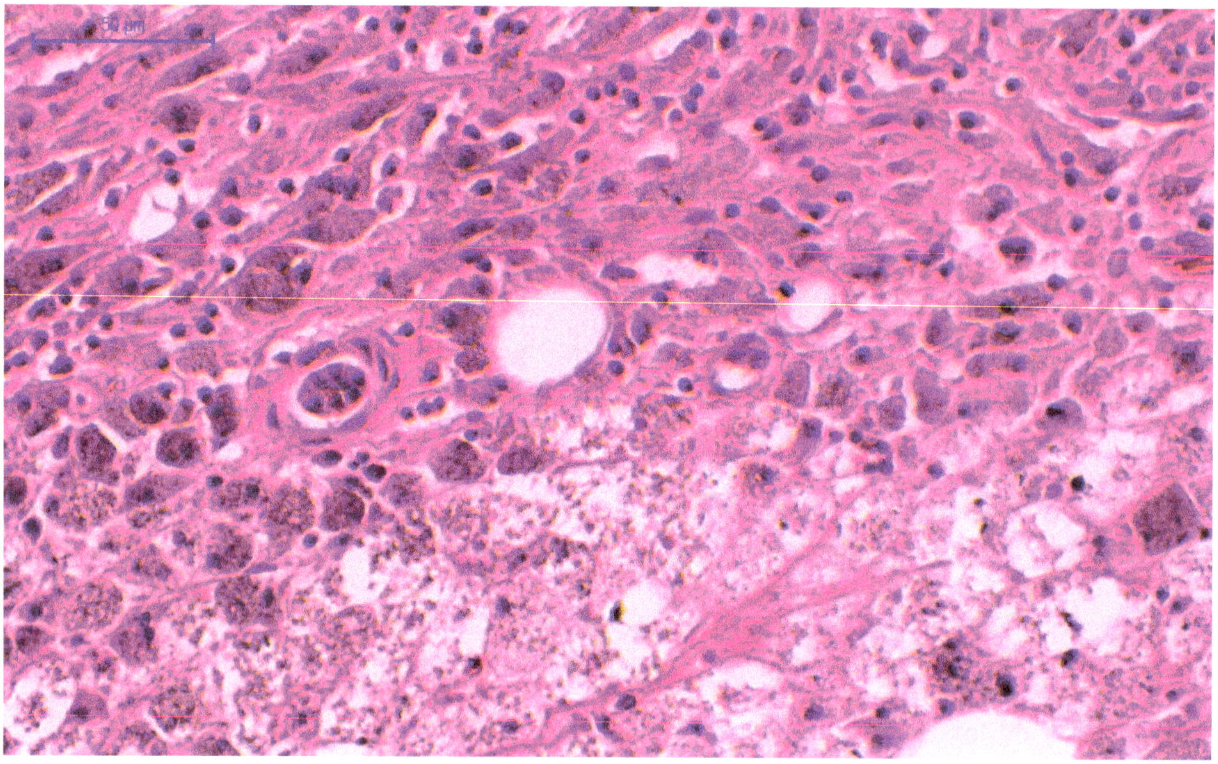

Figure 5. Large number of lymphocytic infiltration with metal particles engulfed macrophages forming multinucleated foreign body Giant cells (H & E 40X)

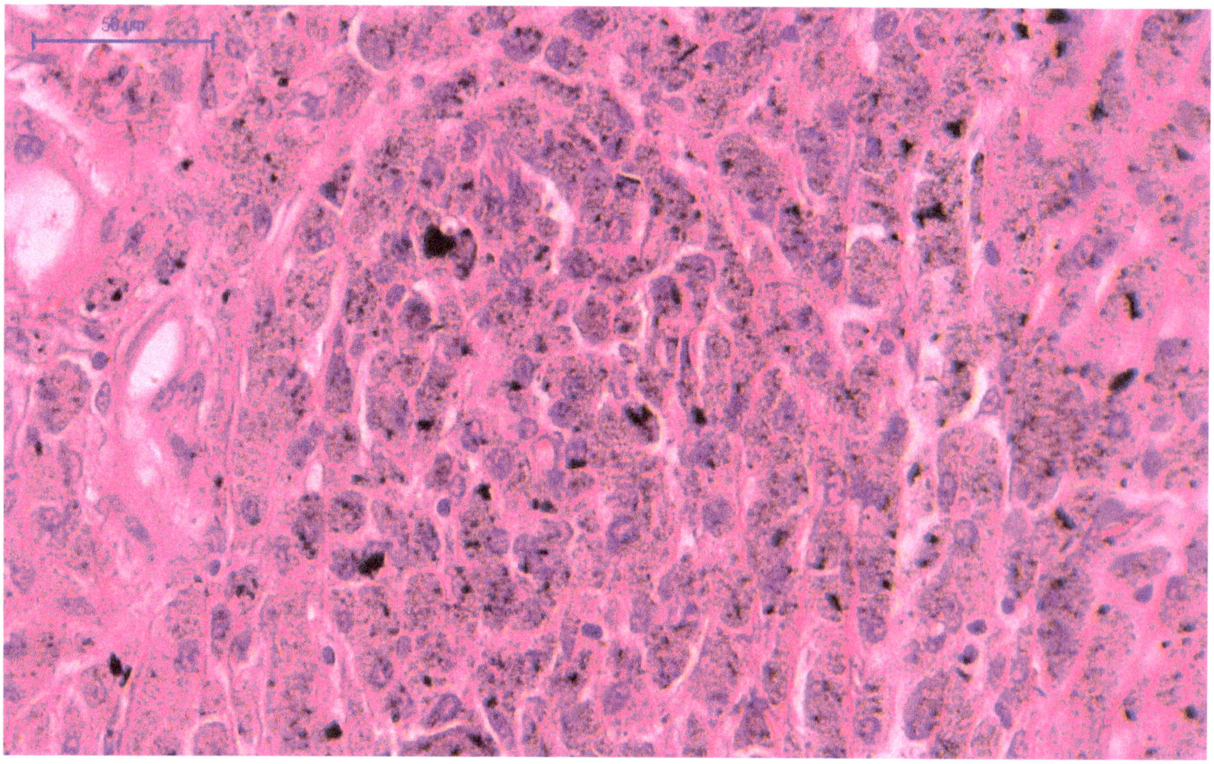

Figure 6. Large number of metal particles (black) seen in bone tissue from a retrieved femoral head (H & E 40X)

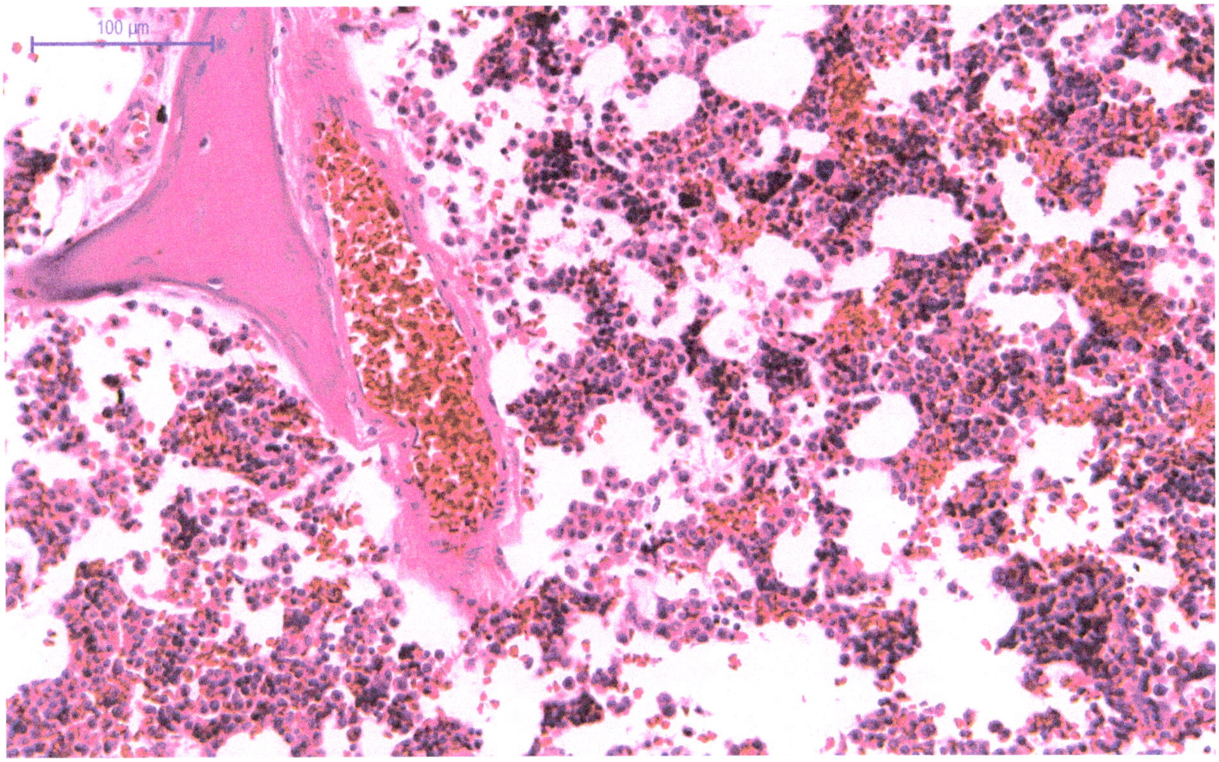

Figure 7. Highly vascular bone in osteolysis and pseudo-tumour formation showing a blood vessel, aggregation of lymphocytes inflammatory cells, and live bone characterised by nucleated lacunae (H & E 20X)

Pseudo-tumours appear to be highly vascular with blood vessels red blood cells, lymphocytes macrophages, and inflammatory cells with live bone until osteolysis occurs. (Figs. 1C, 5–7)

Common cause for aseptic failure of acetabular component is most likely due to osteolysis triggered by the metal particles. [62]

3. Hypothesis of late failure in hip resurfacing

After considering multiple factors that seem to contribute to the eventual failure of the resurfacing implant, I have recognized two possible pathways that may lead to the failure of the implant in the late stages. These are:

3.1. Uncoordinated osteoblast-osteoclast activity

This process seems to be similar to the process seen in fracture healing. However, compared to fracture healing, which occurs in a well-coordinated systematic stepwise manner, here it happens haphazardly. In osteoblastic activity, new bone formation and signs of healing is seen in one part of the bone; simultaneously, osteolysis bone breakdown and remodelling with osteoclastic activity is seen in the other end. Bone remodelling is a process that is essential in the healing of a bone where a fine balance exists between osteoclastic activity and osteoblastic activity. When this fine balance is broken, uncontrolled osteoclastic activity can cause destruction on a large volume of the femoral head leading to complete osteolysis and bone resorption. This is an uncoordinated process and as long as the initial stimuli that triggered remains, the process seems to continue and eventually leading to bone resorption.

This can present as loosening, pain, malpositioning, and femoral neck fractures. Over activity of osteoclasts initially lead to focal areas of destruction (Fig. 10) that eventually leads to osteolysis of the whole femoral head (Fig. 13). However, in patients where osteoclasts and osteoblast act in a normal coordinated way, well-formed new bone growth can occur resulting in a well-fixed and stable metal/cement bone interface (Fig. 12). The factors that cause increased uncontrolled osteoclasts activity are not clearly understood. This is an area that will need further research. In this series, we found both patterns in patients. A hypothesis of the probable pathway is given below (Fig. 8).

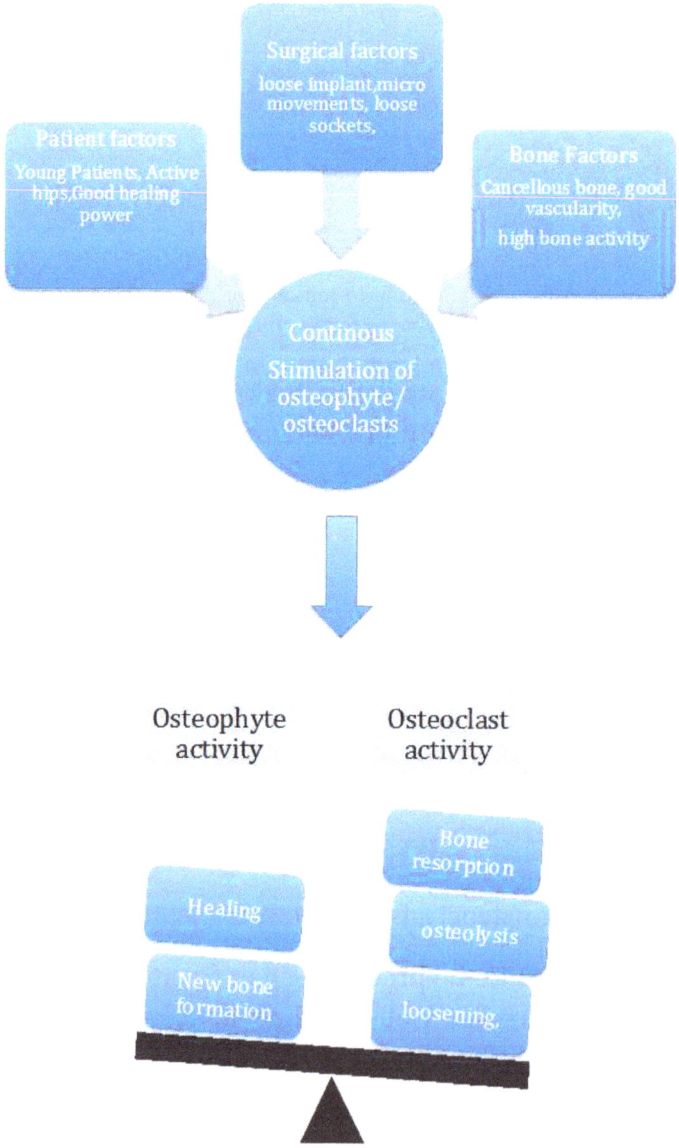

Figure 8. Multiple factors leading to increased bone activity

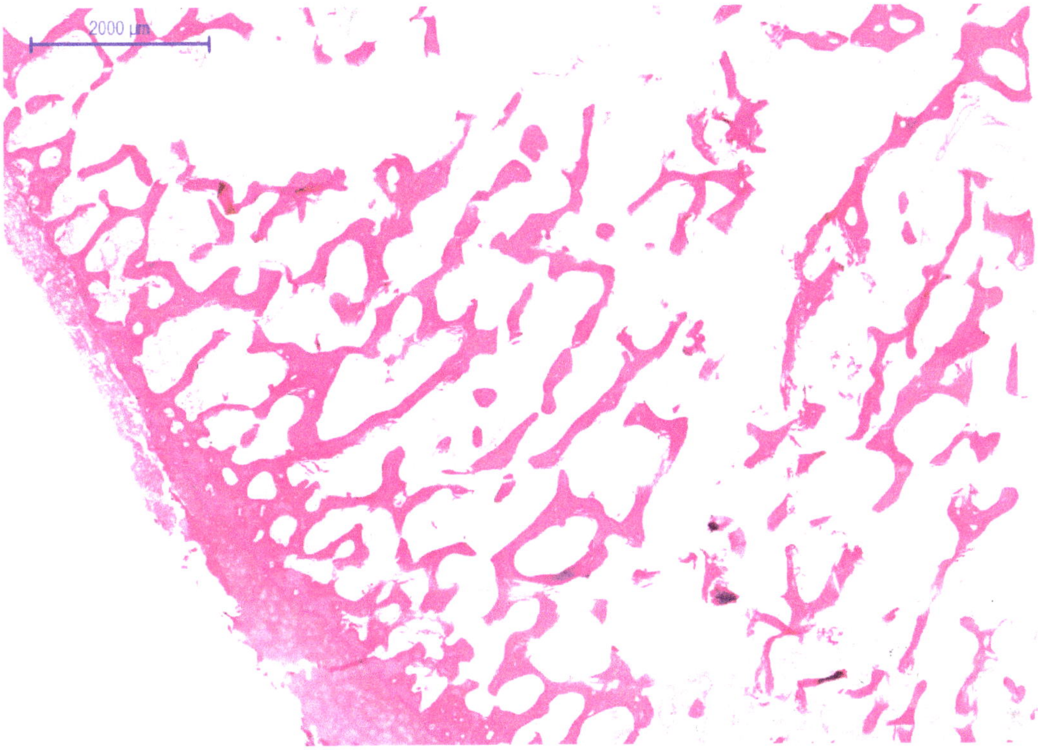

Figure 9. New bone formation from the outer margin while bone remodelling and resorption is shown from a more central area (above). (H & E P 8 ant slice 1X)

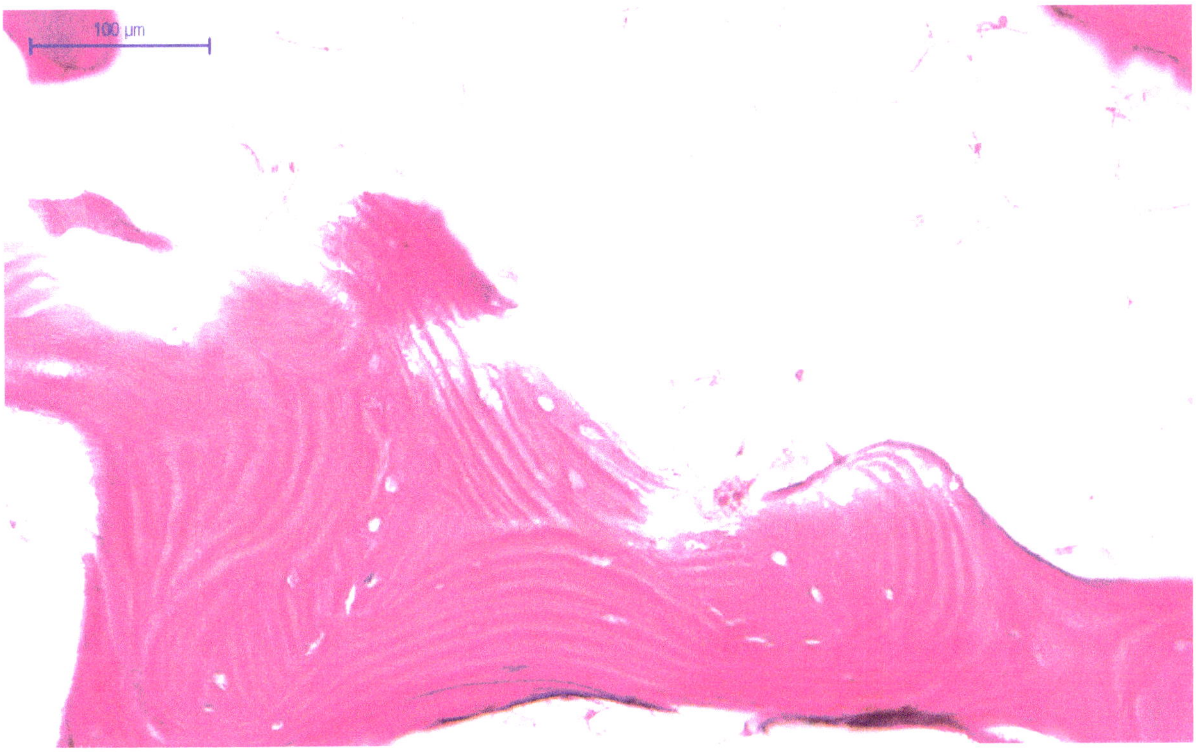

Figure 10. Slide of the central area showing osteoclastic activity with serrated bone margins with an osteoclast causing bone resorption. (H & E 20X)

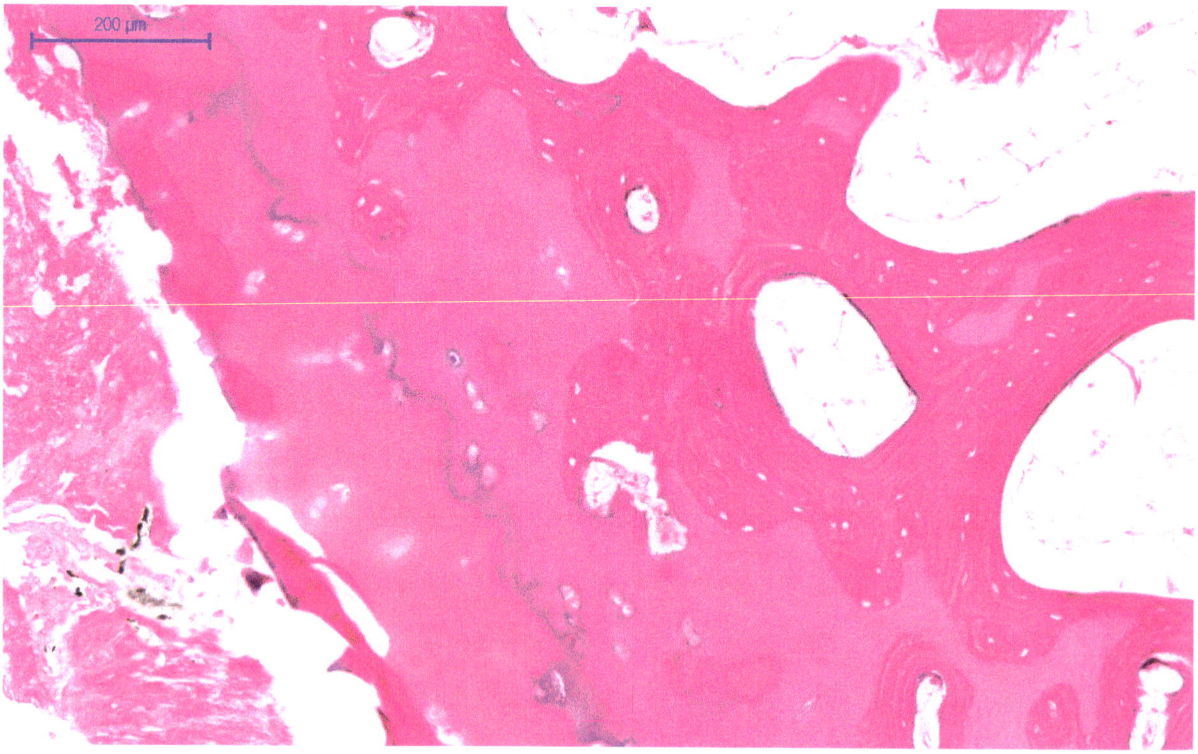

Figure 11. Same slide margin of the bone showing new bone formation (H & E 10X)

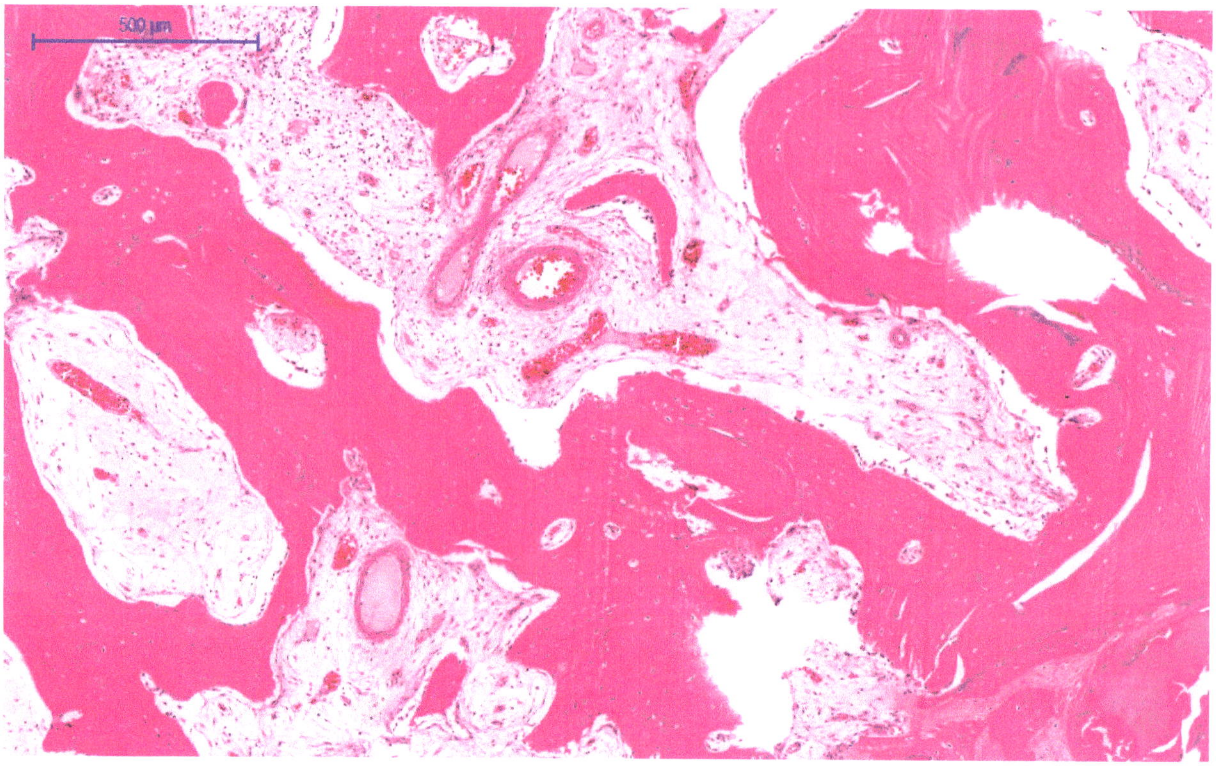

Figure 12. The posterior slice of the same patient (P8) with highly active bone with multiple blood vessels, new bone formation osteoblastic activity, live nucleated lacunae with minimal osteoclasts and bone resorption. (H & E P8 post slice 5x)

In contrast, patients showing loosening, gross osteolysis, bone resorption, show high osteoclastic activity with absence of osteoblastic features or new bone formation.

However, we also noted that both groups show good vascularity with active bones with good blood supply.

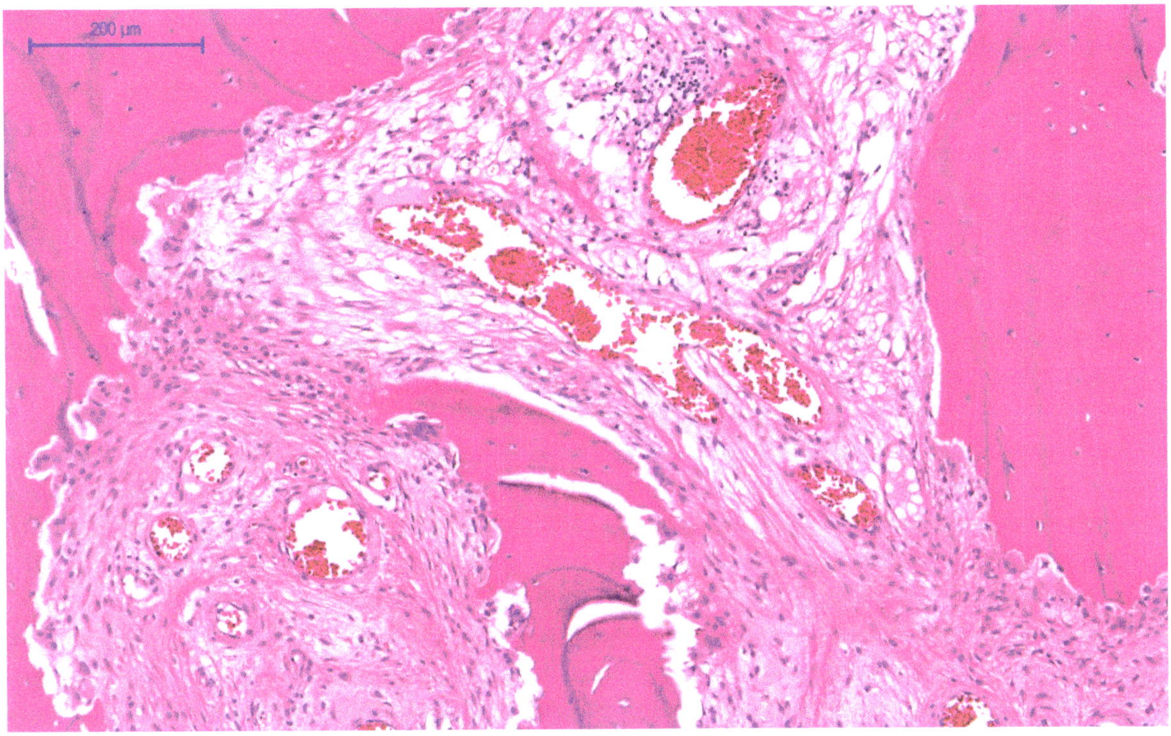

Figure 13. High osteoclastic activity leading to osteolysis along the bone showing serrated bone margin. Note the blood vessels showing good vascularity. (H & E 10x)

3.2. Immune response to foreign bodies leading to delayed hypersensitivity

This mechanism is more established as a number of studies has looked into metal ion release, osteolysis, pseudo-tumour formation, and ALVAL formation.

Metal ions have been implicated as triggering a foreign body type reaction leading to a delayed Type IV hypersensitivity. This has been attributed as a final common pathway leading to osteolysis bone destruction and failure. [51, 52, 57, 60] This may be a cause for unexplained groin pain seen in most of these [63] (Fig 13).

It is also worth mentioning that foreign body granulomas or pseudo-tumours per se may not lead to osteolysis. They can remain asymptomatic. [57, 47] However with time, as they grow in the bone and the under surface of the implant, they can act as a space occupying lesion separating the bone from the metal leading to loosening and malpositioning.

Secondly, they can also trigger immunological reactions that lead to osteolysis and femoral head resorption. As there is no direct evidence for this, this is another area that warrants further investigations and research.

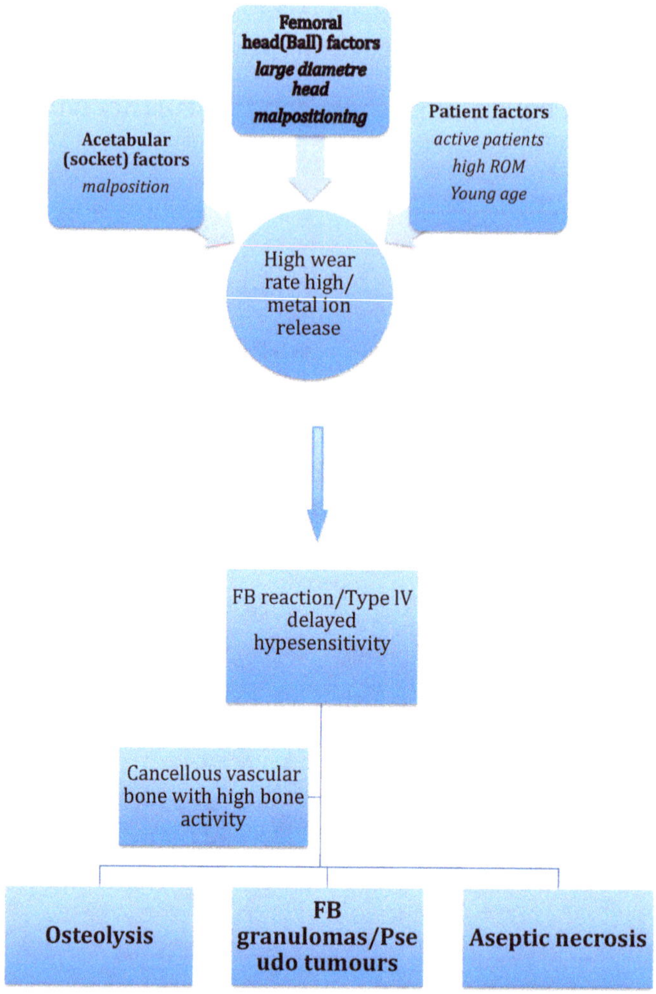

Figure 14. Mechanisms that may lead to immune response seen following hip resurfacing arthroplasty

4. Conclusions

There are many areas where new studies can be done to improve our understanding of the causes and mechanisms of failure of modern metal-on-metal hip arthroplasty.

As we have demonstrated, the causes for failure seem to be multifactorial (Fig. 14) partly due to the mechanisms that are well understood and partly due to mechanisms that at present are ill understood such as persistent groin pain and influence on metal ions.

We might have to rethink the design, taking into account that these biological factors such as femoral head and head neck are developmentally, functionally, structurally, and histologically different bones from the cortical bone. The interaction between metal and bone or cement and bone is different between the two bone types. Secondly, fixing the implant into the most mobile portion (ball of the hip joint) seem to act as a stimulation to trigger many biological responses and inflammatory reactions and immune reactions leading to new bone formation (osteoblastic response) or osteolysis (osteoclastic response).

Micro movement, caused by the loosening and release of high metal particles, made worse by a large diameter head in an environment of high bone activity with good vascularity and healing, in the femoral head seems to trigger ill-understood immune response that is osteoclastic in nature. As the fixation of the femoral component is totally dependant in this area of bone, any microscopic osteolysis can lead to loosening leading to further osteolysis and leading to a vicious cycle (Fig. 15). One option is to break this vicious cycle by having at least a part of the fixation in a less active cortical bone.

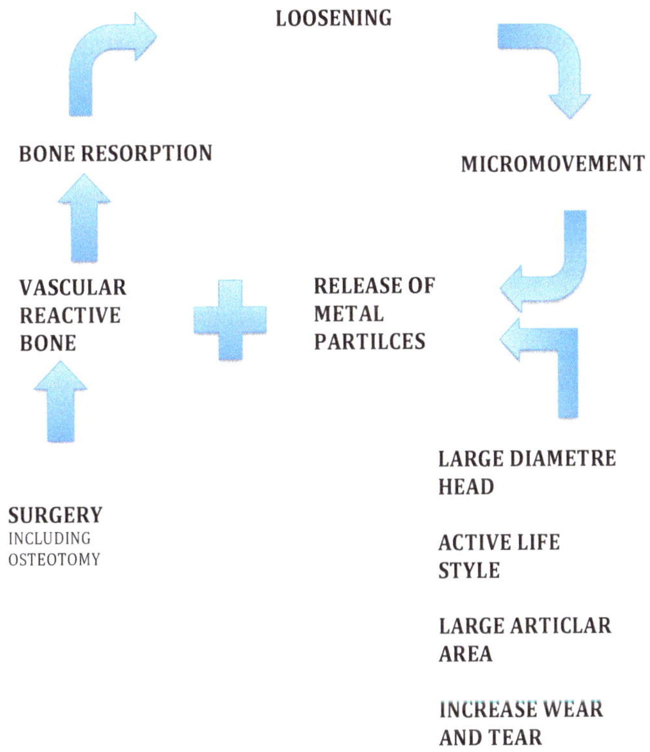

Figure 15. Vicious cycle leading to loosening

The exact relationship between the vascularity of the femoral head and the outcome of resurfacing arthroplasty is not well-established. On one hand, it is argued that vascularity is an essential element for the healing of the resurfaced femoral head to obtain a well-fixed component at the metal bone interface.

However, in spite of good vascularity, cementing can cause thermal necrosis (Fig. 3) at the cement bone interface; but all these implants do not seem to fail. "Does thermal necrosis result in failure of resurfacing arthroplasty?" is a research question that is worth exploring.

Secondly, a good vascular supply can act as a double-edged sword as it enhances bone activity, and with that can stimulate osteoclastic and immune responses (Fig. 13).

These cast doubts whether the trochanteric flip approach is necessarily a good thing as the bone activity in this approach is much higher than other approaches due to the additional osteotomy.

Thirdly, in patients who had AVN caused by non-surgical causes resurfacing arthroplasty [26, 64, 65] or partial resurfacing [66] has been used as a mode of treatment. Therefore, it is worth studying the long-term outcomes in this group in order for us to understand the relationship between vascularity and hip resurfacing.

This retrieval analysis did not demonstrate any relationship between the development of AVN and surgical approach.

One key drawback in finding the exact relationship between vascularity of the bone and AVN is the inability to work out the "critical ischemia" for bone tissue (minimal blood flow needed to keep the bone alive). Experiments that may help us to determine the "critical ischemia" of the femoral head will help us answer this question. [22]

Another limitation is difficulty in finding the bone activity in the femoral head covered by the metal implants. Even though SPECT [67, 68] and Positron Emission Tomography (PET) [69] have been used to study vascularity attenuation caused by the metal implants, they cause difficulty in interpreting the results accurately. [24, 70]

Patient No/Approach Non Posterior (NP) Posterior P	Last follow up since THR (M)	Persistent Problems (Y/N)
1 NP	42	Y (Groin Pain)
2 NP	26	N
3 NP	23	Y (Groin Pain)
4 NP	23	Y (Groin Pain)
5 NP	13	N
6 NP	Loss for follow up	
7 P	28	Died (? CAUSE) Infection
8 P	33	Y (Groin Pain)
9 P	25	Y (Groin Pain)
10 P	30	N
11 P	3.5	Y (Groin Pain)
12 P	21	N

Table 1. Follow up of revision surgery for failed hip resurfacing arthroplasty (note groin pain seem to be persistent even after revision in both groups).

According to this study, patients who had a revision for unexplained groin pain had groin pain even years after conversion to a THR (Table 1). The patients who had only a revision of acetabular component had to be revised within a mean duration of 14.5 months (10-16) to a THR due to persistent problems. These lead us to believe either the damage led to the development of the groin pain that may be irreversible or initial factors that triggered the groin pain persists even after the conversion to a total hip replacement. Therefore, we need to rethink whether THR is the first and the only option in treating patients with persistent unexplained groin pain.

In conclusion, we believe that the failure of hip resurfacing is due to multiple factors, eventually leading to common pathological pathways leading to failure.

The significance of the contribution of each factor to the final pathways is not clear.

The fact that femoral component is fixed in the most mobile area of the joint in a relatively active patient, continuously moving the hip impacting on a relatively weak cancellous bone that constantly attempts to heal, while a large diameter head releasing high levels of metal ions leading to immunological response appear to be a recipe for disaster that finally leads to the failure of metal-on-metal hip resurfacing arthroplasty.

Acknowledgements

Special Thanks to Prof. Pat Campbell, Joint Replacement Centre University of California Los Angeles (UCLA), USA; Prof. Damian Griffin Warwick Orthopaedics, University of Warwick Medical School, University Hospitals of Coventry and Warwickshire, United Kingdom; Dr. Nick Parsons Warwick Orthopaedics, University of Warwick Medical School, University Hospitals of Coventry and Warwickshire, United Kingdom.

Author details

Hiran Wimal Amarasekera[1,2*]

Address all correspondence to: hiruwan@hotmail.com

1 Neville Fernando Teaching Hospital and South Asian Institute of Medicine, Colombo , Sri Lanka

2 Warwick Orthopaedics, University of Warwick,Coventry, United Kingdom

References

[1] Charnley J. Using Teflon in arthroplasty of the hip-joint. The Journal of bone and joint surgery American volume 1966;48(4):819.

[2] McMinn D, Daniel J. History and modern concepts in surface replacement. Proc Inst Mech Eng H 2006;220(2):239-51.

[3] Wagner H. Surface replacement arthroplasty of the hip. Clinical orthopaedics and related research 1978(134):102-30.

[4] Head WC. Wagner surface replacement arthroplasty of the hip. Analysis of fourteen failures in forty-one hips. The Journal of bone and joint surgery American volume 1981;63(3):420-7.

[5] Grujic H, Olerud S, Soreff J. Wagner resurfacing hip arthroplasty: preliminary results. Acta Orthop Scand 1982;53(5):785-9.

[6] McMinn D, Treacy R, Lin K, et al. Metal on metal surface replacement of the hip. Experience of the McMinn prothesis. Clinical orthopaedics and related research 1996(329 Suppl):S89-98.

[7] National joint registry England and Wales, 2004.

[8] Prime MS, Palmer J, Khan WS. The National Joint Registry of England and Wales. Orthopedics 2011;34(2):107-10.

[9] McMinn DJ, Daniel J, Ziaee H, et al. Indications and results of hip resurfacing. International orthopaedics 2011;35(2):231-7.

[10] Rechl H, Pilge H, Rudert M. [Development of hip resurfacing]. Der Orthopade 2008;37(7):626-33.

[11] Gross TP, Liu F. Prevalence of dysplasia as the source of worse outcome in young female patients after hip resurfacing arthroplasty. International orthopaedics 2012;36(1):27-34.

[12] Bose VC, Baruah BD. Resurfacing arthroplasty of the hip for avascular necrosis of the femoral head: a minimum follow-up of four years. The Journal of bone and joint surgery British volume 2010;92(7):922-8.

[13] Underwood RJ, Zografos A, Sayles RS, et al. Edge loading in metal-on-metal hips: low clearance is a new risk factor. Proc Inst Mech Eng H 2012;226(3):217-26.

[14] Beaule PE, Campbell PA, Hoke R, et al. Notching of the femoral neck during resurfacing arthroplasty of the hip: a vascular study. The Journal of bone and joint surgery British volume 2006;88(1):35-9.

[15] Kohan L, Field CJ, Kerr DR. Early complications of hip resurfacing. The Journal of arthroplasty 2012;27(6):997-1002.

[16] Amstutz HC, Le Duff MJ. Eleven years of experience with metal-on-metal hybrid hip resurfacing: a review of 1000 conserve plus. The Journal of arthroplasty 2008;23(6 Suppl 1):36-43.

[17] Morlock MM, Bishop N, Stahmer F, et al. [Reasons for failure of hip resurfacing implants. A failure analysis based on 250 revision specimens]. Der Orthopade 2008;37(7):695-703.

[18] Morlock MM, Bishop N, Zustin J, et al. Modes of implant failure after hip resurfacing: morphological and wear analysis of 267 retrieval specimens. The Journal of bone and joint surgery American volume 2008;90 Suppl 3:89-95.

[19] Amarasekera H, Costa M, Prakash U, et al. FEMORAL BLOOD FLOW DURING HIP RESURFACING: A COMPARISON OF TWO APPROACHES USING LASER DOPPLER FLOW MEASUREMENT. Journal of Bone & Joint Surgery, British Volume 2012;94-B(SUPP III):148.

[20] Beaule PE, Campbell P, Shim P. Femoral head blood flow during hip resurfacing. Clinical orthopaedics and related research 2007;456:148-52.

[21] Griffiths DE, Acton K, Hull JB. Hip resurfacing with preservation of femoral head blood supply. Surgeon 2008;6(2):115-9.

[22] Amarasekera HW, Costa ML, Foguet P, et al. The blood flow to the femoral head/neck junction during resurfacing arthroplasty: A COMPARISON OF TWO APPROACHES USING LASER DOPPLER FLOWMETRY. The Journal of bone and joint surgery British volume 2008;90(4):442-5.

[23] Ganz R, Gill TJ, Gautier E, et al. Surgical dislocation of the adult hip: A TECHNIQUE WITH FULL ACCESS TO THE FEMORAL HEAD AND ACETABULUM WITHOUT THE RISK OF AVASCULAR NECROSIS. The Journal of bone and joint surgery British volume 2001;83-B(8):1119-24.

[24] Amarasekera H, Roberts P, Costa M, et al. Scintigraphic assessment of bone status at one year following hip resurfacing: comparison of two surgical approaches using SPECT-CT scan. Bone and Joint Research 2012;1(1):86-92.

[25] Campbell P, Mirra J, Amstutz HC. Viability of femoral heads treated with resurfacing arthroplasty. The Journal of arthroplasty 2000;15(1):120-2.

[26] Boyd HS, Ulrich SD, Seyler TM, et al. Resurfacing for Perthes disease: an alternative to standard hip arthroplasty. Clinical orthopaedics and related research 2007;465:80-5.

[27] Grecula MJ. Resurfacing arthroplasty in osteonecrosis of the hip. Orthop Clin North Am 2005;36(2):231-42, x.

[28] Schmalzried TP. Total resurfacing for osteonecrosis of the hip. Clinical orthopaedics and related research 2004(429):151-6.

[29] Gerdesmeyer L, Gollwitzer H, Bader R, et al. [Surgical approaches in hip resurfacing]. Der Orthopade 2008;37(7):650-8.

[30] McBryde CW, Revell MP, Thomas AM, et al. The influence of surgical approach on outcome in Birmingham hip resurfacing. Clinical orthopaedics and related research 2008;466(4):920-6.

[31] Beaule PE, Shim P, Banga K. Clinical experience of Ganz surgical dislocation approach for metal-on-metal hip resurfacing. The Journal of arthroplasty 2009;24(6 Suppl):127-31.

[32] Kreuzer S, Leffers K, Kumar S. Direct anterior approach for hip resurfacing: surgical technique and complications. Clinical orthopaedics and related research 2011;469(6): 1574-81.

[33] Jacobs MA, Goytia RN, Bhargava T. Hip resurfacing through an anterolateral approach. Surgical description and early review. The Journal of bone and joint surgery American volume 2008;90 Suppl 3:38-44.

[34] H A. Surgical approaches to the hip joint and its clinical implications in adult hip arthroplasty. In: Knove P, ed. Arthroplasty. 1 ed. Croatia: INTECH, 2013:3-19.

[35] Marker DR, Seyler TM, Jinnah RH, et al. Femoral neck fractures after metal-on-metal total hip resurfacing: a prospective cohort study. The Journal of arthroplasty 2007;22(7 Suppl 3):66-71.

[36] Amanatullah DF, Cheung Y, Di Cesare PE. Hip resurfacing arthroplasty: a review of the evidence for surgical technique, outcome, and complications. Orthop Clin North Am 2010;41(2):263-72.

[37] Amstutz HC, Takamura KM, Le Duff MJ. The effect of patient selection and surgical technique on the results of Conserve(R) Plus hip resurfacing--3.5- to 14-year follow-up. Orthop Clin North Am 2011;42(2):133-42, vii.

[38] Della Valle CJ, Nunley RM, Barrack RL. When is the right time to resurface? Orthopedics 2008;31(12 Suppl 2).

[39] Jameson SS, Langton DJ, Natu S, et al. The influence of age and sex on early clinical results after hip resurfacing: an independent center analysis. The Journal of arthroplasty 2008;23(6 Suppl 1):50-5.

[40] Bitsch RG, Jager S, Lurssen M, et al. Influence of bone density on the cement fixation of femoral hip resurfacing components. Journal of orthopaedic research : official publication of the Orthopaedic Research Society 2010;28(8):986-91.

[41] Kim PR, Beaule PE, Laflamme GY, et al. Causes of early failure in a multicenter clinical trial of hip resurfacing. The Journal of arthroplasty 2008;23(6 Suppl 1):44-9.

[42] Hull P, Baxter JA, Lewis C, et al. Metal-on-metal hip resurfacing with uncemented fixation of the femoral component. A minimum 2 year follow up. Hip international : the journal of clinical and experimental research on hip pathology and therapy 2011.

[43] Ritter MA, Lutgring JD, Berend ME, et al. Failure mechanisms of total hip resurfacing: implications for the present. Clinical orthopaedics and related research 2006;453:110-4.

[44] Beaule PE, Le Duff M, Campbell P, et al. Metal-on-metal surface arthroplasty with a cemented femoral component: a 7-10 year follow-up study. The Journal of arthroplasty 2004;19(8 Suppl 3):17-22.

[45] Campbell P, Takamura K, Lundergan W, et al. Cement technique changes improved hip resurfacing longevity - implant retrieval findings. Bulletin of the NYU hospital for joint diseases 2009;67(2):146-53.

[46] Gill HS, Campbell PA, Murray DW, et al. Reduction of the potential for thermal damage during hip resurfacing. The Journal of bone and joint surgery British volume 2007;89(1):16-20.

[47] Malviya A, Holland JP. Pseudotumours associated with metal-on-metal hip resurfacing: 10-year Newcastle experience. Acta Orthop Belg 2009;75(4):477-83.

[48] A survey on the prevalence of pseudotumors with metal-on-metal hip resurfacing in Canadian academic centers. The Journal of bone and joint surgery American volume 2011;93 Suppl 2:118-21.

[49] Brooks P. Component malposition in hip resurfacing. Orthopedics 2010;33(9):646.

[50] Delaunay C, Petit I, Learmonth ID, et al. Metal-on-metal bearings total hip arthroplasty: the cobalt and chromium ions release concern. Orthop Traumatol Surg Res 2010;96(8):894-904.

[51] Akbar M, Brewer JM, Grant MH. Effect of chromium and cobalt ions on primary human lymphocytes in vitro. J Immunotoxicol 2011;8(2):140-9.

[52] Kwon YM, Thomas P, Summer B, et al. Lymphocyte proliferation responses in patients with pseudotumors following metal-on-metal hip resurfacing arthroplasty. Journal of orthopaedic research : official publication of the Orthopaedic Research Society 2010;28(4):444-50.

[53] Mahendra G, Pandit H, Kliskey K, et al. Necrotic and inflammatory changes in metal-on-metal resurfacing hip arthroplasties. Acta Orthop 2009;80(6):653-9.

[54] Hart AJ, Skinner JA, Henckel J, et al. Insufficient Acetabular Version Increases Blood Metal Ion Levels after Metal-on-metal Hip Resurfacing. Clinical orthopaedics and related research 2011;469(9):2590-7.

[55] Mai MC, Milbrandt JC, Hulsen J, et al. Acetabular cup malalignment after total hip resurfacing arthroplasty: a case for elective revision? Orthopedics 2009;32(11):853.

[56] Kim PR, Beaule PE, Dunbar M, et al. Cobalt and chromium levels in blood and urine following hip resurfacing arthroplasty with the Conserve Plus implant. The Journal of bone and joint surgery American volume 2011;93 Suppl 2:107-17.

[57] Kwon YM, Ostlere SJ, McLardy-Smith P, et al. "Asymptomatic" pseudotumors after metal-on-metal hip resurfacing arthroplasty: prevalence and metal ion study. The Journal of arthroplasty 2011;26(4):511-8.

[58] Antoniou J, Zukor DJ, Mwale F, et al. Metal ion levels in the blood of patients after hip resurfacing: a comparison between twenty-eight and thirty-six-millimeter-head metal-on-metal prostheses. The Journal of bone and joint surgery American volume 2008;90 Suppl 3:142-8.

[59] Beaule PE, Kim PR, Hamdi A, et al. A prospective metal ion study of large-head metal-on-metal bearing: a matched-pair analysis of hip resurfacing versus total hip replacement. Orthop Clin North Am 2011;42(2):251-7, ix.

[60] Moroni A, Savarino L, Hoque M, et al. Do ion levels in hip resurfacing differ from metal-on-metal THA at midterm? Clinical orthopaedics and related research 2011;469(1):180-7.

[61] Matthies A, Underwood R, Cann P, et al. Retrieval analysis of 240 metal-on-metal hip components, comparing modular total hip replacement with hip resurfacing. The Journal of bone and joint surgery British volume 2011;93(3):307-14.

[62] Buechel FF, Drucker D, Jasty M, et al. Osteolysis around uncemented acetabular components of cobalt-chrome surface replacement hip arthroplasty. Clinical orthopaedics and related research 1994(298):202-11.

[63] Campbell P, Shimmin A, Walter L, et al. Metal sensitivity as a cause of groin pain in metal-on-metal hip resurfacing. The Journal of arthroplasty 2008;23(7):1080-5.

[64] Larson AN, McIntosh AL, Trousdale RT, et al. Avascular necrosis most common indication for hip arthroplasty in patients with slipped capital femoral epiphysis. J Pediatr Orthop 2010;30(8):767-73.

[65] Drescher W, Pufe T, Smeets R, et al. [Avascular necrosis of the hip - diagnosis and treatment]. Z Orthop Unfall 2011;149(2):231-40; quiz 41-2.

[66] Siguier T, Siguier M, Judet T, et al. Partial resurfacing arthroplasty of the femoral head in avascular necrosis. Methods, indications, and results. Clinical orthopaedics and related research 2001(386):85-92.

[67] McMahon SJ, Young D, Ballok Z, et al. Vascularity of the femoral head after Birmingham hip resurfacing. A technetium Tc 99m bone scan/single photon emission computed tomography study. The Journal of arthroplasty 2006;21(4):514-21.

[68] Leunig M, Ganz R. Vascularity of the femoral head after Birmingham hip resurfacing. A technetium Tc 99m bone scan/single photon emission computed tomography study. The Journal of arthroplasty 2007;22(5):784-5; author reply 85-6.

[69] Forrest N, Welch A, Murray AD, et al. Femoral head viability after Birmingham resurfacing hip arthroplasty: assessment with use of [18F] fluoride positron emission

tomography. The Journal of bone and joint surgery American volume 2006;88 Suppl 3:84-9.

[70] Amarasekera HW, Costa ML, Parsons N, et al. SPECT/CT bone imaging after hip resurfacing arthroplasty: is it feasible to use CT attenuation correction in the presence of metal implants? Nuclear medicine communications 2011;32(4):289-97.

7

Prevention of Periprosthetic Joint Infection

Hamid Reza Seyyed Hosseinzadeh, Alisina Shahi,
Mohamad Qoreishy and
Mehrnoush Hassas Yeganeh

Abstract

Prosthetic joint infection (PJI) is a serious complication with high morbidity, mortality, and substantial cost. The reported incidence is probably underestimated due to the problems of proper diagnosis. PJI has haunted the orthopedic community for several years and despite all the advances in this field, it is still a demanding issue with a huge impact on patients, surgeons, and healthcare. Numerous elements can predispose patients to PJI. In this chapter, we tried to summarize the effective prevention strategies along with the recommendations of a recent International Consensus Meeting on Surgical Site and Periprosthetic Joint Infection.

Keywords: Prevention, infection, total hip replacement, total knee replacement, total joint arthroplasty, periprosthetic joint infection

1. Introduction

Total joint arthroplasty (TJA) is one of the most effective surgeries in medicine and improves the quality of life and function level in most of the patients suffering from degenerative joint disease. Periprosthetic joint infection (PJI) is still a great challenge to the orthopedic community.

Since there is an escalating increase in the number of total hip and knee arthroplasties all around the world each year, the number of revision knee and hip procedures will also increase correspondingly.

The average incidence of periprosthetic joint infection (PJI) is between 0.25% and 2.0% within two years after primary total hip arthroplasty (THA) or total knee arthroplasty (TKA).[2-4] PJI is a serious complication of TJA; it is the primary indication for revision TKA and the third indication for revision THA.[5-7]

Not only is the diagnosis of PJI very challenging, its management is also very difficult. It requires multiple procedures, antibiotic therapy, and prolonged rehabilitation.[10] Its impact on the medical health system is probably greater than many other diseases.

Therefore, strong efforts to effectively treat PJI are mandatory. Treatment of the infection requires appropriate evaluation of the causing germ, the wound status, and the overall condition of the patient.

In this chapter, we will review PJI, its associated risk factors, and the current evidence available for the prevention of PJI.

2. Definition of PJI

The first Consensus on Periprosthetic Joint Infection (2013) defined PJI as (Figure 1):

- Two positive periprosthetic cultures with phenotypically identical organisms; or
- A sinus tract communicating with the joint; or
- Having three of the following minor criteria:
    - Elevated serum C-reactive protein (CRP) AND erythrocyte sedimentation rate (ESR)
    - Elevated synovial fluid white blood cell (WBC) count OR ++ change on leukocyte esterase test strip
    - Elevated synovial fluid polymorphonuclear neutrophil percentage (PMN%)
    - Positive histological analysis of periprosthetic tissue
    - A single positive culture

When upon histological analysis of periprosthetic tissue, greater than 5 neutrophils per high-power field in 5 high-power fields at ×400 magnification is observed, it is considered positive.

PJI may still be present if fewer than four of these criteria are met. Clinically, PJI may be present without meeting these criteria, in the case of less virulent organisms (e.g., P. acnes). Synovial leukocyte esterase can be performed as a rapid office or intraoperative point of care test using urinalysis strips.

AAOS has provided an algorithmic approach to the diagnosis of PJI. Clinical judgment should not be replaced by diagnostic algorithm or any one individual diagnostic laboratory test. By using this algorithm, preoperative evaluation leading to an aseptic diagnosis should not eliminate suspicion for PJI. If a patient has a history of persistent pain or stiffness in the

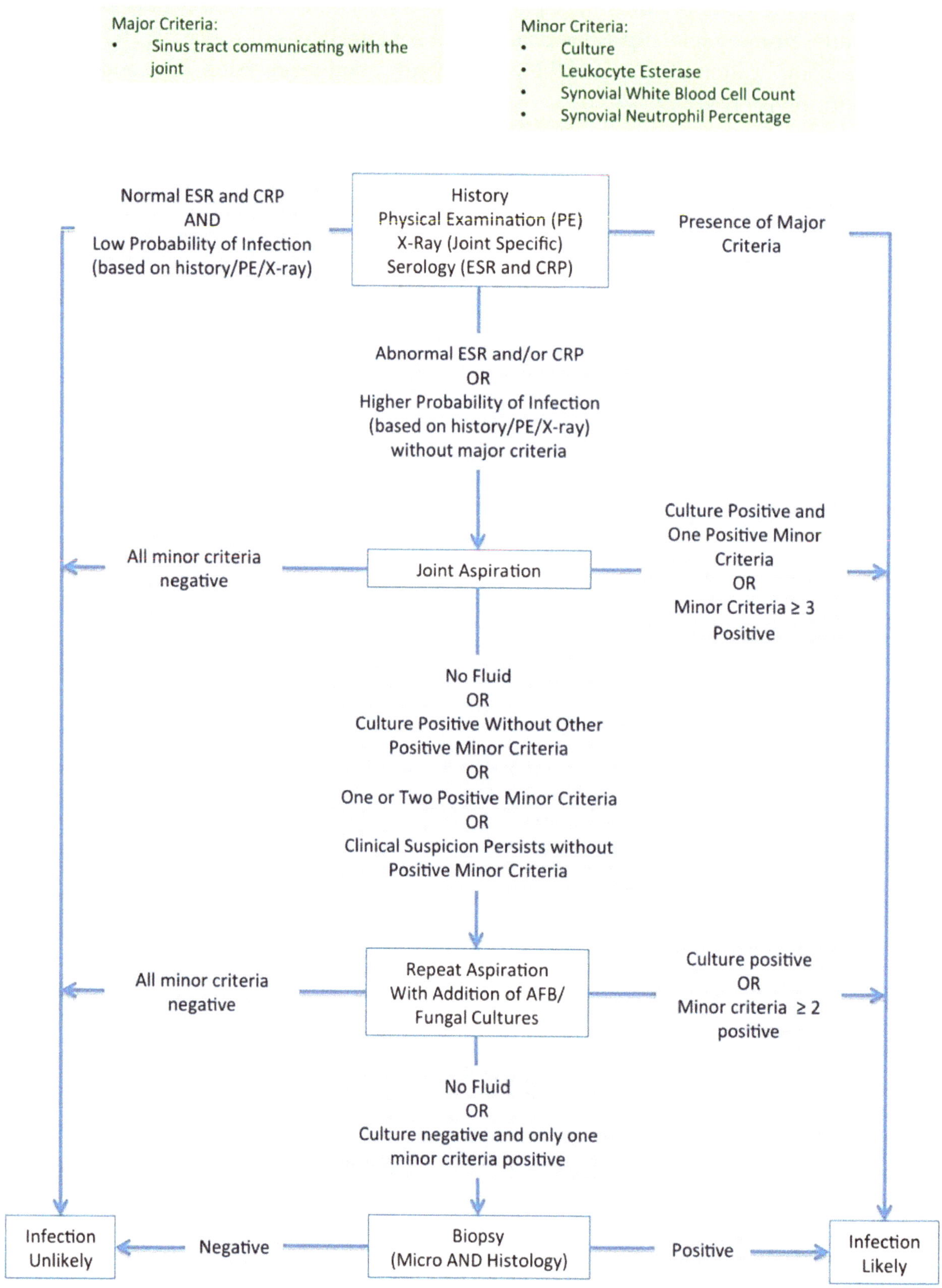

Figure 1. Diagnosis algorithm of periprosthetic joint infection.

prosthetic joint plus any of the following findings, he/she should be considered to have a higher probability of infection:

- Recent bacteremia;
- Multiple surgeries on the same joint;
- History of periprosthetic joint infection;
- Having an immunocompromised state, e.g., diabetes mellitus, inflammatory arthropathy, or malnourishment;
- Factors that increase risk of bacteremia, e.g., intravenous drug use, poor wound conditions, psoriasis, chronic venous stasis, or skin ulceration;
- Superficial surgical site infection in the prosthetic joint.

The following local findings are suggestive of PJI:

- Wound dehiscence
- Joint swelling, warmth, or redness

The following radiographic findings are suggestive of PJI:

- Radiographic findings showing loosening of a previously well-fixed component (especially the loosening seen within the first 5 postoperative years)
- Osteolysis or bone resorption around a component which should not be considered to be the result of wear, particularly if seen within 5 years postoperatively
- Subperiosteal elevation
- Transcortical sinus tracts

It is worth noting that plain radiographs are generally normal in the majority of PJIs.

The following approximate thresholds for the laboratory tests apply to those obtained fewer than 6 weeks from the most recent surgery:

- No threshold for ESR could be determined because this test is not useful in the diagnosis of acute PJI
- CRP > 100 mg/L (knee and hip)
- Synovial WBC count > 10,000 cells/μL
- Synovial PMN% > 90%

But if the tests are obtained more than 6 weeks from the most recent surgery, the following cutoffs apply:

- ESR > 30 mm/hr
- CRP > 10 mg/L

- Synovial WBC count > 3,000 cells per μL
- Synovial PMN% > 80%

There is very limited evidence for the changes of inflammatory markers in patients with an underlying inflammatory arthritis and PJI. But there seems to be no change from the above thresholds for ESR, serum CRP, PMN%, and WBC count for PJI diagnosis in these patients.

In order to accurately analyze synovial fluid cell count, it is recommended that (1) synovial fluid WBC count results be analyzed with respect to the synovial red blood cell (RBC), serum RBC, and serum WBC concentrations to adjust for traumatic aspirations and (2) in joints with metal-on-metal bearing surfaces, a manual WBC analysis be performed.

Routine synovial fluid cultures should be maintained for 5–14 days. In cases of suspension to low virulence organisms or if in spite of high clinical suspension to PJI, the routine preoperative cultures have failed to show bacterial growth (suspected culture-negative PJI) the cultures should be maintained for more than 14 days.

In proven or suspected PJI, AFB and fungal cultures should be limited to those patients at risk for such infections or when other traditional pathogens have not been identified and clinical suspicion persists.

It is recommended that at least three but not more than six distinct intraoperative tissue samples be sent for aerobic and anaerobic culture.

Before obtaining the culture samples, it is not necessary to withhold perioperative prophylactic antibiotics, except only in cases with a high suspicion for PJI in which an infecting organism has not been isolated.

The literature recommends that sonication of explants should be limited to cases of suspected or proven PJI (according to the clinical presentation or laboratory testing) in which preoperative joint aspiration result is not positive or the patient has received within the previous two weeks.

Laboratory tests based on detecting nucleic acids are not currently recommended as a routine diagnostic test for PJI. In patients with high clinical suspicion of PJI but negative cultures or other laboratory tests, molecular techniques may be helpful to identify the unknown pathogens or antibiotic sensitivity.

Although the plain radiographs may be negative, in all cases of suspected PJI, plain radiograph should be performed. But, magnetic resonance imaging (MRI), computed tomography (CT), and nuclear imaging currently do not play a significant role in the diagnosis of PJI but may be helpful in ruling out the other causes of joint pain/failure.

3. Prevention of PJI

Development of PJI depends on both host and environmental factors, and the best way to prevent it is to improve these two factors during the pre-, intra-, and postoperative phases.

Host factors:

Preoperative factors: These factors include, but are not limited to, history of previous surgery, male gender, poorly controlled diabetes mellitus (glucose > 200 mg/L or HbA1C > 7%), diagnosis of posttraumatic arthritis, malnutrition, prior surgical procedure in the affected joint, morbid obesity (BMI > 40 Kg/m2), recent hospitalization, severe immunodeficiency, active liver disease, chronic renal disease, inflammatory arthropathy, excessive smoking (>one pack per day), excessive alcohol consumption (>40 units per week), intravenous drug abuse, and extended stay in a rehabilitation facility.[4, 22, 23]

The impact of various risk factors appears to be accumulative.[24, 25] Lei et al. and Malinzak et al. have shown that any other medical comorbidity accompanied by diabetes leads to a higher risk of infection.[24, 29]

Thus, identifying risk factors and addressing them in the preoperative setting is critical to reduce PJI and other postoperative complications.

4. Preoperative optimization of general health

Reports have shown that the general condition of the patient's health has a direct link with the rate of postoperative complications; and conditions such as ASA > 2, uncontrolled diabetes, and rheumatoid arthritis can significantly increase the risk of PJI. [4, 22, 26-28]

Therefore, it is mandatory to assess all patients in a multidisciplinary approach prior to TJA and to manage comorbidities if required. These assessments have shown to reduce the postoperative mortality rate and per-admission costs significantly in complex orthopaedic surgeries, including TJA.[30]

Marchant et al. found that patients with a higher level of hemoglobin A1c had significantly higher incidence of PJI, at an odds ratio of 2.31.[31]

Furthermore, Mraovic et al.[32] showed that patients with sugar levels of greater than 200 mg/dl on postoperative day one are at a higher risk of developing PJI by two-fold.

Therefore, there is a general consensus in the literature supporting the importance of preoperative health optimization, focusing on the control of blood glucose level.

Preoperative multidisciplinary approach must focus on optimizing the adjustable risk factors in the preoperative phase such as nutrition status, blood sugar level, cardiac and respiratory evaluation, and assessment for possible sources of infection and Methicillin-resistant *Staphylococcus aureus* (MRSA) decolonization (although universal screening for MRSA is not recommended). If MRSA colonization is suspected, short-term nasal application of mupirocin is the most accepted current method of decolonization for MRSA and/or MSSA.

All patients undergoing elective arthroplasty should be screened for evidence of active dental infection. This may be performed by administration of a questionnaire or dental examination.

Routine urine screening is not recommended for all patients undergoing elective arthroplasty and should be reserved for patients with a present history or symptoms of urinary tract infection (UTI).

It seems mandatory to stop the disease-modifying agents prior to elective TJA. The timing of drug cessation before surgery depends on the specific drug pharmacokinetics. The discontinuation of immunosuppressant drugs should be performed in consultation with the treating physician.

All patients with prior septic arthritis should undergo evaluation by serology and aspiration of the joint whenever possible, prior to arthroplasty. In addition to these preoperative assessments, by taking intraoperative cultures, the surgeons must ensure that no evidence of active infection exists.

5. Perioperative patient skin preparation

Many reports have shown that a whole-body bath with an antiseptic agent reduces the bacterial load in the skin and lowers the risk of surgical site infections (SSIs).[34-37]

There is some evidence that applying chlorhexidine gluconate (CHG) twice daily by patients at home prior to TJA could significantly reduce the risk of SSIs.[41, 42]

So we recommend preoperative cleansing of the skin with CHG. In the presence of a sensitivity to CHG, or when it is unavailable, an antiseptic soap is appropriate. After bathing, patients are advised to sleep in clean garments and bedding without the application of any topical products.

The most proper method of hair removal is clipping, as opposed to shaving. There is not enough evidence to advise for or against the use of depilatory cream for hair removal. Literature recommends that hair removal should be performed as close to the time of the surgical procedure as possible.

There is no clear difference between various skin preparation agents. There is some evidence that combinations of antiseptic agents with alcohol may be important for skin antisepsis.

Elective arthroplasty should not be performed in patients with active ulceration of the skin in the vicinity of the surgical site. The incisions should not be placed through active skin lesions. For certain lesions, such as those due to eczema and psoriasis, surgery should be delayed in these patients until their lesions have been optimized.

6. Preoperative surgeon hand scrubbing

The surgeon and operating room personnel should mechanically wash their hands with an antiseptic agent for a minimum of 2 minutes for the first case. A shorter period may be appropriate for subsequent cases. There is no clear difference among various antiseptic agents for hand washing.

7. Preoperative antibiotics

There is a huge amount of evidence in the literature supporting the benefits of preoperative antibiotics in the prevention of PJI.[43-46]

Special care is required for selecting the prophylaxis antibiotic, consistent with the current recommendation of the literature. Patient allergies and resistance issues also need to be taken into account.

The aim of prophylactic antibiotics is to cover the spectrum of the most common organisms of PJI, Staphylococci, and Streptococci.

Therefore, a first- or second-generation cephalosporin (cefazolin or cefuroxime) should be administered for routine perioperative surgical prophylaxis. Isoxazolyl penicillin is used as an appropriate alternative. In a patient with a known anaphylactic reaction to penicillin, vancomycin, or clindamycin should be administered as prophylaxis. Teicoplanin is also an option in countries where it is available. In a patient with a reported non-anaphylactic reaction to penicillin, a second-, third- or fourth-generation cephalosporin can be used safely as there is limited cross-reactivity.

Skin testing in penicillin-allergic patients cannot reliably predict an allergic response to a cephalosporin, particularly to compounds with dissimilar side chains. However, skin testing may be useful in determining whether a true allergy to penicillin exists.

Penicillin has a cross-allergy with first-generation cephalosporins (OR 4.8; CI 3.7-6.2) and a negligible cross-allergy with second-generation cephalosporins (OR 1.1; CI 0.6-2.1). The R1 side chain, not the β-lactam ring, is responsible for this cross-reactivity. So the overall cross-reactivity between penicillin and cephalosporin is lower than previously reported (at 10%) although there is a strong association between amoxicillin and ampicillin with first- and second-generation cephalosporins that share a similar R1 side chain. For penicillin-allergic patients, the use of third- or fourth-generation cephalosporin or cephalosporins (such as cefuroxime and ceftriaxone) with dissimilar side chains than the offending penicillin carries a negligible risk of cross-allergy.

In patients with pre-existing prostheses, such as heart valves, the choice of antibiotics is the same as that for routine elective arthroplasty.

There is always a risk of colonization and infection development of vancomycin-resistant infections due to over-exposure to vancomycin. Routine use of vancomycin for preoperative prophylaxis is not recommended at all. Vancomycin should only be administered to patients who are proven current MRSA carriers or have anaphylactic allergy to penicillins.

The following patients are considered high risk for Methicillin-resistant *Staphylococcus aureus* (MRSA) carrying and should undergo screening:

- Those in regions with a high prevalence of MRSA
- Institutionalized patients (those who have been in the intensive care unit, nursing home residents, and dialysis-dependent patients)
- Healthcare workers

A point to consider is that vancomycin does not have full coverage on methicillin-sensitive *S. aureus*. Therefore, it should always be administered in combination with a cephalosporin.[52]

There is also no evidence to support the routine prophylactic use of dual antibiotics.

Asymptomatic patients with bacteriuria may safely undergo TJA provided that routine prophylactic antibiotics are administered. The presence of urinary tract symptoms should trigger urinary screening prior to TJA. Patients with acute UTI need to be treated prior to elective arthroplasty.

In patients with prior septic arthritis or PJI, the preoperative antibiotic should cover the previous infecting organism of the same joint.

The preoperative dose of antibiotics should be administered within one hour of surgical incision; for antibiotics with longer infusion time, such as vancomycin and fluoroquinolones, this time period should be extended to two hours. In case of tourniquet use, the antibiotic must be fully infused prior to tourniquet inflation. An additional dose of antibiotic should be administered intraoperatively after two half-lives of the prophylactic agent. Re-dosing of antibiotics should also be considered in cases of large blood volume loss (>2000 cc) and fluid resuscitation (>2000cc). As these are independent variables, re-dosing should be considered as soon as the first of these parameters are met.

Antibiotics have different pharmacokinetics based on patient weight, so the preoperative antibiotics should be weight-adjusted.

For current MRSA carriers, vancomycin or teicoplanin is the recommended perioperative antibiotic prophylaxis. Patients with prior history of MRSA should be re-screened preoperatively. If patients are proved to be negative for MRSA, the use of routine perioperative antibiotic prophylaxis is recommended.

For patients undergoing major reconstructions, such as tumor surgeries, revisions and reconstructions with bulk allograft, the use of routine antibiotic prophylaxis the use of routine perioperative prophylactic antibiotics is recommended.

In patients with poorly controlled diabetes, immunosuppression, or autoimmune disease the use of routine antibiotic prophylaxis is recommended.

Perioperative antibiotic prophylaxis should be the same for hips and knees arthroplasties.

The appropriate preoperative antibiotic for the second stage surgeries should include coverage of the prior organism(s).

Intraoperative considerations:

The probability of SSI correlates directly with the number of bacteria that reach the wound. The bacteria shed by personnel are the predominant source of these particles. Accordingly, any strategies to lower particulate and bacterial counts at surgical wounds will lower the incidence of SSI.

8. Operating room environment

Ultraviolet (UV) light can lower infection rates, but this modality can pose a risk to operating room (OR) personnel. However, the benefit of UV might be the inhibition of operating traffic. It might be considered an adjunct but not a replacement for conventional cleaning.

8.1. Laminar flow

Laminar airflow (LAF) was first introduced in the US in 1964. Positive air pressure is created in the surgical field via the directional airflow passing through higher-efficiency particulate air by vertical LAF and can help to reduce the incidence of PJI.[78-81] However, Brandt et al. state that LAF provides no benefits and even increases the risk of SSI after THA.

The LAF is often disrupted by the opening of the OR door, therefore giving pathogens an opportunity to enter the area around the operation site and increasing the risk of PJI.[67, 78, 83]

Nevertheless, there is still controversy about the pros and cons of LAF.[91]

The Centers for Disease Control and Prevention (CDC) has no comment supporting whether LAF may reduce the rate of SSI. There is no specific suggestion for performing arthroplasty procedures under LAF. Nonetheless, the CDC has published the following guidelines:

CDC Guidelines:[92]

1. Maintain positive-pressure ventilation with respect to corridors and adjacent areas.
2. Maintain ≥15 ACH, of which ≥3 ACH should be fresh air.
3. Filter all recirculated and fresh air through the appropriate filters, providing 90% efficiency (dust-spot testing) at a minimum.
4. In rooms not engineered for horizontal LAF, introduce air at the ceiling and exhaust air near the floor.
5. Do not use UV lights to prevent SSIs.
6. Keep OR doors closed except for the passage of equipment, personnel, and patients and limit entry to essential personnel.

Based on the current literature, arthroplasty surgery may be performed in operating theaters without laminar flow. Laminar flow rooms and other strategies that may reduce particulates in operating rooms would be expected to reduce particulate load. But the current evidence does not support the effect of LAF in reducing the incidence of SSI. These are complex technologies that must function in strict adherence to maintenance protocols.

Despite the absence of conclusive studies that show a reduction in SSI when surgical masks are worn properly and uniformly by all staff, adhering to this discipline is expected to reduce the particulate airborne bacteria counts. Until evidence appears that shows an advantage to not wearing a mask, all personnel should wear surgical masks at all time that they are in the OR.

All personnel wear clean theater clothes, including a disposable head covering, when entering an OR. Garments worn outside of the hospital should not be worn during TJA.

8.2. Gloving

Sterile surgical gloves have dual protection responsibilities; on one side it protects the patients from residual bacteria on the surgeon's hands, and on the other side protects the surgeon from the patient's body fluids.

Because double-gloving reduces the risk of perforation, it is highly recommended for orthopedic procedures, where sharp edges are commonly encountered during the surgery.[71-73]

Furthermore, some studies have shown that even double-gloving is not enough and inner gloves could have perforations and contamination. Accordingly, triple-gloving has been recommended during TJA to prevent the risk of contamination and PJI.[75, 76] However, triple gloving has some disadvantages, such as a decrease in tactile sensation and surgical dexterity.[77]

The Consensus on prevention of PJI recommends double gloving and recognizes the theoretical advantage of triple gloving.

The literature supports the advantage of glove changes at least every 90 minutes or more frequently and the necessity of changing perforated gloves. Permeability appears to be compromised by the exposure to methacrylate cement and gloves should be changed after cementation.

The current evidence shows that the timing of opening trays should occur as close to the start of the surgical procedure as possible with the avoidance of any delays between tray opening and the start of surgery.

Dummy Text **When** the surgical trays are not in use for an extended time, they should be covered with a sterile cover, preferably a small one to prevent the drape from passing from contaminated areas across the sterile field.

9. Human exhaust system (personal protection system)

In the 1960s, Sir John Charnley was the first to introduce the idea of the personal protection system (PPS), also known as the human exhaust system, in order to decrease the number of airborne bacteria and contamination in TJA.[93] There is currently no conclusive evidence to support the routine use of space suits in performing TJA. Major issues to consider regarding

PPSs are their bulkiness and susceptibility to contamination. In more than half of the cases, the PPS does not stay sterile externally. Therefore, it is advised that the PPSs not be touched during procedures, and if contact does occur, the gloves should be replaced.[98]

9.1. Operating room traffic

OR personnel, by traffic that creates turbulence and contaminates air and by bacterial shedding, are the major source of air contamination in the OR. Ritter et al. proved that in an OR with 5 personnel, the bacterial counts in OR air increased 34-fold compared to an empty room. Keeping the OR door open significantly increases bacterial contamination in the air of the OR.[17] Andersson et al. showed a direct correlation between the number of people present in the OR and bacterial counts. Some experts propose that passing through a sub-sterile hallway while entering or leaving the OR can increase the OR air contamination, although evidence regarding this concept is lacking. One possible solution to this is to keep the necessary devices and implants in the OR at the start of the surgery.

Another disadvantage of increased OR traffic is the distraction it causes for the surgeon.[106]

Therefore, based on the current literature, OR traffic should be kept to a minimum.

The CDC recommendation for OR traffic is to "keep OR doors closed except for the passage of equipment, personnel, and patients, and limit entry to essential personnel."[92]

9.2. Draping

The literature supports the use of non-permeable paper drapes for draping the surgical site in TJA.[63-66]

Traditional cloth drapes tend to get wet during the surgery and could increase bacterial penetration; to that end, non-permeable paper drapes were introduced to overcome this issue.[63] Ritter et al. have presented that Ioban iodophor-impregnated drapes (3M Health Care) can reduce wound contamination but do not decrease the wound infection rate after TJA.[67]

The penetration of drapes by liquids is believed to be equivalent to contamination; therefore, literature recommends the use of impervious drapes.

Fairclough et al. showed that the rate of wound contamination during hip surgery was reduced from 15% to 1.6% after using plastic adhesive drapes.[68]

The efficacy of plastic adhesive drapes is optimum when the skin preparation is performed using alcohol-based solutions.

Theoretically, the plastic adhesive drapes can provide a sterile operative field at the beginning of the surgery and by immobilization of the bacteria underneath the drape, provide a long-term sterile field during the surgery and by these two, reduce the risk of surgical site contamination.

However, there are controversies about the effectiveness of plastic adhesive drapes in prevention of bacterial contamination.

As the current literature shows, iodine-impregnated skin incise drapes decreased skin bacterial counts but no correlation has been established with SSI.

The traditional practice of covering skin edges with sterile draping may be efficacious.

Light handles can be a source of contamination and literature recommends to minimize handling of lights as much as possible. Other strategies for light control need to be developed in the future to minimize contamination.

Portable electronic devices may be contaminated with bacteria. Besides, increased levels of talking are associated with higher levels of bacteria in the OR environment. Therefore, portable electronic device usage must be limited to that which is necessary for patient care.

The studies do not support the concern regarding risks of transferring infection to a clean surgery following a contaminated surgery. Therefore, when performing a TJA following a contaminated surgery, thorough cleaning before further surgery, as defined by local institutional standards, is recommended.

9.3. Operative time

SSI rates increase directly with the duration of surgery. Perhaps some surgeries present a marked level of complexity that will require more time. But minimizing the duration of surgery is an important goal. To achieve this goal, a coordinated effort must be made to minimize the duration of surgery without technical compromise of the procedure.

The rate of PJI tends to be inversely proportional to the surgeon's volume of surgeries, the lower the surgeon volume, the higher the risk of infection. This seems to be especially statistically significant after TKA. [104]

Literature shows high contamination rates in the scalpel blades that have been used for the skin incision and recommends change of scalpel blade after skin incision.

Since there is no evidence, the literature cannot recommend for or against the necessity and frequency of change of electrocautery disposable tips during elective TJA.

In contrast to electrocautery tip, literature supports changing suction tips every 60 minutes based on studies showing higher rates of contamination. Suction tips can be introduced into the femoral canal to evacuate fluid but should not be left in the canal, where they can circulate large amounts of air and particles that may contaminate femoral canal.

Studies confirm that the use of fluid filled basins that sit open during the surgery is associated with increased infection rates.

There is at least some theoretical basis for irrigation to dilute contamination and nonviable tissue and that a greater volume of irrigation would be expected to achieve greater dilution. However, literature cannot support any recommendation for one method over another. The only proved mechanism of action for irrigation is the mechanical effect of the solution. But there exists conflicting evidence supporting the use of one agent over the other.

10. Wound closure and surgical dressing

Numerous techniques such as skin staples, absorbable sutures, and knotless barbed sutures are used for skin closure in TJA. Despite the lack of evidence supporting the superiority of one technique of skin closure over others (staples, suture, adhesive, or tapes), the use of monofilament suture for wound closure is recommended to decrease the SSI. Literature does not support the effect of staples on decreasing the rate of SSI.

The kind of dressing applied after the procedure may have an essential role in the wound healing process.[120, 121] The re-epithelization and collagen synthesis rates are increased in wounds that have the wound dressing applied to them when compared to wounds that are allowed to be exposed to air.[122, 123]

Following TJA, the use of occlusive dressings with alginated hydrofiber is strongly recommended. Silver-impregnated dressings have not been conclusively shown to reduce SSI/PJI.

Persistent wound drainage after TJA is defined as continued drainage from the operative incision site for greater than 72 hours. This persistent wound drainage should be managed by wound care. According to various studies, the first line treatment for persistent wound drainage is nonsurgical management prior to surgical intervention. Other treatment modalities, such as antibiotics, are highly discouraged because they can mask an underlying infection. Since the cause and effect relationship between persistent wound drainage and PJI has been proven, observation alone is strongly discouraged.[17, 21, 24, 26] One of these measures is negative pressure wound therapy (NPWT), which has proved to decrease the size of postoperative seromas.[27]

It is discouraged to use greater than 24 hours of postoperative antibiotics to treat persistent wound drainage after TJA because there is no evidence that it decreases PJI.[18, 20]

If wound care measures are not effective and the wound drainage has persisted for greater than 5 to 7 days from the time of diagnosis, reoperation should be performed without delay. The surgical management should consist of opening the fascia, performing a thorough irrigation and debridement (I&D) with exchange of modular components. When performing I&D, intraoperative cultures (minimum of three) should be taken. In these situations, the administration of perioperative antibiotics given within one hour prior to I&D reoperation should not be withheld prior to skin incision.

As literature shows, allogeneic blood transfusions is associated with an increased risk of SSI/PJI. However, the role of autologous transfusion in the risk of SSI/PJI remains inconclusive. The female gender, higher Charlson comorbidity index, use of general anesthesia, and longer duration of surgery are predictors of the potential need for allogeneic blood transfusion in patients undergoing TJA. There is no defined benefit for the use of cell salvage systems, reinfusion drains, biopolar sealers, and hemodilution for management of PJI.

There is no evidence to demonstrate that the use of closed drains increases the risk of SSI/PJI following TJA. And there is no conclusive evidence for the optimal timing of drain removal yet.

The evidences show that blood salvage should be utilized with caution during the second stage surgery for PJI.

The literature supports that the type of prosthesis (cemented versus uncemented) or coating with hydroxyapatite does not influence the incidence of SSI or PJI. However, antibiotic-impregnated polymethylmethacrylate cement (ABX-PMMA) reduces the incidence of PJI following TJA and should be used in patients at high risk for PJI following elective arthroplasty, whether in primary or revision arthroplasties.

Observational data suggest that metal-on-metal bearing may be associated with a higher risk of PJI.

The bulk of prosthesis has a direct effect on the incidence of PJI. The incidence of infection is higher following the use of mega-prostheses.

The incidence of SSI/PJI may be lower with the use of porous metal (tantalum) implants during revision arthroplasty compared to titanium.

There is no study in the literature to prove that adding the vancomycin powder to the wound in the vicinity of an implant can reduce the incidence of PJI. This effect of vancomycin has been shown in nonarthroplasty surgeries in a few studies.

11. Postoperative antibiotic prophylaxis

Postoperative antibiotics should not be administered for greater than 24 hours after surgery. In patients with a suspected infection when culture results are pending, empiric antibiotic coverage, depending on the local microbiological epidemiology, should be continued until the results of culture are ready. Then, the antibiotic choice and timing should be based on the culture data.

Recommendations:

- Until final cultures become available, we recommend to treat the acute hematogenous infections with cefazolin and gentamicin.
- We recommend vancomycin to treat all chronic and acute postoperative infections with gram-positive bacteria and all cases in which a gram stain fails to identify.
- The recommended antibiotics for infections with gram-negative bacteria are third or fourth generation cephalosporin.
- The recommended regimen to treat the infections with mixed gram-positive and gram-negative bacteria is a combination of vancomycin and third or fourth generation cephalosporin.
- As 93% cultures tested positive by the fourth postoperative day, the authors recommend that if culture results are not positive by the fourth postoperative day, termination of empiric antibiotic therapy should be considered. But the culture must continue for 14 days.

There is no evidence to support the continued use of postoperative antibiotics when urinary catheter or surgical drains are in place.

As mentioned earlier PJI can occur any time after the surgery. Episodic bacteremia could be a potential risk for PJI and certain medical procedures are more likely to cause bacteremia. Therefore, in 2012, the American Academy of Orthopaedic Surgeons (AAOS) released a new guideline on "The Prevention of Orthopaedic Implant Infections in Patients Undergoing Dental Procedures." It has three main recommendations:[126]

1. "The practitioner might consider discontinuing the practice of routinely prescribing prophylactic antibiotics for patients with hip and knee prosthetic joint implants undergoing dental procedures."
2. "The guideline does not recommend for or against the use of topical oral antimicrobials in patients with prosthetic joint implants or other orthopaedic implants undergoing dental procedures."
3. "Although there is not reliable evidence linking poor oral health to prosthetic joint infection, it is the opinion of the work group that patients with prosthetic joint implants or other orthopedic implants maintain appropriate oral hygiene."

The evidence shows that the use of prophylactic antibiotics prior to dental procedures in patients who underwent TJA should be based on individual patient risk factors and the complexity of the dental procedure.

Furthermore, in cases of viral infection, it is recommended that there is no role for oral antibiotics, even for patients at higher risk.

The literature confirmed that for other minor surgical procedures such as endoscopy and colonoscopy, transient bacteremia could be minimized by administration of prophylactic antibiotics, especially in high-risk patients.[127]

12. Conclusion

PJI is a serious complication with significant morbidity and mortality. Several factors in the pre-, intra-, and postoperative phases are involved that can predispose a patient to PJI. It is always better to focus on prevention rather than treatment. One of the most important preoperative factors to reduce the risk of PJI is optimization of the patient's health. Administration of preoperative prophylactic antibiotics should always be considered. It is crucial to follow the recommendations of the Consensus on the prevention of PJI to minimize the risk of infection intraoperatively. Finally, patients who undergo TJA are always at risk of infection; therefore, it is very important to prescribe prophylactic antibiotics prior to certain medical procedures.

Author details

Hamid Reza Seyyed Hosseinzadeh, Alisina Shahi*, Mohamad Qoreishy and Mehrnoush Hassas Yeganeh

*Address all correspondence to: alisina.ir@gmail.com

Thomas Jefferson University, USA

References

[1] Kurtz S, Ong K, Lau E, Mowat F, Halpern M. Projections of primary and revision hip and knee arthroplasty in the United States from 2005 to 2030. J Bone Joint Surg Am. 2007 Apr;89(4):780–5.

[2] Berbari EF, Hanssen AD, Duffy MC, Steckelberg JM, Ilstrup DM, Harmsen WS, et al. Risk factors for prosthetic joint infection: case-control study. Clin Infect Dis. 1998 Nov;27(5):1247–54.

[3] Kurtz SM, Lau E, Schmier J, Ong KL, Zhao K, Parvizi J. Infection burden for hip and knee arthroplasty in the United States. J Arthroplasty. 2008 Oct;23(7):984–91.

[4] Pulido L, Ghanem E, Joshi A, Purtill JJ, Parvizi J. Periprosthetic joint infection: the incidence, timing, and predisposing factors. Clin Orthop Relat Res. 2008 Jul;466(7): 1710–5.

[5] Bozic KJ, Kurtz SM, Lau E, Ong K, Chiu V, Vail TP, et al. The Epidemiology of Revision Total Knee Arthroplasty in the United States. Clin Orthop Relat Res. 2010 Jan; 468(1):45–51.

[6] Clohisy JC, Calvert G, Tull F, McDonald D, Maloney WJ. Reasons for revision hip surgery: a retrospective review. Clin Orthop Relat Res. 2004 Dec;(429):188–92.

[7] Vessely MB, Whaley AL, Harmsen WS, Schleck CD, Berry DJ. The Chitranjan Ranawat Award: Long-term survivorship and failure modes of 1000 cemented condylar total knee arthroplasties. Clin Orthop Relat Res. 2006 Nov;452:28–34.

[8] Della Valle C, Parvizi J, Bauer TW, Dicesare PE, Evans RP, Segreti J, et al. Diagnosis of periprosthetic joint infections of the hip and knee. J Am Acad Orthop Surg. 2010 Dec;18(12):760–70.

[9] Parvizi J, Adeli B, Zmistowski B, Restrepo C, Greenwald AS. Management of periprosthetic joint infection: the current knowledge: AAOS exhibit selection. J Bone Joint Surg Am. 2012 Jul 18;94(14):e104.

[10] Parvizi J, Zmistowski B, Adeli B. Periprosthetic joint infection: treatment options. Orthopedics. 2010 Sep;33(9):659.

[11] Kurtz SM, Lau E, Watson H, Schmier JK, Parvizi J. Economic burden of periprosthetic joint infection in the United States. J Arthroplasty. 2012 Sep;27(8 Suppl):61–65.e1.

[12] Parvizi J, Zmistowski B, Berbari EF, Bauer TW, Springer BD, Della Valle CJ, et al. New definition for periprosthetic joint infection: from the Workgroup of the Musculoskeletal Infection Society. Clin Orthop Relat Res. 2011 Nov;469(11):2992–4.

[13] Zimmerli W, Trampuz A, Ochsner PE. Prosthetic-joint infections. N Engl J Med. 2004 Oct 14;351(16):1645–54.

[14] ELEK SD, CONEN PE. The virulence of Staphylococcus pyogenes for man; a study of the problems of wound infection. Br J Exp Pathol. 1957 Dec;38(6):573–86.

[15] Zimmerli W, Waldvogel FA, Vaudaux P, Nydegger UE. Pathogenesis of foreign body infection: description and characteristics of an animal model. J Infect Dis. 1982 Oct; 146(4):487–97.

[16] Sendi P, Banderet F, Graber P, Zimmerli W. Clinical comparison between exogenous and haematogenous periprosthetic joint infections caused by Staphylococcus aureus. Clin Microbiol Infect Off Publ Eur Soc Clin Microbiol Infect Dis. 2011 Jul;17(7):1098–100.

[17] Murdoch DR, Roberts SA, Fowler Jr VG Jr, Shah MA, Taylor SL, Morris AJ, et al. Infection of orthopedic prostheses after Staphylococcus aureus bacteremia. Clin Infect Dis. 2001 Feb 15;32(4):647–9.

[18] Fitzgerald RH Jr, Nolan DR, Ilstrup DM, Van Scoy RE, Washington JA 2nd, Coventry MB. Deep wound sepsis following total hip arthroplasty. J Bone Joint Surg Am. 1977 Oct;59(7):847–55.

[19] Tsukayama DT, Estrada R, Gustilo RB. Infection after total hip arthroplasty. A study of the treatment of one hundred and six infections. J Bone Joint Surg Am. 1996 Apr; 78(4):512–23.

[20] Zimmerli W, Moser C. Pathogenesis and treatment concepts of orthopaedic biofilm infections. FEMS Immunol Med Microbiol. 2012 Jul;65(2):158–68.

[21] Maderazo EG, Judson S, Pasternak H. Late infections of total joint prostheses. A review and recommendations for prevention. Clin Orthop Relat Res. 1988 Apr;(229): 131–42.

[22] Bozic KJ, Lau E, Kurtz S, Ong K, Berry DJ. Patient-related risk factors for postoperative mortality and periprosthetic joint infection in medicare patients undergoing TKA. Clin Orthop Relat Res. 2012 Jan;470(1):130–7.

[23] Garvin KL, Konigsberg BS. Infection following total knee arthroplasty: prevention and management. Instr Course Lect. 2012;61:411–9.

[24] Malinzak RA, Ritter MA, Berend ME, Meding JB, Olberding EM, Davis KE. Morbidly obese, diabetic, younger, and unilateral joint arthroplasty patients have elevated total joint arthroplasty infection rates. J Arthroplasty. 2009 Sep;24(6 Suppl):84–8.

[25] Fletcher N, Sofianos D, Berkes MB, Obremskey WT. Prevention of perioperative infection. J Bone Joint Surg Am. 2007 Jul;89(7):1605–18.

[26] Buller LT, Sabry FY, Easton RW, Klika AK, Barsoum WK. The preoperative prediction of success following irrigation and debridement with polyethylene exchange for hip and knee prosthetic joint infections. J Arthroplasty. 2012 Jun;27(6):857–864.e1–4.

[27] Jämsen E, Huhtala H, Puolakka T, Moilanen T. Risk factors for infection after knee arthroplasty. A register-based analysis of 43,149 cases. J Bone Joint Surg Am. 2009 Jan;91(1):38–47.

[28] Jämsen E, Nevalainen P, Eskelinen A, Huotari K, Kalliovalkama J, Moilanen T. Obesity, diabetes, and preoperative hyperglycemia as predictors of periprosthetic joint infection: a single-center analysis of 7181 primary hip and knee replacements for osteoarthritis. J Bone Joint Surg Am. 2012 Jul 18;94(14):e101.

[29] Lai K, Bohm ER, Burnell C, Hedden DR. Presence of medical comorbidities in patients with infected primary hip or knee arthroplasties. J Arthroplasty. 2007 Aug; 22(5):651–6.

[30] Kamal T, Conway RM, Littlejohn I, Ricketts D. The role of a multidisciplinary preassessment clinic in reducing mortality after complex orthopaedic surgery. Ann R Coll Surg Engl. 2011 Mar;93(2):149–51.

[31] Marchant MH Jr, Viens NA, Cook C, Vail TP, Bolognesi MP. The impact of glycemic control and diabetes mellitus on perioperative outcomes after total joint arthroplasty. J Bone Joint Surg Am. 2009 Jul;91(7):1621–9.

[32] Mraovic B, Suh D, Jacovides C, Parvizi J. Perioperative hyperglycemia and postoperative infection after lower limb arthroplasty. J Diabetes Sci Technol. 2011 Mar;5(2): 412–8.

[33] Mangram AJ, Horan TC, Pearson ML, Silver LC, Jarvis WR. Guideline for Prevention of Surgical Site Infection, 1999. Centers for Disease Control and Prevention (CDC) Hospital Infection Control Practices Advisory Committee. Am J Infect Control. 1999 Apr;27(2):97–132; quiz 133–134; discussion 96.

[34] Rao N, Cannella B, Crossett LS, Yates AJ Jr, McGough R 3rd. A preoperative decolonization protocol for staphylococcus aureus prevents orthopaedic infections. Clin Orthop Relat Res. 2008 Jun;466(6):1343–8.

[35] Bleasdale SC, Trick WE, Gonzalez IM, Lyles RD, Hayden MK, Weinstein RA. Effectiveness of chlorhexidine bathing to reduce catheter-associated bloodstream infections in medical intensive care unit patients. Arch Intern Med. 2007 Oct 22;167(19): 2073–9.

[36] Climo MW, Sepkowitz KA, Zuccotti G, Fraser VJ, Warren DK, Perl TM, et al. The effect of daily bathing with chlorhexidine on the acquisition of methicillin-resistant Staphylococcus aureus, vancomycin-resistant Enterococcus, and healthcare-associated bloodstream infections: results of a quasi-experimental multicenter trial. Crit Care Med. 2009 Jun;37(6):1858–65.

[37] Rao N, Cannella BA, Crossett LS, Yates AJ Jr, McGough RL 3rd, Hamilton CW. Preoperative screening/decolonization for Staphylococcus aureus to prevent orthopedic surgical site infection: prospective cohort study with 2-year follow-up. J Arthroplasty. 2011 Dec;26(8):1501–7.

[38] Darouiche RO, Wall MJ Jr, Itani KMF, Otterson MF, Webb AL, Carrick MM, et al. Chlorhexidine-Alcohol versus Povidone-Iodine for Surgical-Site Antisepsis. N Engl J Med. 2010 Jan 7;362(1):18–26.

[39] Hidron AI, Edwards JR, Patel J, Horan TC, Sievert DM, Pollock DA, et al. NHSN annual update: antimicrobial-resistant pathogens associated with healthcare-associated infections: annual summary of data reported to the National Healthcare Safety Network at the Centers for Disease Control and Prevention, 2006-2007. Infect Control Hosp Epidemiol. 2008 Nov;29(11):996–1011.

[40] Ramos N, Skeete F, Haas JP, Hutzler L, Slover J, Phillips M, et al. Surgical site infection prevention initiative - patient attitude and compliance. Bull NYU Hosp Jt Dis. 2011;69(4):312–5.

[41] Johnson AJ, Daley JA, Zywiel MG, Delanois RE, Mont MA. Preoperative chlorhexidine preparation and the incidence of surgical site infections after hip arthroplasty. J Arthroplasty. 2010 Sep;25(6 Suppl):98–102.

[42] Zywiel MG, Daley JA, Delanois RE, Naziri Q, Johnson AJ, Mont MA. Advance preoperative chlorhexidine reduces the incidence of surgical site infections in knee arthroplasty. Int Orthop. 2011 Jul;35(7):1001–6.

[43] Fogelberg EV, Zitzmann EK, Stinchfield FE. Prophylactic penicillin in orthopaedic surgery. J Bone Joint Surg Am. 1970 Jan;52(1):95–8.

[44] Pavel A, Smith RL, Ballard A, Larsen IJ. Prophylactic antibiotics in clean orthopaedic surgery. J Bone Joint Surg Am. 1974 Jun;56(4):777–82.

[45] Meehan J, Jamali AA, Nguyen H. Prophylactic antibiotics in hip and knee arthroplasty. J Bone Joint Surg Am. 2009 Oct;91(10):2480–90.

[46] Mauerhan DR, Nelson CL, Smith DL, Fitzgerald RH Jr, Slama TG, Petty RW, et al. Prophylaxis against infection in total joint arthroplasty. One day of cefuroxime compared with three days of cefazolin. J Bone Joint Surg Am. 1994 Jan;76(1):39–45.

[47] Engesaeter LB, Lie SA, Espehaug B, Furnes O, Vollset SE, Havelin LI. Antibiotic prophylaxis in total hip arthroplasty: effects of antibiotic prophylaxis systemically and in bone cement on the revision rate of 22,170 primary hip replacements followed 0-14

years in the Norwegian Arthroplasty Register. Acta Orthop Scand. 2003 Dec;74(6): 644–51.

[48] Van Kasteren MEE, Manniën J, Ott A, Kullberg B-J, de Boer AS, Gyssens IC. Antibiotic prophylaxis and the risk of surgical site infections following total hip arthroplasty: timely administration is the most important factor. Clin Infect Dis. 2007 Apr 1;44(7): 921–7.

[49] Recommendations for the Use of Intravenous Antibiotic Prophylaxis in Primary Total Joint Arthroplasty. AAOS website. Available from: http://www.aaos.org/about/papers/advistmt/1027.asp. Last updated June 2004. Last accessed March 9 2014.

[50] vancomycin prophylaxis (Clinical Practice Guidelines for Antimicrobial Prophylaxis in Surgery) [Internet]. Available from: http://www.ashp.org/DocLibrary/BestPractices/TGSurgery.aspx.

[51] Southorn PA, Plevak DJ, Wright AJ, Wilson WR. Adverse effects of vancomycin administered in the perioperative period. Mayo Clin Proc. 1986 Sep;61(9):721–4.

[52] Antimicrobial prophylaxis in surgery. Med Lett Drugs Ther. 2001 Oct 29;43(1116-1117):92–7.

[53] Tanner J, Norrie P, Melen K. Preoperative hair removal to reduce surgical site infection. Cochrane Database Syst Rev. 2011;(11):CD004122.

[54] Von Eiff C, Becker K, Machka K, Stammer H, Peters G. Nasal carriage as a source of Staphylococcus aureus bacteremia. Study Group. N Engl J Med. 2001 Jan 4;344(1):11–6.

[55] Lee J, Singletary R, Schmader K, Anderson DJ, Bolognesi M, Kaye KS. Surgical site infection in the elderly following orthopaedic surgery. Risk factors and outcomes. J Bone Joint Surg Am. 2006 Aug;88(8):1705–12.

[56] Prokuski L. Prophylactic antibiotics in orthopaedic surgery. J Am Acad Orthop Surg. 2008 May;16(5):283–93.

[57] Edwards PS, Lipp A, Holmes A. Preoperative skin antiseptics for preventing surgical wound infections after clean surgery. Cochrane Database Syst Rev. 2004;(3):CD003949.

[58] Ostrander RV, Brage ME, Botte MJ. Bacterial skin contamination after surgical preparation in foot and ankle surgery. Clin Orthop Relat Res. 2003 Jan;(406):246–52.

[59] Keblish DJ, Zurakowski D, Wilson MG, Chiodo CP. Preoperative skin preparation of the foot and ankle: bristles and alcohol are better. J Bone Joint Surg Am. 2005 May; 87(5):986–92.

[60] Ostrander RV, Botte MJ, Brage ME. Efficacy of surgical preparation solutions in foot and ankle surgery. J Bone Joint Surg Am. 2005 May;87(5):980–5.

[61] Tanner J, Swarbrook S, Stuart J. Surgical hand antisepsis to reduce surgical site infection. Cochrane Database Syst Rev. 2008;(1):CD004288.

[62] Larson EL, Butz AM, Gullette DL, Laughon BA. Alcohol for surgical scrubbing? Infect Control Hosp Epidemiol. 1990 Mar;11(3):139–43.

[63] French ML, Eitzen HE, Ritter MA. The plastic surgical adhesive drape: an evaluation of its efficacy as a microbial barrier. Ann Surg. 1976 Jul;184(1):46–50.

[64] Johnston DH, Fairclough JA, Brown EM, Morris R. Rate of bacterial recolonization of the skin after preparation: four methods compared. Br J Surg. 1987 Jan;74(1):64.

[65] Blom AW, Gozzard C, Heal J, Bowker K, Estela CM. Bacterial strike-through of reusable surgical drapes: the effect of different wetting agents. J Hosp Infect. 2002 Sep; 52(1):52–5.

[66] Blom A, Estela C, Bowker K, MacGowan A, Hardy JR. The passage of bacteria through surgical drapes. Ann R Coll Surg Engl. 2000 Nov;82(6):405–7.

[67] Ritter MA, Campbell ED. Retrospective evaluation of an iodophor-incorporated antimicrobial plastic adhesive wound drape. Clin Orthop Relat Res. 1988 Mar;(228):307–8.

[68] Fairclough JA, Johnson D, Mackie I. The prevention of wound contamination by skin organisms by the pre-operative application of an iodophor impregnated plastic adhesive drape. J Int Med Res. 1986;14(2):105–9.

[69] Jacobson C, Osmon DR, Hanssen A, Trousdale RT, Pagnano MW, Pyrek J, et al. Prevention of wound contamination using DuraPrep solution plus Ioban 2 drapes. Clin Orthop Relat Res. 2005 Oct;439:32–7.

[70] Webster J, Alghamdi AA. Use of plastic adhesive drapes during surgery for preventing surgical site infection. Cochrane Database Syst Rev. 2007;(4):CD006353.

[71] Guo YP, Wong PM, Li Y, Or PPL. Is double-gloving really protective? A comparison between the glove perforation rate among perioperative nurses with single and double gloves during surgery. Am J Surg. 2012 Aug;204(2):210–5.

[72] Tanner J, Parkinson H. Double gloving to reduce surgical cross-infection. Cochrane Database Syst Rev. 2006;(3):CD003087.

[73] Ersozlu S, Sahin O, Ozgur AF, Akkaya T, Tuncay C. Glove punctures in major and minor orthopaedic surgery with double gloving. Acta Orthop Belg. 2007 Dec;73(6): 760–4.

[74] Beldame J, Lagrave B, Lievain L, Lefebvre B, Frebourg N, Dujardin F. Surgical glove bacterial contamination and perforation during total hip arthroplasty implantation: when gloves should be changed. Orthop Traumatol Surg Res. 2012 Jun;98(4):432–40.

[75] Carter AH, Casper DS, Parvizi J, Austin MS. A prospective analysis of glove perforation in primary and revision total hip and total knee arthroplasty. J Arthroplasty. 2012 Aug;27(7):1271–5.

[76] Demircay E, Unay K, Bilgili MG, Alataca G. Glove perforation in hip and knee arthroplasty. J Orthop Sci. 2010 Nov;15(6):790–4.

[77] Pieper SP, Schimmele SR, Johnson JA, Harper JL. A prospective study of the efficacy of various gloving techniques in the application of Erich arch bars. J Oral Maxillofac Surg. 1995 Oct;53(10):1174–1176; discussion 1177.

[78] Evans RP. Current concepts for clean air and total joint arthroplasty: laminar airflow and ultraviolet radiation: a systematic review. Clin Orthop Relat Res. 2011 Apr; 469(4):945–53.

[79] Lidwell OM, Elson RA, Lowbury EJ, Whyte W, Blowers R, Stanley SJ, et al. Ultraclean air and antibiotics for prevention of postoperative infection. A multicenter study of 8,052 joint replacement operations. Acta Orthop Scand. 1987 Feb;58(1):4–13.

[80] Dharan S, Pittet D. Environmental controls in operating theatres. J Hosp Infect. 2002 Jun;51(2):79–84.

[81] Ayliffe GA. Role of the environment of the operating suite in surgical wound infection. Rev Infect Dis. 1991 Oct;13 Suppl 10:S800–804.

[82] Gastmeier P, Breier A-C, Brandt C. Influence of laminar airflow on prosthetic joint infections: a systematic review. J Hosp Infect. 2012 Jun;81(2):73–8.

[83] Parikh SN, Grice SS, Schnell BM, Salisbury SR. Operating room traffic: is there any role of monitoring it? J Pediatr Orthop. 2010 Sep;30(6):617–23.

[84] Panahi P, Stroh M, Casper DS, Parvizi J, Austin MS. Operating room traffic is a major concern during total joint arthroplasty. Clin Orthop Relat Res. 2012 Oct;470(10):2690–4.

[85] Ritter MA. Operating room environment. Clin Orthop Relat Res. 1999 Dec;(369):103–9.

[86] Salvati EA, Robinson RP, Zeno SM, Koslin BL, Brause BD, Wilson PD Jr. Infection rates after 3175 total hip and total knee replacements performed with and without a horizontal unidirectional filtered air-flow system. J Bone Joint Surg Am. 1982 Apr; 64(4):525–35.

[87] Knobben BAS, van Horn JR, van der Mei HC, Busscher HJ. Evaluation of measures to decrease intra-operative bacterial contamination in orthopaedic implant surgery. J Hosp Infect. 2006 Feb;62(2):174–80.

[88] Pasquarella C, Sansebastiano GE, Ferretti S, Saccani E, Fanti M, Moscato U, et al. A mobile laminar airflow unit to reduce air bacterial contamination at surgical area in a conventionally ventilated operating theatre. J Hosp Infect. 2007 Aug;66(4):313–9.

[89] Talon D, Schoenleber T, Bertrand X, Vichard P. [Performances of different types of airflow system in operating theatre]. Ann Chir. 2006 May;131(5):316–21.

[90] Stocks GW, O'Connor DP, Self SD, Marcek GA, Thompson BL. Directed air flow to reduce airborne particulate and bacterial contamination in the surgical field during total hip arthroplasty. J Arthroplasty. 2011 Aug;26(5):771–6.

[91] Lidwell OM, Lowbury EJ, Whyte W, Blowers R, Stanley SJ, Lowe D. Effect of ultraclean air in operating rooms on deep sepsis in the joint after total hip or knee replacement: a randomised study. Br Med J Clin Res Ed. 1982 Jul 3;285(6334):10–4.

[92] Sehulster L, Raymond Y.W. Chinn. Guidelines for Environmental Infection Control in Health-Care Facilities; Recommendations of CDC and the Healthcare Infection Control Practices Advisory Committee (HICPAC). CDC website. Available from: http://www.cdc.gov/mmwr/preview/mmwrhtml/rr5210a1.htm. Last updated June 6 2003. Last accessed April 9 2014.

[93] Charnley J, Eftekhar N. Penetration of gown material by organisms from the surgeon's body. Lancet. 1969 Jan 25;1(7587):172–3.

[94] Der Tavitian J, Ong SM, Taub NA, Taylor GJS. Body-exhaust suit versus occlusive clothing. A randomised, prospective trial using air and wound bacterial counts. J Bone Joint Surg Br. 2003 May;85(4):490–4.

[95] Howard JL, Hanssen AD. Principles of a clean operating room environment. J Arthroplasty. 2007 Oct;22(7 Suppl 3):6–11.

[96] Pasquarella C, Pitzurra O, Herren T, Poletti L, Savino A. Lack of influence of body exhaust gowns on aerobic bacterial surface counts in a mixed-ventilation operating theatre. A study of 62 hip arthroplasties. J Hosp Infect. 2003 May;54(1):2–9.

[97] Sanzén L, Carlsson AS, Walder M. Air contamination during total hip arthroplasty in an ultraclean air enclosure using different types of staff clothing. J Arthroplasty. 1990 Jun;5(2):127–30.

[98] Kearns KA, Witmer D, Makda J, Parvizi J, Jungkind D. Sterility of the personal protection system in total joint arthroplasty. Clin Orthop Relat Res. 2011 Nov;469(11):3065–9.

[99] Ong KL, Lau E, Manley M, Kurtz SM. Effect of procedure duration on total hip arthroplasty and total knee arthroplasty survivorship in the United States Medicare population. J Arthroplasty. 2008 Sep;23(6 Suppl 1):127–32.

[100] Urquhart DM, Hanna FS, Brennan SL, Wluka AE, Leder K, Cameron PA, et al. Incidence and risk factors for deep surgical site infection after primary total hip arthroplasty: a systematic review. J Arthroplasty. 2010 Dec;25(8):1216–1222.e1–3.

[101] Ong KL, Kurtz SM, Lau E, Bozic KJ, Berry DJ, Parvizi J. Prosthetic joint infection risk after total hip arthroplasty in the Medicare population. J Arthroplasty. 2009 Sep;24(6 Suppl):105–9.

[102] Peersman G, Laskin R, Davis J, Peterson M. Infection in total knee replacement: a retrospective review of 6489 total knee replacements. Clin Orthop Relat Res. 2001 Nov;(392):15–23.

[103] Kurtz SM, Ong KL, Lau E, Bozic KJ, Berry D, Parvizi J. Prosthetic joint infection risk after TKA in the Medicare population. Clin Orthop Relat Res. 2010 Jan;468(1):52–6.

[104] Muilwijk J, van den Hof S, Wille JC. Associations between surgical site infection risk and hospital operation volume and surgeon operation volume among hospitals in the Dutch nosocomial infection surveillance network. Infect Control Hosp Epidemiol. 2007 May;28(5):557–63.

[105] Andersson AE, Bergh I, Karlsson J, Eriksson BI, Nilsson K. Traffic flow in the operating room: an explorative and descriptive study on air quality during orthopedic trauma implant surgery. Am J Infect Control. 2012 Oct;40(8):750–5.

[106] Young RS, O'Regan DJ. Cardiac surgical theatre traffic: time for traffic calming measures? Interact Cardiovasc Thorac Surg. 2010 Apr;10(4):526–9.

[107] Cassar Gheiti AJ, Baker JF, Brown TE, Mulhall KJ. Management of total femoral bone loss using a hybrid cement spacer surgical technique. J Arthroplasty. 2013 Feb;28(2):347–51.

[108] Dairaku K, Takagi M, Kawaji H, Sasaki K, Ishii M, Ogino T. Antibiotics-impregnated cement spacers in the first step of two-stage revision for infected totally replaced hip joints: report of ten trial cases. J Orthop Sci. 2009 Nov;14(6):704–10.

[109] Romanò CL, Romanò D, Logoluso N, Meani E. Long-stem versus short-stem preformed antibiotic-loaded cement spacers for two-stage revision of infected total hip arthroplasty. Hip Int J. 2010 Mar;20(1):26–33.

[110] Hanssen AD, Spangehl MJ. Practical applications of antibiotic-loaded bone cement for treatment of infected joint replacements. Clin Orthop Relat Res. 2004 Oct;(427):79–85.

[111] Chiu FY, Lin CF, Chen CM, Lo WH, Chaung TY. Cefuroxime-impregnated cement at primary total knee arthroplasty in diabetes mellitus. A prospective, randomised study. J Bone Joint Surg Br. 2001 Jul;83(5):691–5.

[112] Wenke JC, Owens BD, Svoboda SJ, Brooks DE. Effectiveness of commercially-available antibiotic-impregnated implants. J Bone Joint Surg Br. 2006 Aug;88(8):1102–4.

[113] Jaeblon T. Polymethylmethacrylate: properties and contemporary uses in orthopaedics. J Am Acad Orthop Surg. 2010 May;18(5):297–305.

[114] Smith TO, Sexton D, Mann C, Donell S. Sutures versus staples for skin closure in orthopaedic surgery: meta-analysis. BMJ. 2010;340:c1199.

[115] Newman JT, Morgan SJ, Resende GV, Williams AE, Hammerberg EM, Dayton MR. Modality of wound closure after total knee replacement: are staples as safe as sutures? A retrospective study of 181 patients. Patient Saf Surg. 2011;5(1):26.

[116] Eggers MD, Fang L, Lionberger DR. A comparison of wound closure techniques for total knee arthroplasty. J Arthroplasty. 2011 Dec;26(8):1251–1258.e1–4.

[117] Patel RM, Cayo M, Patel A, Albarillo M, Puri L. Wound complications in joint arthroplasty: comparing traditional and modern methods of skin closure. Orthopedics. 2012 May;35(5):e641–646.

[118] Stephens S, Politi J, Taylor BC. Evaluation of Primary Total Knee Arthroplasty Incision Closure with the Use of Continuous Bidirectional Barbed Suture. Surg Technol Int. 2011 Dec 1;XXI:199–203.

[119] Eickmann T, Quane E. Total knee arthroplasty closure with barbed sutures. J Knee Surg. 2010 Sep;23(3):163–7.

[120] Clarke JV, Deakin AH, Dillon JM, Emmerson S, Kinninmonth AWG. A prospective clinical audit of a new dressing design for lower limb arthroplasty wounds. J Wound Care. 2009 Jan;18(1):5–8, 10–1.

[121] Cosker T, Elsayed S, Gupta S, Mendonca AD, Tayton KJJ. Choice of dressing has a major impact on blistering and healing outcomes in orthopaedic patients. J Wound Care. 2005 Jan;14(1):27–9.

[122] Cho CY, Lo JS. Dressing the part. Dermatol Clin. 1998 Jan;16(1):25–47.

[123] Mertz PM, Marshall DA, Eaglstein WH. Occlusive wound dressings to prevent bacterial invasion and wound infection. J Am Acad Dermatol. 1985 Apr;12(4):662–8.

[124] Dumville JC, Walter CJ, Sharp CA, Page T. Dressings for the prevention of surgical site infection. Cochrane Database Syst Rev. 2011;(7):CD003091.

[125] Burke NG, Green C, McHugh G, McGolderick N, Kilcoyne C, Kenny P. A prospective randomised study comparing the jubilee dressing method to a standard adhesive dressing for total hip and knee replacements. J Tissue Viability. 2012 Aug;21(3): 84–7.

[126] Gross L. AAOS, ADA Release CPG for Prophylactic Antibiotics. AAOS website. Available from: http://www.aaos.org/news/aaosnow/jan13/cover1.asp. Last updated December 7 2012. Last accessed April 9 2014.

[127] Chen A, Haddad F, Lachiewicz P, Bolognesi M, Cortes LE, Franceschini M, et al. Prevention of late PJI. J Arthroplasty. 2014 Feb;29(2 Suppl):119–28.

8

X-ray Digital Tomosynthesis Imaging — Comparison of Reconstruction Algorithms in Terms of a Reduction in the Exposure Dose for Arthroplasty

Tsutomu Gomi

Abstract

Aims The purpose of this review was (1) to identify indications for volumetric X-ray digital tomosynthesis by using a conventional reconstruction technique [the filtered back-projection (FBP) algorithm] and modern reconstruction techniques [the maximum likelihood expectation maximization (MLEM) and simultaneous iterative reconstruction techniques (SIRT)] and (2) to compare the conventional and modern reconstruction techniques in terms of a reduction in the exposure dose.

Review The methods included the following: (1) an overview and analysis of the characteristics of the FBP, MLEM, and SIRT algorithms; (2) an overview of the properties of phantom imaging for arthroplasty when imaging overlying structures and the effect of those properties on various artifacts in images; and (3) a review of each method regarding exposure reductions.

Summary In the phantom study, the MLEM and SIRT techniques can suppress streak artifacts; therefore, they warrant further evaluation in comparison with FBP. With the FBP technique, the exposure dose may be decreased to half of the reproducibility for a reconstructed prosthesis phantom image. The results show the characteristics of each technique that need to be considered in clinical practice (better suppression of streak artifacts: MLEM and SIRT; better reproducibility: FBP). In addition, understanding the advantages of each reconstruction technique during digital tomosynthesis imaging will improve diagnostic accuracy in clinical applications.

Keywords: Tomosynthesis, arthroplasty, exposure dose, reconstruction algorithm

1. Introduction

Digital tomosynthesis is a limited-angle image reconstruction method where a dataset of projections acquired at regular intervals during a single acquisition pass is used to reconstruct planar sections posteriori. Digital tomosynthesis also provides the additional benefits of digital imaging [1-17], as well as the tomographic benefits of computed tomography (CT) at decreased radiation doses and lower costs using an approach that can easily be implemented in conjunction with radiography. Digital tomosynthesis is a promising technique for improving early detection rates of cancer [6-7, 9-10, 13-14] because it can provide three-dimensional (3D) structural information by reconstructing an entire image volume from a sequence of projection-view radiograms acquired at a small number of projection angles over a limited angular range; the total radiation dose is comparable with that used during conventional radiography.

X-ray CT has continually matured, and it now constitutes a powerful tool in medical diagnostics. Metal artifacts influence image quality by reducing contrast and obscuring detail, thus impairing the detectability of structures of interest; in the worst case, this can make diagnosis impossible (Fig. 1).

Various digital tomosynthesis reconstruction methods have been explored previously [17]. Nevertheless, image quality assessments have been based on the use of phantoms with features that did not address radiation doses. In fact, to date, no studies have quantitatively compared digital tomosynthesis algorithms in terms of image quality and radiation doses. One recently developed CT technique, iterative reconstruction (IR), was found to effectively decrease quantum noise and radiation exposure [18]. IR may yield improvements in image quality and a reduction in the exposure dose in comparison with the conventional filtered back-projection (FBP) technique.

We chose to focus on the conventional FBP, statistical reconstruction technique [maximum likelihood expectation maximization (MLEM) [19]], and the algebraic reconstruction technique [simultaneous IR technique (SIRT) [20]]. We evaluated and compared the characteristics of the reconstructed images and the possible reduction in the radiation dose associated with FBP, MLEM, and SIRT algorithms for hip prosthesis phantoms. The algorithms were implemented using a digital tomosynthesis system and were experimentally evaluated by obtaining measurements using a phantom.

2. Tomosynthesis system

The tomosynthesis system (SonialVision Safire II, Shimadzu Co., Kyoto, Japan, Fig. 2) comprised an X-ray tube with a 0.4 mm focal spot and a 362.88 × 362.88 mm digital flat-panel detector composed of amorphous selenium. Each detector element was 150 × 150 μm in size. Tomography was performed linearly with a total acquisition time of 6.4 s {80 kVp, 250 mA, 20 ms/view, reference effective dose: 0.69 mSv [International Commission on Radiological Protection (ICRP) 103], half effective dose: 0.42 mSv (80 kVp, 250 mA, 14 ms/view), quarter

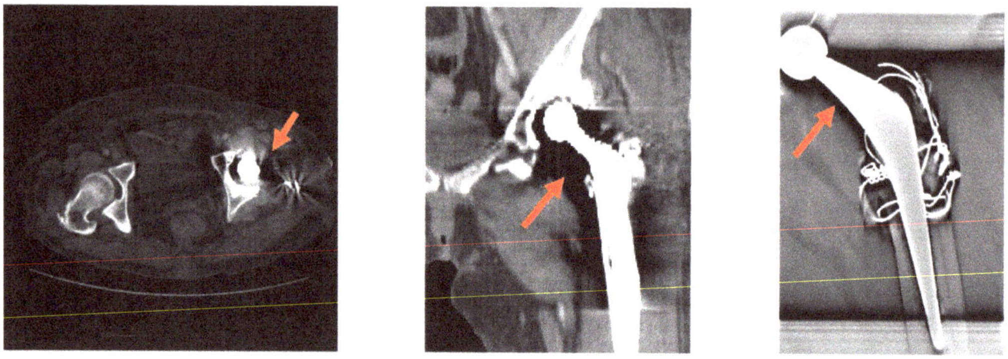

Figure 1. Comparison of metal artifact images with images obtained from each modality [CT (axial and coronal images) and conventional FBP tomosynthesis image].

effective dose: 0.24 mSv (80 kVp, 250 mA, 7 ms/view), and an acquisition angle of 40° (74 projections). The reconstructed images (0.272 mm/pixel) were obtained at 1 mm reconstruction intervals. (Table 1, Fig. 3)

Tomosynthesis system	SonialVision Safire II (Shimadzu Co., Japan)
X-ray focal spot	0.4 mm
Detector area	362.88 × 362.88 mm
Detector type	Direct conversion-type flat-panel detector (amorphous selenium)
Detector element	150 × 150 μm
X-ray tube voltage	80 kVp
X-ray tube current	250 mA
Acquisition time	Reference dose: 20 ms/view
	Half dose: 14 ms/view
	Quarter dose: 7 ms/view
Acquisition angle	40°
Projections	74
Reconstruction interval	1 mm

Table 1. The detailed estimates of the acquisition parameters.

3. Phantom specifications

A hip prosthesis phantom (PerFix HA CMT91006; Japan Medical Materials Co., Tokyo, Japan; Fig. 4) was used in a polymethyl methacrylate (PMMA) case filled with water (case φ, 200 × 300 mm). The prosthetic phantom were designed to evaluate image reconstruction quality for in-plane (x-y plane) and out-plane (z-axis) images.

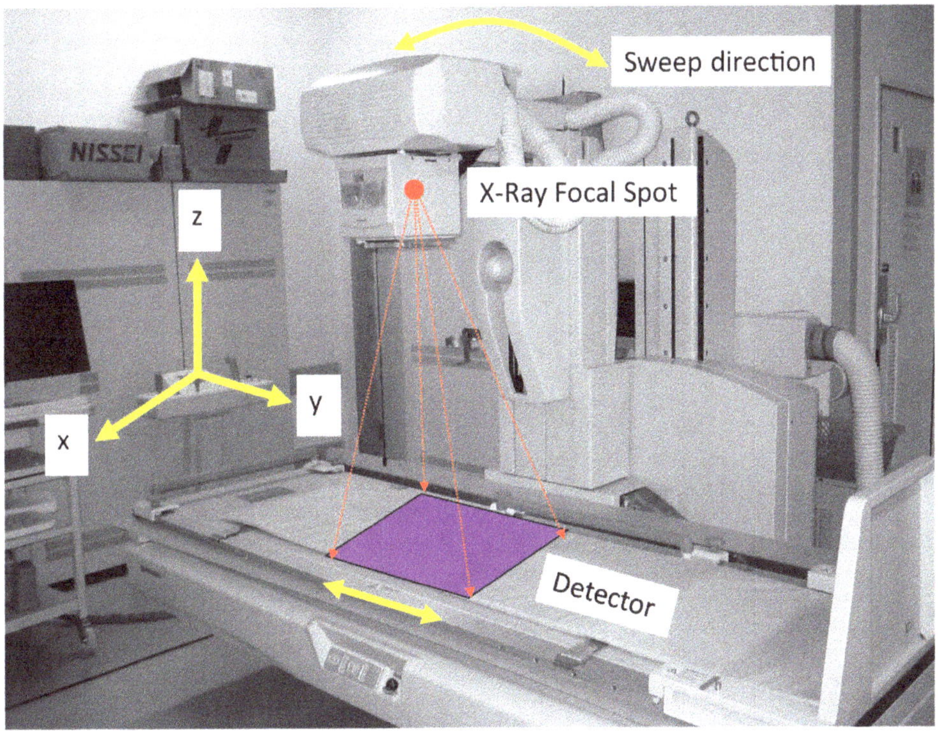

Figure 2. Illustration of a SonialVision Safire II tomosynthesis system (Shimadzu Co., Kyoto, Japan). This system acquires 3D projection data by linear motion in the y-axis direction. The detector uses a direct conversion-type flat-panel detector (FPD).

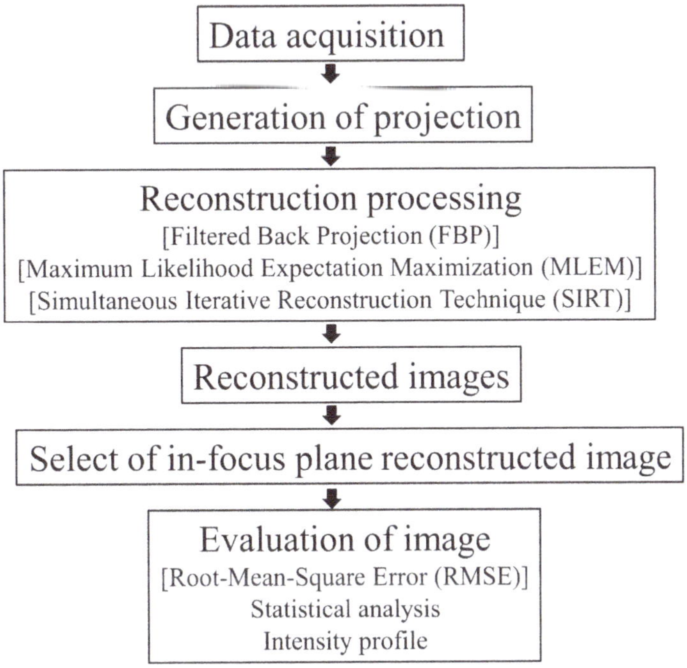

Figure 3. Flow chart of image reconstruction processing and image evaluation.

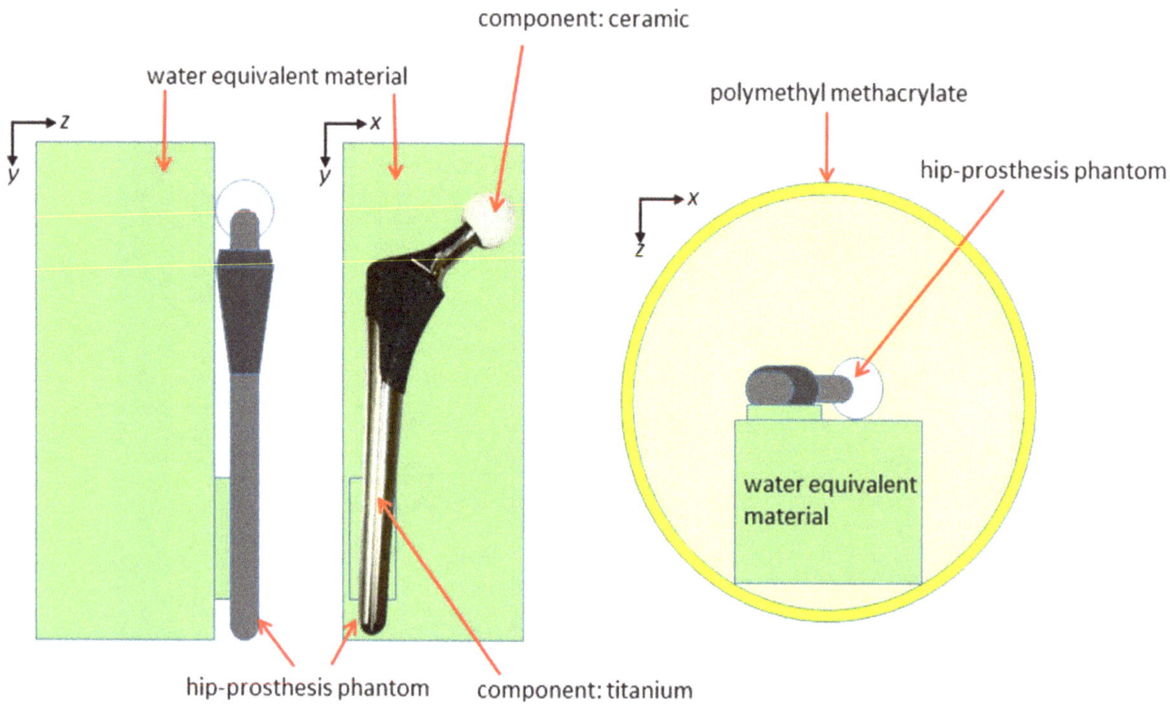

Figure 4. Illustration of the hip-prosthesis phantom used in this study.

4. Image reconstruction for digital tomosynthesis

In FBP algorithms, which are widely used in tomography, many projections are acquired for cross-sectional image reconstruction. The relationship between the radon transform and cone-beam projections has been thoroughly studied, and cone-beam reconstruction solutions have been obtained previously [14]. Two-dimensional (2D) image filtering via multiplication of the Fourier transform by means of a Ramp or Shepp-Logan (SL) filter kernel restores the proper impulse shape for the reconstructed image. The FBP algorithm generally provides highly precise 3D reconstruction images [14]. In this study, a conventional SL filter kernel was used to reconstruct FBP images (Fig. 5).

IR algorithms perform reconstruction recursively [21-22], unlike the one-step operation used in back projection and FBP algorithms. Instead, reconstruction is accomplished by iteratively updating unknown linear attenuation coefficients by minimizing the error between the measured and calculated projection data.

The original method in this family of algebraic reconstruction techniques (ARTs) [20] has already been determined. ART features fast convergence speed because only a single projection value is used to update linear attenuation coefficients at a given time point, but it converges to a least-squares solution that can result in considerable noise when severely ill-posed inverse problems, such as limited-angle reconstruction, are being solved. Variations have been proposed regarding ART implementation for facilitating improvements. ART can be modified according to other methods such as SIRT [20], depending on the amount of projection data and the method used to update the current estimation (Fig. 6).

On the other hand, MLEM methods consisting of two steps per iteration (in which the tomosynthesis acquisition process is modeled in a forward step and the reconstructed object is updated in a backward step) have also been proposed for digital tomosynthesis. The most commonly studied method in digital tomosynthesis is MLEM introduced for digital tomosynthesis by Wu et al. [19]. MLEM and SIRT are applied iteratively such that the reconstructed volume projections, which are computed using an image formation model, resemble the experimental projections (Figs. 6-7). In this chapter, seventeen MLEM and SIRT iterations were used to improve image quality (to attain highest contrast and to minimize metal artifacts). The FBP, MLEM, and SIRT image reconstruction calculations from real projection data of a digital tomosynthesis system were performed using MATLAB (Mathworks, Natick, MA, USA).

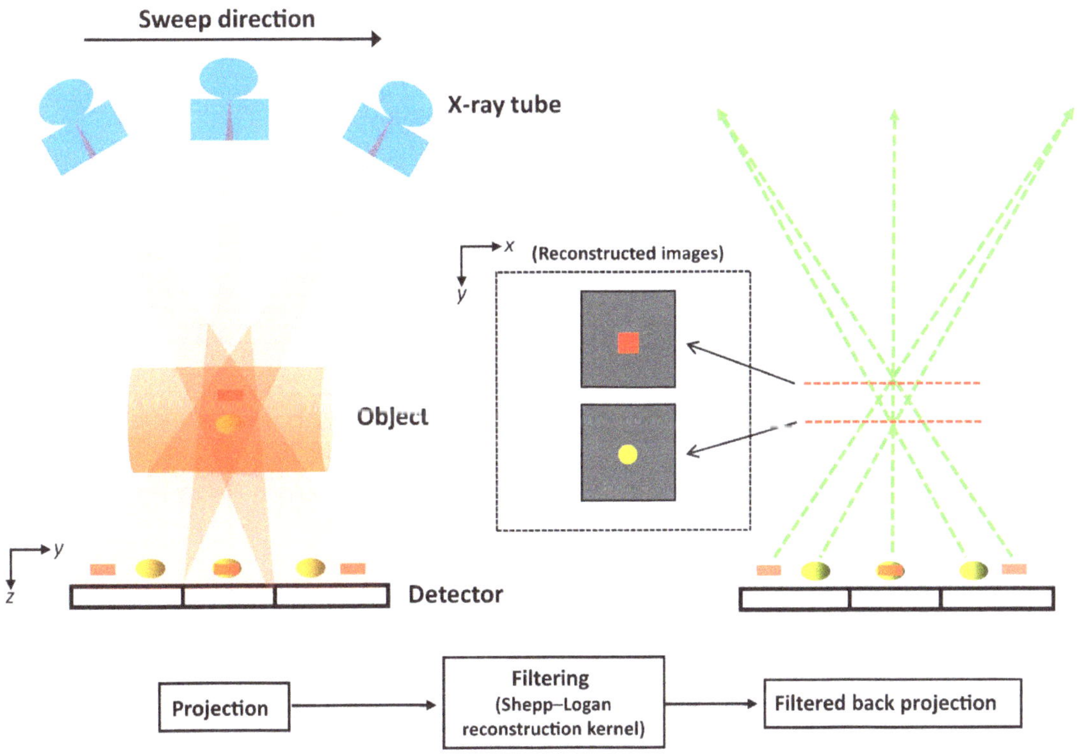

Figure 5. Concept of the FBP-processing method for tomosynthesis.

5. Evaluation

In the chapter, the metal artifact-reduction and image quality performance was evaluated using the intensity profile and root-mean-square error (RMSE). The intensity profiles were

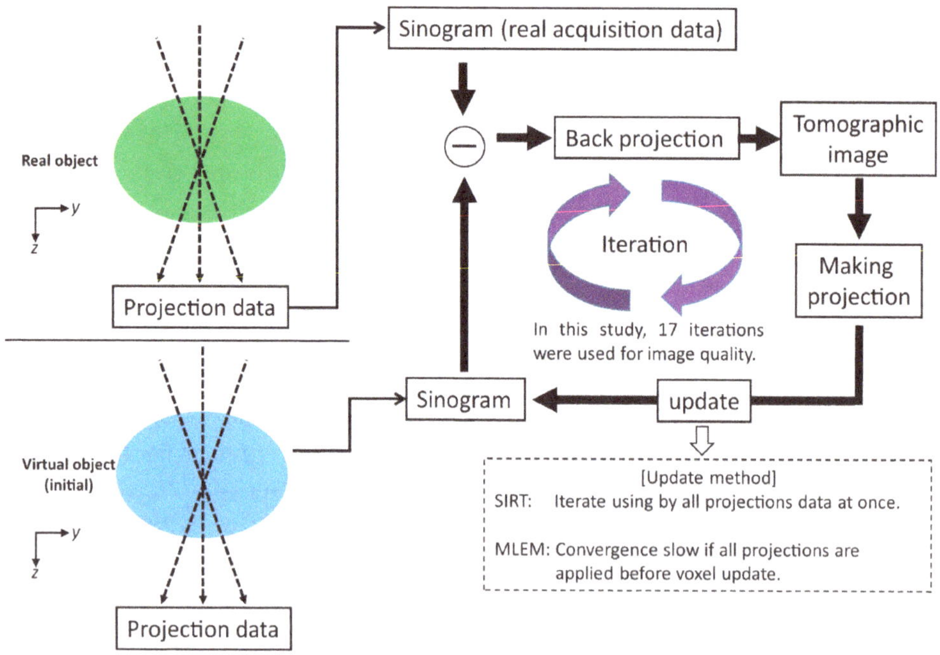

Figure 6. Concept of the IR-processing method (MLEM and SIRT) for tomosynthesis.

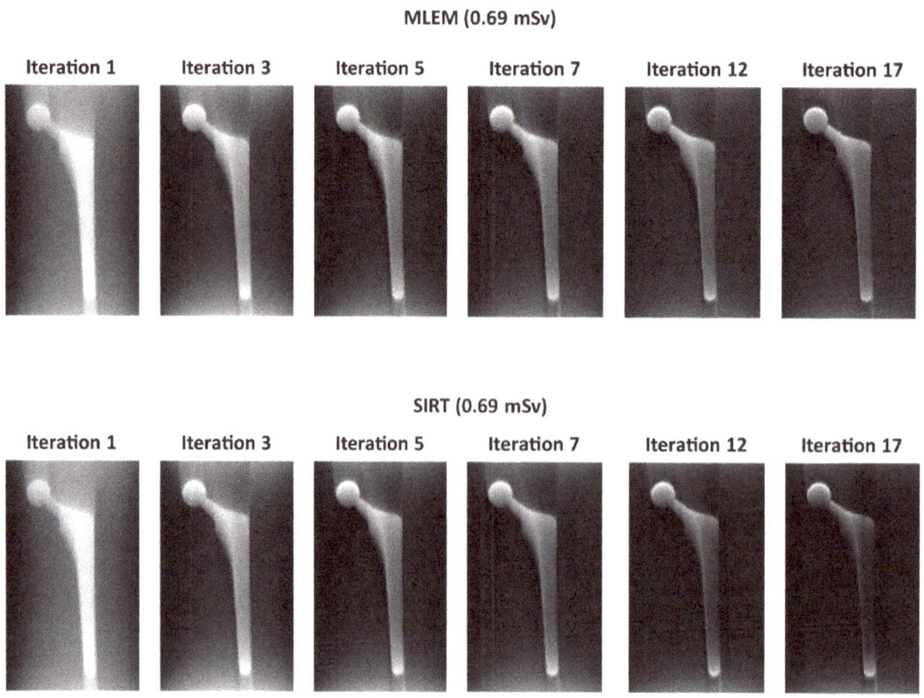

Figure 7. Comparison between tomosynthesis images (different iteration) and those obtained from the imaging algorithms of MLEM and SIRT technique in the in-focus plane. The MLEM and SIRT tomosynthesis images for the corresponding prosthesis phantom are displayed with the same window width and window level. The x-ray source moved in the vertical direction relative to the image shown. Image quality (reproducibility and artifact) is improved by increasing the number of iterations.

compared using different reconstruction methods in the in-focus plane. Another important metric to be considered is RMSE, which can be computed by obtaining the root of the summation of the square of the standard deviation and the square of the bias. The errors in the image plane are defined in terms of RMSE as

$$RMSE = \sqrt{\sum_{i=1}^{n} \left(X - x_i \right)^2 / n} \tag{1}$$

where X is the observed image, x_i is the referenced image, and n is the number of compounds in the analyzed set.

The effects of image artifacts and quality were assessed in paired *t*-test. Statistical tests were used to assess differences between pixel values (from intensity profile) of FBP, MLEM, and SIRT. We performed the tests on a total of 84 samples. The statistical analysis was performed in SPSS for Windows, version 21.0 (SPSS Inc., Chicago, IL, USA). All probability (*P*) values <0.05 were assumed to denote statistical significance.

6. Results

A comparison of the intensity profiles and RMSEs of the tomosynthesis images revealed that tomosynthesis (IR algorithm) decreased the number of metal and beam hardening artifacts in the reconstructed images. Furthermore, this IR technique can reduce quantum noise, and the noise structure was slightly smoother. The MLEM and SIRT techniques can suppress streak artifacts; therefore, they warrant further evaluation in comparison with FBP (Figs. 8-10).

The comparison of the reference exposure dose (0.69 mSv for the FBP image) with the reduced exposure dose (0.42 mSv for the FBP image) involved the paired *t*-test: p = 0.112 (not a statistically significant difference), t = −1.664, degrees of freedom (DF) = 20, 95% confidence interval (CI): −0.120 to 0.013. The comparison of the reference exposure dose (0.69 mSv for the MLEM image) and the reduced exposure dose (0.42 mSv for the MLEM image) was also based on the paired *t*-test: p < 0.05 (statistically significant difference), t = −7.386, DF = 20, 95% CI: -0.108 to -0.060. The comparison of the reference exposure dose (0.69 mSv for the SIRT image) with the reduced exposure dose (0.42 mSv for the SIRT image) involved the paired *t*-test: p < 0.05 (statistically significant difference), t = −7.372, DF = 20, 95% CI: −0.126 to −0.070. With the FBP technique, it was possible to maybe maintain the reproducibility of a reconstructed image with an approximately 50% reduction in the radiation dose. The results show the characteristics of each technique that need to be considered in clinical practice (better suppression of streak artifacts: MLEM and SIRT; better reproducibility: FBP).

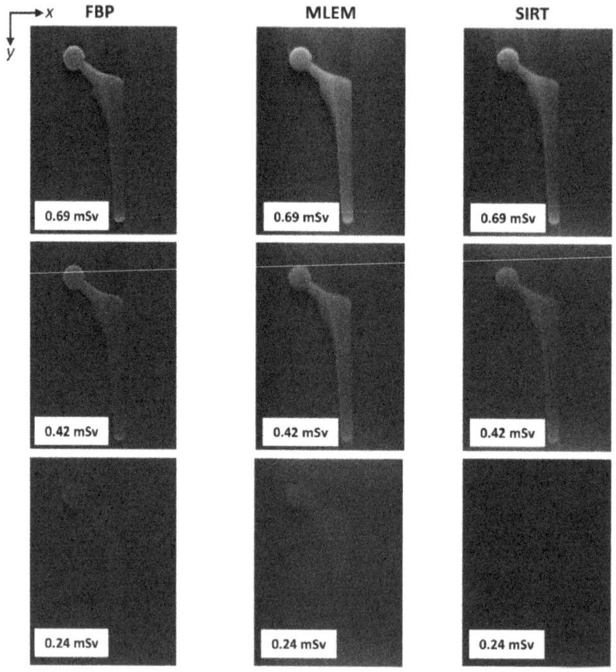

Figure 8. Comparison between tomosynthesis images (different reconstruction technique and different exposure dose, FBP filter kernel: Shepp-Logan, IR iteration: 17) and those obtained from the imaging algorithms of FBP, MLEM, and SIRT techniques in the in-focus plane. The FBP, MLEM, and SIRT tomosynthesis images for the corresponding prosthesis phantom are displayed with the same window width and window level. The x-ray source moved in the vertical direction relative to the image shown.

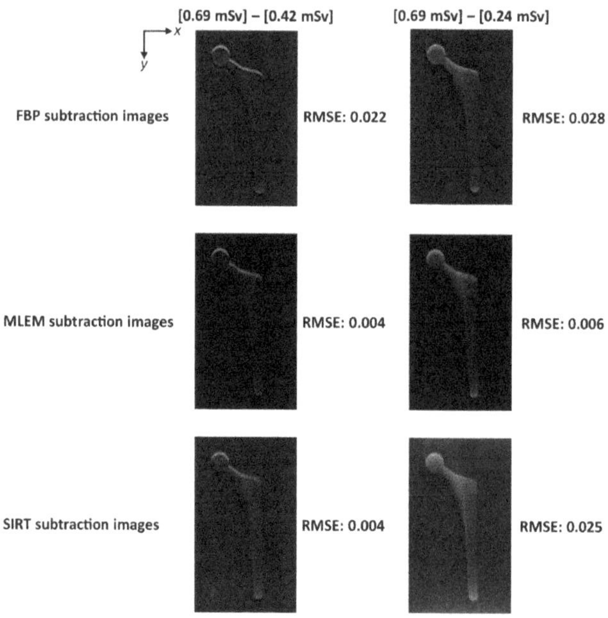

Figure 9. Comparison between tomosynthesis subtraction images (FBP filter kernel: Shepp-Logan, IR iteration: 17) and those obtained from the imaging algorithms of FBP, MLEM, and SIRT techniques in the in-focus plane. The FBP, MLEM, and SIRT tomosynthesis images for the corresponding prosthesis phantom are displayed with the same window width and window level. The x-ray source moved in the vertical direction relative to the image shown.

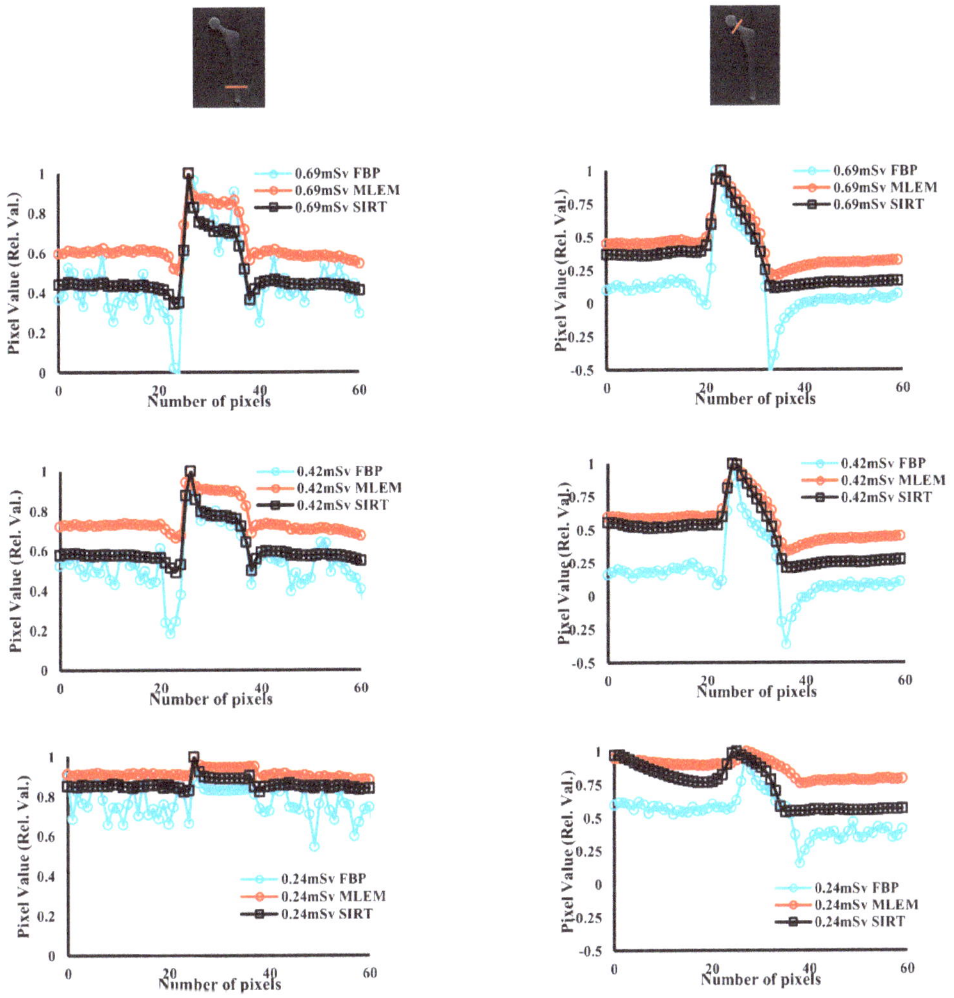

Figure 10. Comparison between intensity profiles using tomosynthesis (different exposure dose) in the in-focus plane. Artifacts (part of undershooting) are reduced by the IR technique for tomosynthesis.

7. Conclusion

In this study, the results of a prosthesis phantom study suggest that digital tomosynthesis (IR algorithm) can produce improved image quality compared with that by conventional FBP tomosynthesis by the same exposure dose level. In addition, the IR algorithm apparently facilitates the significant improvement of images corrupted by metal artifacts.

With the FBP technique, the exposure dose may be decreased to half of the reproducibility for a reconstructed prosthesis phantom image.

In addition, understanding the advantages of each reconstruction technique during digital tomosynthesis imaging (better suppression of streak artifacts: IR algorithm; better reproducibility: FBP) will improve diagnostic accuracy in clinical applications.

Author details

Tsutomu Gomi

Address all correspondence to: gomi@kitasato-u.ac.jp

School of Allied Health Sciences, Kitasato University, Japan

References

[1] Ziedses des, Plante BG. Eine neue methode zur differenzierung in der roentgenographie (planigraphie). Acta radiologica 1932; 13 182-192.

[2] Miller ER, McCurry EM, Hruska B. An infinite number of laminagrams from a finite number of radiographs. Radiology 1971; 98 249-255.

[3] Grant DG. Tomosynthesis. A three-dimensional radiographic imaging technique. IEEE transactions on bio-medical engineering 1972; 19 20-28.

[4] Baily NA, Lasser EC, Crepeau RL. Electrofluoro-plangigraphy. Radiology 1973; 107 669-671.

[5] Kruger RA, Nelson JA, Ghosh-Roy D, Miller FJ, Anderson RE, Liu PY. Dynamic tomographic digital subtraction angiography using temporal filteration. Radiology 1983; 147 863-867.

[6] Sone S, Kasuga T, Sakai S, Aoki J, Izuno I, Tanizaki Y, Shigeta H, Shibata K. Development of a high-resolution digital tomosynthesis system and its clinical application. Radiographics 1991; 11 807-822.

[7] Sone S, Kasuga T, Sakai F, Kawai T, Oguchi K, Hirano H, Li F, Kudo K, Honda T, Hanouda M. Image processing in the digital tomosynthesis for pulmonary imaging. European Radiology 1995; 5 96-101.

[8] Machida H, Yuhara T, Mori T, Ueno E, Moribe Y, Sabol JM. Optimizing parameters for flat-panel detector digital tomosynthesis. Radiographics 2010; 30 549-562.

[9] Vikgren J, Zachrisson S, Svalkvist A, Johnsson AA, Boijsen M, Flinck A, Kheddache S, Båth M. Comparison of chest tomosynthesis and chest radiography for detection of pulmonary nodules: Human observer study of clinical cases. Radiology 2008; 217 251-256.

[10] Skaane P, Bandos AI, Gullien R, Eben EB, Ekseth U, Haakenaasen U, Izadi M, Jebsen IN, Jahr G, Krager M, Niklason LT, Hofvind S, Gur D. Comparison of digital mammography alone and digital mammography plus tomosynthesis in a population-based screening program. Radiology 2013; 267 47-56.

[11] Stiel G, Stiel LG, Klotz E, Nienaber CA. Digital flashing tomosynthesis: A promising technique for angiographic screening. IEEE transactions on medical imaging 1993; 12 314-321.

[12] Duryea J, Dobbins JT, Lynch JA. Digital tomosynthesis of hand joints for arthritis assessment. Medical Physics 2003; 30 325-33.

[13] Niklason LT, Christian BT, Niklason LE, Kopans DB, Castleberry DE, Opsahl-Ong BH, Landberg CE, Slanetz PJ, Giardino AA, Moore R, Albagli D, DeJule MC, Fitzgerald PF, Fobare DF, Giambattista BW, Kwasnick RF, Liu J, Lubowski SJ, Possin GE, Richotte JF, Wei CY, Wirth RF. Digital tomosynthesis in breast imaging. Radiology 1997; 205 399-406.

[14] Dobbins JT III, Godfrey DJ. Digital x-ray tomosynthesis: Current state of the art and clinical potential. Physics in medicine and biology 2003; 48 R65-106.

[15] Gomi T, Hirano H. Clinical potential of digital linear tomosynthesis imaging of total joint arthroplasty. Journal of Digital Imaging 2008; 21 312-322.

[16] Gomi T, Hirano H, Umeda T. Evaluation of the x-ray digital linear tomosynthesis reconstruction processing method for metal artifact reduction. Computerized Medical Imaging and Graphics 2009; 33 257-274.

[17] Gomi T, Hirano H, Nakajima M. Recent advance in arthroplasty. In: X-ray digital linear tomosynthesis imaging of arhtoroplasty. Rijeka: InTech 2012; 95-108.

[18] Marin D, Nelson RC, Schindera ST, Richard S, Youngblood RS, Yoshizumi TT, Samei E. Low-tube-voltage, high-tube-current multidetector abdominal CT: Improved image quality and decreased radiation dose with adaptive statistical iterative reconstruction algorithm-initial clinical experience. Radiology 2010; 254 145-153.

[19] Wu T, Stewart A, Stanton M, McCauley T, Phillips W, Kopans DB, Moore RH, Eberhard JW, Opsahl-Ong B, Niklason L, Williams MB. Tomographic mammography using a limited number of low-dose cone-beam projection images. Medical Physics 2003; 30 365-380.

[20] Gordon R, Bender R, Hermen GT. Algebraic reconstruction techniques (ART) for three-dimensional electron microscopy and x-ray photography. Journal of theoretical biology 1970; 29 471-481.

[21] Bleuet P, Guillemaud R, Magnin I, Desbat L. An adapted fan volume sampling scheme for 3D algebraic reconstruction in linear tomosynthesis. IEEE Trans Nucl Sci 2001; 3 1720-1724.

[22] Wu T, Zhang J, Moore R, Rafferty E, Kopans D, Meleis W, Kaeli D. Digital tomosynthesis mammography using a parallel maximum-likelihood reconstruction method. Proc SPIE 2004; 5368 1-11.

9

Importance of Bone Markers and Radiological Status on Clinical Signs of Temporomandibular Joint Disorders

Oksana Ivask, Ülle Voog-Oras and Edvitar Leibur

Abstract

This chapter describes the diagnostics of temporomandibular joint disorders (TMDs) with the main focus on the radiographic changes and the role of different bone markers as procollagen type I N-terminal propeptide (P1NP), C-telopeptide crosslaps of type I collagen (CTX-1) as well as vitamin D (25(OH)D) in the pathogenesis of TMDs. From our population-based study, 47% subjects had TMJ problems where pain is commonly accompanied by stiffness, sounds and functional limitations, resulting in a decreased quality of life, and thus exert a significant negative impact on activities of daily living (ADL). Assessment of individual pain level is important in the evaluation of TMD. Radiographic examination is commonly used for assessment of TMJ problems. Orthopantomograph (OPTG) is the most routine method for assessment of bone structural changes as erosions, flattening and osteophytes of the condyle and temporal part of TMJ. It is found that subjects with increased levels of P1NP, CTX-1 have less TMJ pain/discomfort. Increased levels of CTX-1 would probably cause an immediate increase of P1NP which is known as a sensitive marker of bone formation. TMJ radiographic changes seem to be related to the low level of 25(OH)D level.

Hence, the aim of this chapter is to critically review the evidence of possible association between TMJ pain and bone radiographic changes with main focus on the role of different bone markers and vitamin D.

Keywords: Activities of daily living, biochemical markers, OPTG, osteoporosis, pain measurement, temporomandibular joint disease, vitamin D

1. Introduction

Temporomandibular joint disorders (TMDs) present an important health problem. It has been estimated that approximately 20% to 30% of the adult population will experience temporomandibular joint (TMJ) dysfunction [1,2].

The most signs and symptoms include facial and jaw pain which can be initiated by jaw movements, TMJ sounds and functional disability. Radiological investigation often shows the displacement of the disc from its normal location, or osteoarthritic changes in the TMJ. Many researches focus on the role of biochemical mediators in development and progression of TMJ pain and dysfunction. There has been found association between bone markers (procollagen type I N-terminalpropeptide (P1NP), C-telopeptide crosslaps of type I collagen (CTX-1) as well as vitamin D (25(OH)D) and TMD [3,4,5]. Several biochemical markers of bone turnover can be used to predict individual bone loss on risk for TMJ pathologies [6].

The globally increasing prevalence of TMD calls for a more detailed knowledge on the relationship between bone markers and vitamin D in the pathogenesis of TMJ disorders. The Northern Europe population has a high risk for D-hypovitaminosis [7]. There is still a lack of the knowledge of the specific impact of TMJ pain on daily activities in patients with clinical involvement of the TMJ. Hopefully, the new knowledge of the TMJ etiopathogenesis will help predict TMJ bone destruction. Additional vitamin D consumption might be suggested to avoid TMJ dysfunctions and thereby reduce pain level. A multidimensional understanding of the etiopathogenesis of TMJ pathologies detected at an earlier stage would help improve diagnostics and apply evidence-based treatment.

2. Temporomandibular joint disorders and pain

2.1. TMJ pain

Pain in the jaw musculature is the most commonly reported pain of nondental origin in the orofacial region [8]. The TMJ pain is common among all age groups [9]. Chronic craniofacial pain conditions with a prevalence of approximately 10 15% are increasing in the adult population [10,11,12]. The prevalence of TMJ pain across lifetime is still debated, but there seems to be a peak of the pain at approximately 45 years of age for women, although also elderly people may suffer from TMD pain [13]. Pain is always a subjective experience, and the impact of chronic pain is not just a sensory experience but also an emotional experience [14,15,16].

Chronic pain may be nociceptive, neuropathic, ischemic, visceral or exhibit a combination of different etiologies. Nociceptive pain may result from the stimulation of nociceptors at the nerve endings and is characteristically present in TMDs. Stress, somatic distress and depression may be potential etiological risk factors for TMDs-related pain. In chronic pain, psychological factors may become more obvious and prominent [17]. In a population-based study, 47% subjects had TMJ problems where pain is commonly accompanied by stiffness, sounds and functional limitations, which result in a decreased quality of life, and thus exert a significant negative impact on activities of daily living (ADL) [5]. The following everyday activities such as eating, talking, yawning and laughing were more disturbed [18,19,20]. It was found that the impact of TMJ pain/discomfort was the greatest on eating (ADL 9) in 68% of the men and 77% of the women and smallest on performing daily household chores (ADL 3) in 37% of the men and in 61% of the women (Table 1) [5].

	Median	IQR	% pos.	Median	IQR	% pos.
ADL questions		Male			Female	
ADL1	0	4	45	3	5	74
ADL2	0	3	37	2	4	68
ADL3	0	3	37	2	4	61
ADL4	1	5	50	4	6	68
ADL5	0	3	37	2	5	74
ADL6	0	3	45	3	5	67
ADL7	1	5	50	3	6	67
ADL8	2	5	53	3	5	74
ADL9	3	7	68	3	4	77
ADL11	0	3	50	3	6	68
ADL12	1	4	58	3	4	75

IQR = interquartile range, % pos: percentage of observations exceeding zero, ADL scale: 0–12, socialize with family and close friends? (ADL 1), perform daily work? (ADL 2), perform daily household chores (preparing meals, cleaning, taking care of small children)? (ADL 3), sit in a company or participate in other social activities (e.g. parties)? (ADL 4), exercise (walk, bicycle, jogging, etc.)? (ADL 5), perform hobbies (read, fish, knit, play an instrument)? (ADL 6), sleep at night? (ADL 7), concentrate (ADL 8), eat (chew, swallow)? (ADL 9), talking (laughing, singing)? (ADL 10), yawn, open mouth wide? (ADL 11), how much does the pain/discomfort affect your daily activities? (ADL 12) where 0 = activity without any pain/discomfort at all and 12 = activity impossible due to pain/ discomfort.

Table 1. The influence of temporomandibular joint pain/discomfort on activities of daily living

2.2. Temporomandibular joint Disorders (TMD)

Temporomandibular joint disorders refer to several clinical conditions that involve muscles of mastication and TMJ or both [21]. Also, TMD are associated with disc displacement [22]. The etiology of TMD is multifactorial, being related to factors such as stress, muscle hyperactivity, arthrogenous factors, parafunctions or the anatomy of the TMJ [23]. The knowledge of the pathogenesis on a molecular level of disorders of the TMJ has been improved by allowing a possibility to use these data for the evidence-based treatment [24-26].

Signs and symptoms of TMD may include pain, impaired jaw function, malocclusion, deviation or deflection, limited range of motion, joint noise and locking. Headache, tinnitus, visual changes and other neurologic complaints may also accompany TMD. It has been found that 28% of the adult population have signs of temporomandibular joint disorder, with higher prevalence in women at reproductive ages [11,27–29]. Women report more pain, TMJ pain of longer duration, higher clinical and experimental pain intensity and lower pain thresholds [30]. Together with arthralgia of the temporomandibular joints, it is collectively referred to as 'temporomandibular disorder' [8].

The TMJ involvement may occur in systemic rheumatic diseases (rheumatoid arthritis, psoriatic arthritis, etc.), secondary from the neighbouring regions (otitis, maxillary sinusitis, tonsillitis), trauma (chronic), prevalence of dental arch defects, e.g. missing of molar teeth, malocclusion, endocrinological disturbances, odontogenic infections [31]. Many specific bacteria and several inflammatory mediators play an important role in the pathogenesis of TMJ diseases [32-34]. These inflammatory mediators drive catabolic pathways, inhibit matrix synthesis and promote cellular apoptosis. The bone loss at the TMJ condyle involves a common resorptive pathway: cytokine-activated osteoblasts promote activity of osteoclasts, which in turn result in the secretion of enzymes that are responsible for the breakdown of hydroxyapatite and collagen [35].

The most common form of TMJ arthritis is osteoarthritis (OA). It is one of the chronic diseases that involves TMJ [2]. The OA is classified as follows: (a) primary, which is idiopathic, i.e. factors are unknown; (b) secondary, where local and systemic factors are identified. It is mentioned that in secondary OA systemic causes are related to ethnicity, nutritional factors, genetics, hormonal status and bone metabolism, where as local causes include obesity, mechanical environment, overloading of articular cartilage and acute joint injury [36,37]. Most scientists regard osteoarthritis as an inflammatory process, being the most frequent TMJ disorder, characterized by proliferative changes in the synovia and primary degeneration of the cartilage and surrounding tissues with destruction of the bone structures and causing TMJ pain [24,38]. Nowadays, it is increasingly recognized that OA is a disease of the whole joint that affects all articular structures, including articular cartilage, subchondral bone, synovium, tendons, ligaments and menisci. The role of bone and articular soft tissues in the pathophysiology of OA has been widely overlooked [39].

3. Diagnostics of temporomandibular joint disorders

3.1. Activities of Daily Living (ADL) and the Visual Analogue Scale (VAS)

The impact of pain on the health status and quality of life in patients with chronic inflammatory joint diseases has been recognized, but there is a lack of knowledge about the specific impact of TMJ pain on daily activities in patients with clinical involvement of the TMJ [18]. Assessment of the individual level of daily activities is important in the evaluation of TMD. There are several scales for assessing patients' TMJ functions and for describing the particulars of their disability and the fact how their current status reflects in their day-to-day activities.

The term 'activities of daily living'(ADL) has been used to denote activities undertaken as part of a person's daily functions [40]. The ADL scale by Katz et al. [41] was primarily designed to measure the ability to carry out every day activities necessary for daily living. It has been validated and modified for specific use in patients with TMJ disorders [18,42–44]. Use of an ADL questionnaire is a very convenient method for pain assessment. This questionnaire is very simple and easy to handle and it can be recommended for future clinical trials in patients with TMJ disorders [45,46]. Only a few systematic reviews have addressed to daily activities or quality of life in relation to management of TMJ disorders. It is concluded that the use of specific questionnaires is justified for assessment of the character of TMJ pain [5].

The visual analogue scale (VAS) is a single-item scale to measure pain intensity [47]. The VAS is a continuous scale comprised of a horizontal or vertical line, usually 10 cm (100 mm) in length, anchored by two verbal descriptors, one for each symptom extreme. For pain intensity, the scale is most commonly anchored by 'no pain' (score of 0) and 'pain as bad as it could be' or 'worst imaginable pain' (score of 100 [100-mm scale; 48,49]. The VAS was initially used in psychology by Freud in the early 1900s and was elaborated in rheumatology through a series of investigations by Huskisson et al. in the late 1970s [50]. The scale has a high degree of sensitivity and validity because slight changes in pain intensity can be detected; however, it can also be confusing in a way for both very young and elderly patients [51,52]. The VAS scale has been used in several TMJ studies [53–56].

3.2. Radiographic imaging

Radiographic examination is commonly used for assessment of TMJ problems. Radiographic changes of the TMJ can be evaluated by orthopantomography, computed tomography and magnet resonance imaging [57,58] among other techniques, as well as by ultrasonography [59].

3.2.1. Orthopantomography (OPTG)

Orthopantomography (OPTG) is most commonly used for assessment of bone changes in the TMJ. By evaluating OPTGs, the following radiographic signs of bone structural changes can be detected, such as presence of erosions, flattening and osteophytes of the TMJ condyle as well as of temporal bone [60,61]. OPTGs give the possibility to describe structural changes in bone in different regions as alveolar cortical thickness of the mandible, lamina dura width, alveolar bone hight, mandibular bone mineral density (BMD) and status of teeth [62–66]. The studies have shown that mandibular cortical shape on OPTGs may be an indicator of bone turnover and spine BMD [67–70].

The most visible radiographic sign in the TMJ by OPTG is erosion (Figure 1).

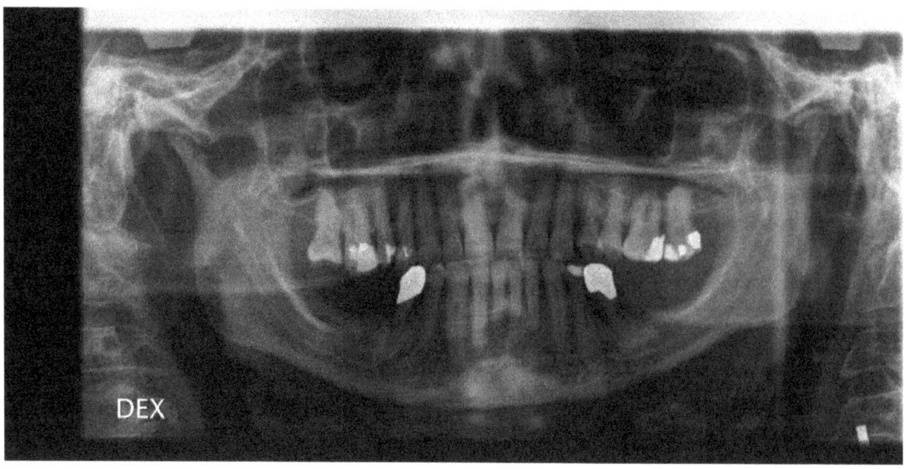

Figure 1. Ortopantomograph. Subchondral bony erosions of the right mandibular condyles are visible. Narrowing of both temporomandibular joint spaces and an irregularity of joint surfaces is observed.

The mandibular cortical erosion has been significantly associated with increased N-telopeptide cross-links of type I collagen and alkaline phosphatase levels [71]. Recent investigations have shown that radiographic examination including OPTG may be an effective tool as primary changes appear in alveolar bone for the early diagnosis of osteoporosis [4,72–75]. OPTGs could be useful as a simple screening method to estimate bone structure changes in the TMJ as well as to provide valuable information about the quality of the jaw bone such as joint space narrowing, osteophytes, subchondral sclerosis and subchondral cysts [76].

The total sum of radiographic changes in the TMJ is observed in 57% of the participants. Erosions occurred in 80%, flattening occurred in 37% and osteophytes occurred in 5% of the participants (Figure 2) [77].

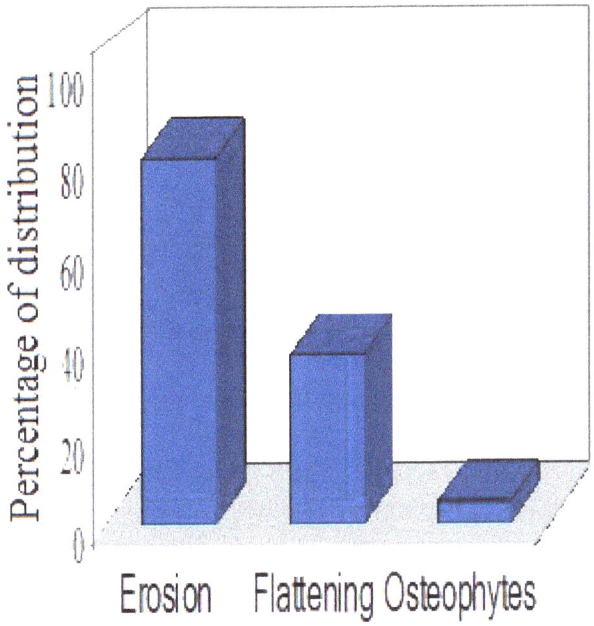

Figure 2. Distribution of radiographic changes.

3.2.2. Computed Tomography (CT)

The first report of TMJ computed tomography (CT) was published by Suarez et al. in 1980 [78] and this method is superior to plain transcranial or transmaxillary imaging for detecting bone changes. CT allows detailed three-dimensional examination of the TMJ and it is capable to detect even small bone changes not demonstrable by conventional tomographic procedures [2,79]. According to Rohlin and Petersson [80], the changes can be investigated by CT as follows: erosion – a local area with decreased density of the cortical joint surface including or not including adjacent subcortical bone, sclerosis – a local area with increased density of the cortical bony joint surface that may extend into the subcortical bone, subchondral pseudocyst (a well-defined local area of bone rarefication underneath an intact cortical outlining of the joint surface; Figure 3) and flattening (a flat bony contour deviating from the convex form osteophyte – a marginal bony outgrowth; Figure 4).

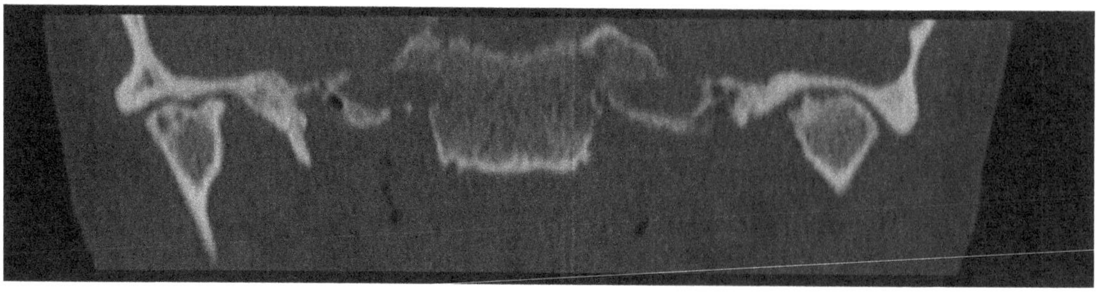

Figure 3. Osteoarthritis of TMJ. Bilateral signs of erosions on the surfaces of the condyles in a coronal view of the CT. Subchondral cyst in the right condyle. The joint spaces are asymmetric.

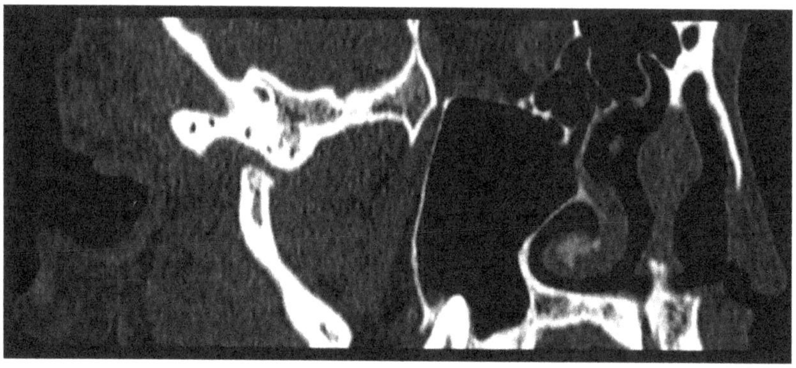

Figure 4. Sagittal view of the CT, right TMJ in an open mouth position. Sign of flattening of the mandibular condyle.

The CT allows to diagnose TMJ fractures, ankylosis, dislocation, neoplasms and growth abnormalities such as condylar hyperplasia [81]. The first choice for TMJ pathology diagnostics is OPTG; the CT imaging must improve treatment planning and prognosis.

4. The role of bone markers, vitamin D and osteoporosis in the pathogenesis of TMD

4.1. C-Telopeptidecrosslaps of type I collagen (CTX-1) and procollagen type I N-terminal Propeptide (P1NP)

Although several markers have been described to measure bone metabolism, it has been difficult to differ between the different mechanisms of bone resorption. These assays measure, in serum or in urine, enzymes or matrix proteins synthesized or degraded by bone cells [6]. It is stated that the most sensitive markers of bone resorption are C-telopeptidecrosslaps of type I collagen (CTX-1) and C-terminal telopeptide of type I collagen (1CTP), which are released from bone by different enzymatic pathways. The key osteoclastic enzyme for systemic bone resorption is generated by cathepsin K. The 1CTP is generated by matrix-metalloproteinases which plays an important role in collagen degradation associated with systemic inflammatory disease [82]. Procollagen type I N-terminal propeptide (P1NP) is a sensitive marker of bone formation. P1NP is synthesized by osteoblasts from type I procollagen precursor proteins. These precursors have large extension domains at both ends. While type I collagen is being synthesized, type I aminoterminal and carboxyterminal propeptides, PINP and PICP, respectively, are enzymatically removed and released into the circulation [83]. As bone is the major structure synthesizing type I collagen, PINP and PICP reflect bone formation [84]. Bone markers provide information beyond that of a single bone density measurement and on the cellular process leading to bone loss [85]. However, some of the few studies have not reported relationship between biomarkers and BMD [86]. Serum bone biomarkers are associated not only with systemic BMD loss but also with alveolar bone loss [87]. Biomarkers have the potential to provide an early warning of the initiation of breakdown of the articular matrix, which in future could lead to earlier treatment to prevent joint destruction that leads to disability [88].

The markers of joint tissue metabolism have opened new possibilities for earlier diagnosis of radiographic changes in joints and of OA [89,90]. It is found [77] that subjects with increased levels of P1NP, CTX-1 have less TMJ pain/discomfort. Increased levels of CTX-1 would probably cause an immediate increase of P1NP, which is known as a sensitive marker of bone formation. Subjects with a lower BMD had significantly less occluding pairs of teeth (Figure 5).

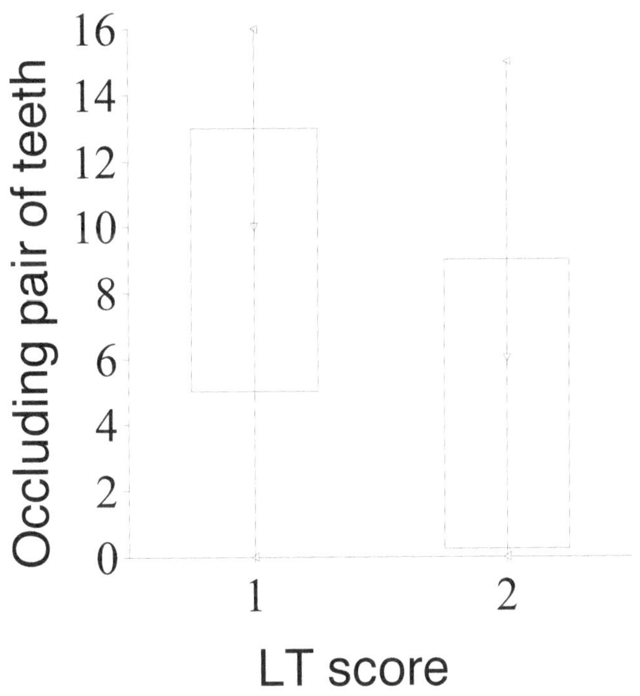

Figure 5. Relationship between occluding pair of teeth and LT score. Box plot showing the relationship between occluding pair of teeth and LT score. Box number 1 – subjects with normal mineral density. Box number 2 – subjects with lower LT score.

There are not enough data about the bone characteristics of patients with TMJ disorders. There still remains the question whether osteopenia in the TMJ area of the mandible is a local manifestation of osteoporosis having similar aetiology and risk factors, or it is an independent process depending primarily on factors that cause bone structural changes in the TMJ [75]. All these points to the need for additional studies which would evaluate the influence of potential contributing factors to further define the relationship between bone markers and TMJ disorders in population.

4.2. Vitamin D (25(OH)D)

Vitamin D (25(OH)D) plays an important role in calcium and bone metabolism inhibiting cytokine production and cell proliferation in various tissues [91]. Low levels of vitamin D lead to compensatory elevation of parathyroid hormone, which can cause lowering of BMD and eventually osteoporosis [92,93]. Vitamin D is related to musculoskeletal functioning and has been associated with a lower incidence of several cancers and autoimmune diseases. Studies have also shown that vitamin D has a role in neuromuscular function [94-96].

A majority of studies examined the association between serum 25(OH)D concentration and physical performance in community-dwelling older adults [93,95,97–99]. In particular, elderly people have a higher risk of vitamin D insufficiency, but it affects all age groups [100,101]. Low levels of 25(OH)D in young people can be partly explained by inadequate dietary sources and low activity in the daytime. It is estimated that vitamin D inadequacy is present in 36% of healthy young adults and in 57% of general medicine inpatients in the United States [102,103]. Vitamin D insufficiency seems a common health problem for people who live in countries at high latitudes where sunshine hours are short in the winter. Also Vitamin D levels are affected by modifiable and non-modifiable factors such as diet, time outdoors, skin pigmentation, sunbathing habits and medications [104,105,106]. Limited clinical research has focused on the specific effects of vitamin D deficiency on jaw pain. It is reported that vitamin D deficiency can cause predisposition to TMJ disorders [5,77,107,108].

A number of studies have addressed the relationship between sex hormones and TMDs and between low levels of vitamin D and pain all over the body but have not described the relationship between vitamin D and TMDs.

It was found [5] that lowering of 25(OH)D correlated negatively with activities of daily living such as social life with family (ADL 1), other social activities (ADL 4), exercising (ADL 5), performing hobbies (ADL 6), concentrating (ADL 8), eating (ADL 9), how much the pain/discomfort affects daily activities (ADL 12; Fig. 6). The women had lower 25(OH)D level compared to the men.

4.3. Osteoporosis

Osteoporosis is one of the most common human bone diseases affecting millions of people, including over one-third of females above the age of 65 years and generally characterized by low bone mass, with increase in bone fragility and susceptibility to fracture. According to the World Health Organization, osteoporosis is considered to be present when BMD is 2.5 standard deviations (SD) below the young normal. Osteopenia is defined as bone density levels between 1 SD and 2.5 SD below normal BMD. Osteopenia is a reduction in bone mass due to imbalance

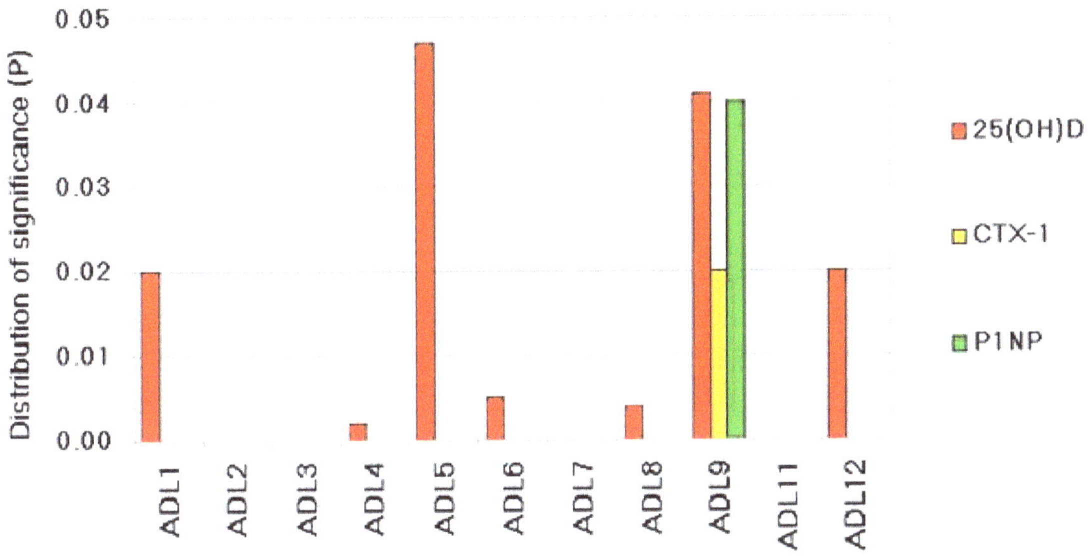

Figure 6. Distribution of significance between ADL data and bone characteristics. Relationship between bone characteristics and activities of daily living.

between bone resorption and formation, favouring resorption, resulting in demineralization and leading to osteoporosis [109]. The risk factors for osteoporosis are: sex, age, low body mass, early menopause, race, heredity, physical inactivity, lack of calcium intake, smoking and alcohol consumption [66].

The association between osteoporosis and oral bone disease was found already in 1960 [110]. Osteoporosis can affect all craniofacial and oral structures [76]. Osteoporosis is reported to cause bone loss in the alveolar processes of the maxilla and the mandible, which provides bony framework for tooth anchorage [111]. Some researchers have investigated whether dental radiographs could play a role in the detection of individuals with osteoporosis [112]. Bone mass in the jaw might be related to that of other skeletal sites in which osteoporosis was a significant problem [113,114]. The association between systemic osteoporosis and oral health remains controversial [115] while studies in this area are limited. Therefore, the relationship between systemic osteoporosis and oral health is still a complex problem of great interest for a large number of researchers and clinicians. Some epidemiological studies found that non-osteoporotic women's mandibular bone mass was not affected by age but was significantly associated with skeletal bone mass at the spine and wrist. The trabecular pattern was a highly significant predictor of future skeletal fracture risk [63,116]. Biochemical markers of bone turnover can be used to predict individual bone loss and therefore, they may help to alert patients to the risk of pathologies in the TMJ [4]. Thus, studies which evaluate the above mentioned contributing factors to define relationship between TMJ pain and several bone characteristics and ADL in population are justified.

The radiographic changes in the TMJ seem to be related to BMD. The patients with severe erosion of the cortex had significantly lower BMD values. In a population-based study was found out of 95 participants, 42% had abnormally low values of LT score. Among them osteoporosis was observed in 10.4% and osteopenia in 31.6% [77].

5. Conclusion

It is demonstrated that pain/discomfort originating from the TMJ is influenced by the biochemical markers of bone turnover. TMJ radiographic changes and teeth loss seem to be related to the low levels of BMD and 25(OH)D. The finding leads to the possible role of 25(OH)D in lowering of BMD in the TMJ and eventually osteoporosis. These findings indicate that presence of lowering BMD seems to be as one of the predictors for TMJ bone destruction.

Associations between TMJ pain/discomfort with vitamin D with the activities of daily living is evident. Subjects with lower 25(OH)D values experienced difficulties in performing physical exercises, engaging hobbies, they have problems with eating, participating in static social gatherings or other social activities. The social life of these persons is disrupted to a considerable degree. The median value of TMJ pain in the male as well as in the female group was relatively high considering that the study sample consisted of voluntary participants. Comparing the different sexes, we found highly significant correlations between female gender in following activities of daily living: social life, performing daily work, performing daily household chores, exercising, performing hobbies and yawning and opening the mouth wide. The same correlations in male were less significant.

Low 25(OH)D level can predict TMJ bone destruction and additional vitamin D consumption might be suggested to avoid TMJ dysfunction.

It is found that subjects with increased levels of P1NP, CTX-1 have less TMJ pain/discomfort. Increased levels of CTX-1 would probably cause an immediate increase of P1NP, which is known as a sensitive marker of bone formation.

Correlation between these two markers is probably due to equal shift / balance in a normal bone metabolism, where osteoblasts are acting simultaneously with osteoclasts.

The tight interaction and coordination between different aspects of TMD can be as a puzzle for health professionals. Based on obtained knowledge, the accuracy of diagnosis, quality of treatment as well as care for TMD can improve in the nearest future.

Acknowledgements

The study was financially supported by targeted funding project IUT2-8, by grant 6591 of the Estonian Science Foundation, by the European Union through the European Social Fund and by Ermst Jaakson Memorial Scholarship.

Author details

Oksana Ivask[1*], Ülle Voog-Oras[1] and Edvitar Leibur[2]

*Address all correspondence to: oksana.ivask@kliinikum.ee

1 Department of Stomatology, University of Tartu, Estonia

2 Departments of Stomatology and InternalMedicine, University of Tartu, Estonia

References

[1] Guo C, Shi Z, Revington P. Arthrocentesis and lavage for treating temporomandibular joint disorders. Cochrane Database Systemat Rev 2009;7(4):CD004973.

[2] Lee JY, Kim DJ, Lee SG, Chung JW. A longitudinal study on the osteoarthritic change of the temporomandibular joint based on 1-year follow-up computed tomography. J Cranio-Maxillo-Facial Surg 2012;40(8):e223–8.

[3] Israel HA, Langevin CJ, Singer MD, Behrman DA. The relationship between temporomandibular joint synovitis and adhesions: pathogenic mechanisms and clinical implications for surgical management. J Oral Maxillofacial Surg 2006;64(7):1066–74.

[4] Vlasiadis KZ, Damilakis J, Velegrakis GA, Skouteris CA, Fragouli I, Goumenou A, Matalliotakis J, Koumantakis EE. Relationship between BMD, dental panoramic radiographic findings and biochemical markers of bone turnover in diagnosis of osteoporosis. Maturitas 2008;59(3):226–33.

[5] Jagur O, Kull M, Leibur E, Kallikorm R, Lember M, Voog-Oras U. The associations of TMJ pain and bone characteristics on the activities of daily living. Open J Stomatol 2012;2(12):237–43.

[6] Garnero P, Ferreras M, Karsdal MA, Nicamhlaoibh R, Risteli J, Borel O, Qvist P, Delmas PD, Foged NT, Delaisse JM. The type I collagen fragments ICTP and CTX reveal distinct enzymatic pathways of bone collagen degradation. J Bone Miner Res 2003;18(5):859–67.

[7] Kull M Jr, Kallikorm R, Tamm A, Lember M. Seasonal variance of 25-(OH) vitamin D in the general population of Estonia, a Nothern European country. BMC Public Health 2009;9:22–33.

[8] Okeson JP. Management of Temporomandibular Disorders and Occlusion. In: St. Louis. Mosby; 2003; pp. 413–435.

[9] Helkimo M. Studies on function and dysfunction of the masticatory system. I. An epidemiological investigation of symptoms of dysfunction in Lapps in the north of Finland. Acta Odontol Scandinav 1974;32(4):225–65.

[10] Dworkin SF, Huggins KH, LeResche L, Von Korff M, Howard J, Truelove E, et al. Epidemiology of signs and symptoms in temporomandibular disorders: clinical signs in cases and controls. J Am Dental Assoc 1990;120(3):273–81.

[11] LeResche L. Epidemiology of temporomandibular disorders: implications for the investigation of etiologic factors. Crit Rev Oral Biol Med 1997;8(3):291–305.

[12] John MT, Dworkin SF, Mancl LA. Reliability of clinical temporomandibular disorder diagnoses. Pain 2005;118(1–2):61–9.

[13] Svensson P, Jadidi F, Arima T, Baad H, Sessle BJ. Relationships between craniofacial pain and bruxism. J Oral Rehab 2008;35(7):524–47.

[14] Kelley P, Clifford P. Coping with chronic pain: assessing narrative approaches. Social Work 1997;42(3):266–77.

[15] Thomas SP. A phenomenologic study of chronic pain. West J Nurs Res 2000;22(6): 6836–99.

[16] Tjakkes GH, Reinders JJ, Tenvergert EM, Stegenga B. TMD pain: the effect on health related quality of life and the influence of pain duration. Health Quality Life Outcomes 2010;28:46.

[17] Zakrzewska JM. Trigeminal neuralgia. In: Zakrzewska JM, Harrison SD. (Eds.) Assessment and Management of Orofacial Pain, 1st edn. Amsterdam: Elsevier Sciences; 2002; pp. 267–370.

[18] Voog U, Alstergren P, Leibur E, Kallikorm R, Kopp S. Impact of temporomandibular joint pain on activities of daily living in patients with rheumatoid arthritis. Acta Odontol Scandinav 2003a;61(5):278–82.

[19] Bessa-Nogueira RV, Vasconcelos B, Niederman R. The methodological quality of systematic reviews comparing temporomandibular joint disorder surgical and non-surgical treatment. BMC Oral Health 2008;26:8–27.

[20] De Boever JA, Carlsson GE, Klineberg IJ. Need for occlusal therapy and prosthodontic treatment in the management of temporomandibular disorders. Part I. Occlusal interferences and occlusal adjustment. J Oral Rehab 2000;27(5):367–79.

[21] Peck CC, Goulet JP, Lobbezoo F, Schiffman EL,Alstergren P, Anderson GC, de Leeuw R, Jensen R, Michelotti A, Ohrbach R, Petersson A, List T. Expanding the taxonomy of the diagnostic criteria for temporomandibular disorders. J Oral Rehab 2014;41(1):2–23.

[22] Barkin S, Weinberg S. Internal derangements of the temporomandibular joint: the role of arthroscopic surgery and arthrocentesis. J (Canad Dental Assoc) 2000;66(4): 199–203.

[23] Yáñez-Vico RM, Iglesias-Linares A, Torres-Lagares D, Gutiérrez-Pérez JL, Solano-Reina E. Association between condylar asymmetry and temporomandibular disorders using 3D-CT. Med Oral, Patol Oral y Cirugia Bucal 2012;17(5):e852–8.

[24] Holmlund AB, Axelsson S. Temporomandibular arthropathy: correlation between clinical signs and symptoms and arthroscopic findings. Int J Oral Maxillofacial Surg 1996;25(3):266–71.

[25] Kumagai K, Hamada Y, DDS, Holmlund AB, Gotoh A, Nakaoka K, et al. The levels of vascular endothelial growth factor in the synovial fluid correlated with the severity of arthroscopically observed synovitis and clinical outcome after temporomandibular joint irrigation in patients with chronic closed lock. Oral Surg Oral Med Oral Pathol Oral Rad Endodontics 2010;109(2):185–90.

[26] Guarda-Nardini L, PavanCk, Arveda N, Ferronato G, Manfredini D. Psychometric features of temporomandibular disorders patients in relation to pain diffusion, location, intensity and duration. J Oral Rehab 2012a;(39):737–73.

[27] Bagis Bhttp://www.medsci.org/v09p0539.htm – coraddress, Aydogan E, Turgut S, Durkan R, Özcan M. Gender difference in prevalence of signs and symptoms of temporomandibular joint disorders: a retrospective study on 243 consecutive patients. Int J Med Sci 2012;9(7):539–44.

[28] Rezaii T, Hirschberg AL, Carlström K, Ernberg M. The influence of menstrual phases on pain modulation in healthy women. J Pain 2012;13(7):646–55.

[29] Sipila K, Näpänkangas R, Könönen M, Alanen P, Siominen AL. The role of dental loss and denture status on clinical signs of temporomandibular disorders. J Oral Rehab 2013;40(1):15–23.

[30] Rezaii T, Ernberg M. Infuence of oral contraceptives on endogenous pain control in healthy women. Experiment Brain Res 2010;203(2):329–38.

[31] Tallents RH, Macher DJ, Kyrkanides S, Katzberg RW, Moss ME. Prevalence of missing posterior teeth and intraarticular temporomandibular disorders. J Prosthet Dentist 2002;87(1):45–50.

[32] Kim SJ, Park YH, Hong SP, Cho BO, Park JW, Kim SG. The presence of Bacteria in the synovial fluid of the temporomandibular joint and clinical significance: preliminary study. J Oral Maxillofacial Surg 2003;61(10):1156–61.

[33] Voog Ü, Alstergren P, Eliasson S, Leibur E, Kallikorm R, Kopp S. Inflammatory mediators and radiographic changes in temporomandibular joints with rheumatoid arthritis. Acta Odontol Scandinav 2003b;60:57–65.

[34] Hamada Y, Holmlund AB, Kondoh T, Nakaoka K, Sekiya H, Shiobara N, et al. Severity of arthroscopically observed pathology and levels of inflammatory cytokines in the synovial fluid before and after visually guided temporomandibular joint irrigation correlated with the clinical outcome in patients with chronic closed lock. Oral Surg Oral Med Oral Pathol Oral Radiol Endodontics 2008;106(3):343–9.

[35] Gunson MJ, Arnett GW, Milam SB. Pathophysiology and pharmacologic control of osseous mandibular condylar resorption. J Oral Maxillofacial Surg 2012;70(8):1918–34.

[36] Jordan JM, Kingtom RS, LaneNe, Nevitt MC, Zhang Y, Sowers MF, et al. Systemic risk factors for osteoarthritis. In: Felson DT, conference chair. Osteoarthritis: new insights. Part I: The disease and its risk factors. Annal Internal Med 2000;133(8):637–9.

[37] Kang SC, Lee DG, Choi JH, Kim ST, Kim YK, Ahn HJ. Association between estrogen receptor polymorphism and pain susceptibility in female temporomandibular joint osteoarthritis patients. Int J Oral Maxillofacial Surg 2007;36:391–4.

[38] Emshoff R. Clinical factors affecting the outcome of arthrocentesis and hydraulic distension of the temporomandibular joint. Oral Surg Oral Med Oral Pathol Oral Radiol Endodontics 2005;100(4):409–14.

[39] Brandt KD, Doherty M, Lohmander LS. Definition and classification of osteoarthritis.In: Brandt KD, Doherty M, Lohmander LS. (Eds.) Osteoarthritis. New York: Oxford University Press; 2003.

[40] Bucks SR, Haworth J. Bristol activities of daily living scale: a critical evaluation. Expert Rev Neurotherapeutics 2002;2(5):669–76.

[41] Katz S, Ford AB, Moskowitz RW, Jackson BA, Jaffe MW. Studies of illness in the aged. The index of ADL: a standardized measure of biological and psychological function. JAMA 1963;185:914–9.

[42] List T, Helkimo M. A scale for measuring the activities of daily living (ADL) of patients with craniomandibular disorders. Swed Dental J 1995;19(1–2):33–40.

[43] Kaselo E, Jagomägi T, Voog Ü. Malocclusion and the need for orthodontic treatment in patients with temporomandibular dysfunction. Stomatologija, Baltic Dental Maxillofacial J 2007;9(3):79–85.

[44] Karibe H, Goddard G, Aoyagi K, Kawakami T, Warita S, Shimazu K, Rudd PA, McNeill C. Comparison of subjective symptoms of temporomandibular disorders in young patients by age and gender.Cranio 2012;30(2):114–20.

[45] Murakami K, Segami N, Okamoto I, Takahashi K, Tsuboi Y. Outcome of arthroscopic surgery for internal derangement of the temporomandibular joint: long-term results covering 10 years. J Cranio-Maxillo-Facial Surg 2000;28(5):264–71.

[46] Undt G, Murakami K, Clark GT, Ploder O, Dem A, Lang T, et al. Cross–cultural adaptation of the JPF-Questionnarie for German speaking patients with functional temporomandibular joint disorders. J Cranio-Maxillo-Facial Surg 2006;34(4):226–33.

[47] McCormack HM, Horne DJ, Sheather S. Clinical applications of visual analogue scales: a critical review. Psychol Med 1988;18(4):1007–19.

[48] Burckhardt CS, Jones KD. Adult measures of pain: The McGill Pain Questionnaire (MPQ), Rheumatoid Arthritis Pain Scale (RAPS), Short-Form McGill Pain Questionnaire (SF-MPQ), Verbal Descriptive Scale (VDS), Visual Analog Scale (VAS), and West Haven-Yale Multidisciplinary Pain Inventory (WHYMPI). Arthritis Care Res 2003;49:S96–104.

[49] Hawker GA, Mian S, Kendzerska T, French M. Measures of adult pain: Visual Analog Scale for Pain (VAS Pain), Numeric Rating Scale for Pain (NRS Pain), McGill Pain Questionnaire (MPQ), Short-Form McGill Pain Questionnaire (SF-MPQ), Chronic Pain Grade Scale (CPGS), Short Form-36 Bodily Pain Scale (SF-36BPS), and Measure of Intermittent and Constant Osteoarthritis Pain (ICOAP). Arthritis Care Res 2011;63(11):S240–52.

[50] Sokka T. Assessment of pain in patients with rheumatic diseases. Best Practise Res Clin Rheumatol 2003;17(3):427–49.

[51] Gagliese L, Weizblit N, Ellis W, et al. The measurement of postoperative pain: a comparison of intensity scales in younger and older surgical patients. Pain 2005;117(3): 412–20.

[52] Williamson A, Hoggart B. Pain: a review of three commonly used pain rating scales. J Clin Nurs 2005;14(7):798–804.

[53] Ahn HJ, Lee YS, Jeong SH, Kang SM, Byun YS, KIM BI. Objective and subjective assessment of masticatory function for patients with temporomandibular disorder in Korea. J Oral Rehab 2011;38(7):475–81.

[54] Rusanen J, Silvola AS, Tolvanen M, Pirttiniemi P, Lahti S, Sipilä K. Pathways between temporomandibular disorders, occlusal characteristics, facial pain, and oral health-related quality of life among patients with severe malocclusion. Eur J Orthodontics 2012;34(4):512–7.

[55] Edefonti V, Bravi F, Cioffi I, Capuozzo R, Ammendola L, Abate G, Decarli A, Ferraroni M, Farella M, Michelotti A. Chronic pain and weather conditions in patients suffering from temporomandibular disorders: a pilot study. Commun Dentist Oral Epidemiol 2012;40(1):56–64.

[56] Guarda-Nardini L, Cadorin C, Frizziero A, Ferronato A, Manfredini D. Comparison of 2 hyaluronic acid drugs for the treatment of temporomandibular joint osteoarthritis. J Oral Maxillofacial Surg 2012b;70(11):2522–30.

[57] Ohnuki T, Fukuda M, Iino M, Takahashi T. Magnetic resonance evaluation of the disk before and after arthroscopic surgery for temporomandibular disorders. Oral Surg Oral Med Oral Pathol Oral Radiol Endodontics 2003;96(2):141–8.

[58] Whyte AM, McNamara D, Rosenberg I, Whyte AW. Magnetic resonance imaging in the evaluation of temporomandibular joint disc displacement. Int J Oral Maxillofacial Surg 2006;35(8):696–703.

[59] Landes CA, Sader R. Sonographic evaluation of the ranges of condylar translation and of temporomandibular joint space as well as first comparison with symptomatic joints. J Cranio-Maxillo-Facial Surg 2007;35(8):374–81.

[60] Rohlin M. Åkerman S, Kopp S. Tomography as an aid to detect macroscopic changes of the temporomandibular joint. Acta Odontol Scandinav 1986;44(3):131–40.

[61] Helenius L, Hallikainen D, Meurman J, Koskimies S, Tervahartiala P, Kivisaari L, Hietanen J, Suuronen R, Lindqvist C, Lerisalo-Repo M. HLA-DRB1 alleles and temporomandibular joint erosion in patientes with rheumatic disease. Scand J Rheumatol 2004;33:24–9.

[62] Leibur E, Jian JL, Söder PÖ. Alveolar bone level on intraoral and panoramic radiographs analysed by a computerized image system. Oral Surg Oral Diag 1995;6(2):13–7.

[63] Jeffcoat MK, Lewis CE, Reddy MS, Wank CY, Redford M. Post-menopausal bone loss and its relationship to oral bone loss. Periodontology 2000;23:94–102.

[64] Jonasson G, Bankvall G, Kiliaridis S. Estimation of skeletal bone mineral density by means of the trabecular pattern of the alveolar bone, its interdental thickness and the bone mass of the mandible. Oral Surg Oral Med Oral Pathol Oral Radiol Endodontics 2001;92(3):346–52.

[65] Krejc CB, Bissada NF. Womens health issues and their relationship to periodontitis. J Am Dental Assoc 2002;133(3):323–8.

[66] Hardanti S, Azhari, Oscandar F. Description of mandibular bone quality based on measurements of cortical thickness using Mental Index of male and female patients between 40-60 years old. Imaging Sci Dentist 2011;41(4):151–3.

[67] Balcikonyte E, Balciuniene I, Alekna V. Panoramic radiographs in assessment of the bone mineral density. Stomatologija, Baltic Dental and Mafillofacial J 2004;6:17–9.

[68] Vlasiadis KZ, Skouteris CA, Velegrakis GA, Fragouli I, Neratzoulakis JM, Damilakis J, et al. Mandibular radiomorphometric measurements as indicators of possible osteoporosis in postmenopausal women. Maturitas 2007;58(3):226–35.

[69] Taguchi A. Panoramic radiographs for identifying individuals with undetected osteoporosis. Jap Dental Sci Rev 2009;45(2):109–20.

[70] Hastar E, Yilmaz HH, Orhan H. Evaluation of mental index, mandibular cortical index and panoramic mandibular index on dental panoramic radiographs in the elderly. Eur J Dentist 2011;5(1):60–7.

[71] Taguchi A, Tsuda M, Ohtsuka M, Kodama I, Sanada M, Nakamoto T, et al. Use of dental panoramic radiographs in identifying younger postmenopausal women with osteoporosis. Osteoporosis Int 2006;17(3):387–94.

[72] Bonnick SL, Shulman L. Monitoring osteoporosis therapy: bone mineral density, bone turnover markers, or both? Am J Med 2006;119(4 Suppl 1):25–31.

[73] Jagelaviciene E, Kubilius R. The relationship between general osteoporosis of the organism and periodontal diseases. Medicina 2006;42(8):613–8.

[74] Miliuniene E, Alekna V, Peciuliene V, Tamulaitiene M, Maneliene R. Relationship between mandibular cortical bone height and bone mineral density of lumbar spine. Stomatologija. Baltic Dental Maxillofacial J 2008;10(2):72–5.

[75] Khatoonabad MJ, Aghamohammadzade N, Taghilu H, Esmaeili HF, Khamnei J. Relationship among panoramic radiography findings, biochemical markers of bone turnover and hip BMD in the diagnosis of postmenopausal osteoporosis. Iran J Radiol 2011;8(1):23–8.

[76] Aggarwal A, Panat SR. Identification of postmenopausal women at risk of osteoporosis using panoramic and intraoral radiographs – a review. Minerva Stomatol 2012;61(7–8):323–8.

[77] Jagur O, Kull M, Leibur E, Kallikorm R, Loorits D, Lember M, Voog-Oras U. Relationship between radiographic changes in the temporomandibular joint and bone mineral density: a population based study. Stomatologija 2011;13(2):42–8.

[78] Suarez FR, Bhussry BR, Neff PA, Huang HK, Vaughn D (1980). A preliminary study of computerized tomographs of the temporomandibular joint. Compend Continuing Edu Gen Dentist 1980;1(3):217–22.

[79] Larheim TA, Westesson P, Sano T. Temporomandibular joint disk displacement: comparison in asymptomatic volunteers and patients. Radiology 2001;218(2):428–32.

[80] Rohlin M, Petersson A. Rheumatoid arthritis of the temporomandibular joint:radiologic evaluation based on standard reference films. Oral Surg Oral Med Oral Pathol 1989;67(5):594–9.

[81] Barghan S, Tetradis S, Mallya SM. Application of cone beam computed tomography for assessment of the temporomandibular joints. Austral Dental J 2012;57(Suppl 1): 109–18.

[82] Chopin F, Garnero P, le Henanff A, Debiais F, Daragon A, Roux C, Sany J, Wendling D, Zarnitsky C, Ravaud P, Thomas T. Long term effects of infliximab on bone and

cartilage turnover markers in patients with rheumatoid arthritis. Annal Rheumatic Dis 2008;67(3):353–7.

[83] Calvo MS, Eyre DR, Gundberg CM. Molecular basis and clinical application of biological markers of bone turnover. Endocrine Rev 1996;17(4):333–68.

[84] Delmas PD. Clinical use of biochemical markers of bone remodeling in osteoporosis. Bone 1992;13(suppl 1):S17–21.

[85] Åkesson K, Vergnaud P, Gineyts E, Delmas Obrant KJ. Impairment of bone turnover in elderly women with hip fracture. Calcif Tissue Int 1993;53(3):162–9.

[86] Cosman F, Nieves J, Wilkinson C, Schnering D, ShenV, Lindsay R. Bone density change and biochemical indices of skeletal turnover. Calcif Tissue Int 1996;58(4):236–43.

[87] Payne JB,Stoner JA, Lee HM, Nummikoski PV, Reinhardt RA, Golub LM. Serum bone biomarkers and oral/systemic bone loss in humans. J Dental Res 2011;90(6):747–51.

[88] Kraus VB, Burnett B, Coindreau J, Cottrell S, Eyre D, Gendreau M, Gardiner J, et al. Application of biomarkers in the development of drugs intended for the treatment of osteoarthritis. Osteoarthritis Cartilage 2011;19(5):515–42.

[89] Garnero P, Ayral X, Rousseau JC, Christgau S, Sandell LJ, Dougados M, et al.Uncoupling of type II collagen synthesis and degradation predicts progression ofjoint damage in patients with knee osteoarthritis. Arthritis Rheumatism 2002;46(10):2613–24.

[90] Kumm J, Tamm A, Lintrop M, Tamm A. The value of cartilage biomarkers in progressive knee osteoarthritis: cross-sectional and 6-year follow-up study in middle-aged subjects. Rheumatol Int 2012;33(4) 903–11.

[91] Dietrich T, Joshipura K. Association between serum concentrations of 25-hydroxyvitamin D 3 and periodontal disease in the US population. Am J Clin Nutrit 2004;80(1): 108–13.

[92] Kwon J, Suzuki T, Yoshida H, Kim H, Yoshida Y, Iwasa H. Concomitant lower serum albumin and vitamin D levels are associated with decreased objective physical performance among Japanese community-dwelling elderly. Gerontology 2007;53(5):322–8.

[93] Annweiler C, Beauchet O, Berrut G, Couris C, Fantino B, Bonnefoy M, Herrmann FR, Schott AM. Is there a relationship between serum vitamin D insufficiency and reduced muscle strength among older women? Results from baseline assessment of EPIDOS study. J Nutrit Health Aging 2009;13:90–5.

[94] Bischoff HA, Borchers M, Gudat F, Duermueller U, Theiler R, Stahelin HB, et al. In situ detection of 1,25-dihydroxyvitamin D3 receptor in human skeletal muscle tissue. Histochem J 2001;33(1):19–24.

[95] Bischoff-Ferrari HA, Dietrich T, Orav EJ, Dawson-Hughes B. Positive association between 25-hydroxy vitamin D levels and bone mineral density: a population-based study of younger and older adults. Am J Med 2004;116(9):634–9.

[96] Bischoff-Ferrari HA. The 25-hydroxyvitamin D threshold for better health. J Steroid Biochem Molecul Biol 2007;103(3–5):614–9.

[97] Dukas L, Staehelin HB, Schacht E, Bischoff HA. Better functional mobility in community-dwelling elderly is related to D-hormone serum levels and to daily calcium intake. J Nutrition Health Aging 2005;9(5):347–51.

[98] Gerdhem P, Ringsberg KA, Obrant KJ, Akesson K. Association between 25-hydroxy vitamin D levels, physical activity, muscle strength and fractures in the prospective population-based OPRA Study of Elderly Women. Osteoporos Int 2005;16:1425–31.

[99] Houston DK, Cesari M, Ferrucci L, Cherubini A, Maggio D, Bartali B, Johnson MA, Schwartz GG, Kritchevsky SB. Association between vitamin D status and physical performance: the InCHIANTI study. J Gerontol Ser A Biol Sci Med Sci 2007;62(4): 440–6.

[100] Chapuy MC, Preziosi P, Maamer M, Arnaud S, Galan P, Hercberg S, et al. Prevalence of vitamin D insufficiency in an adult normal population. Osteoporos Int 1997;7(5): 439–43.

[101] Lappe JM, Davies KM, Travers-Gustafson D, Heaney RP. Vitamin D status in a rural postmenopausal female population. J Am College Nutrit 2006;25(5):395–402.

[102] Holick MF. High prevalence of vitamin D inadequacy and implications for health. Mayo Clin Proc 2006;81(3):353–73.

[103] Holick MF. Vitamin D deficiency. New Engl J Med 2007;357(3):266–81.

[104] Sherman SS, Hollis BW, Tobin JD. Vitamin D status and related parameters in a healthy population: the effects of age, sex, and season. J Clin Endocrinol Metabolism 1990;71(2):405–13.

[105] Budak N, Çiçek B, Sahin H, Tutus A. Bone mineral density and serum 25-hydroxyvitamin D level: is there any difference according to the dressing style of the female university students. Int J Food Sci Nutrit 2004;55(7):569–75.

[106] Bolek-BerquistJ, Elliott ME, Ronald E,Gemar D, Engelke J, Lawrence SJ, Hansen KE. Use of a questionnaire to assess vitamin D status in young adults. Public Health Nutrit 2009;12(2):236–43.

[107] Abdel-Fattah RA. Evaluating TMJ Injuries, Volume 1. New York: Wiley Law Publications; 1992; pp. 105–112.

[108] Shen M, Luo Y, Niu Y, Chen L, Yuan X, Goltzman D, Chen N, Miao D. 1,25 (OH) 2D deficiency induces temporomandibular joint osteoarthritis *via* secretion of senescence – associated inflammatory cytokines. Bone 2013;55(2):400–9.

[109] Wactawski-Wende J, Grossi SG, Trevisan M, Genco RJ, et al. The role of osteopenia in oral bone loss and periodontal disease. J Periodontol 1996;67(10):1076–84.

[110] Groen JJ, Duyvensz F, Halsted JA. Diffuse alveolar atrophy of the jaw (non-inflammatory form of paradental disease) and presenile osteoporosis. Gerontol Clin 1960;2:68–86.

[111] Wactawski-Wende J, Hausmann E, Hovey K, Trevisan M, Grossi S, Genco RJ. The association between osteoporosis and alveolar crestal height in postmenopausal women. J Periodontol 2005;76(11):116–1124.

[112] Nackaerts O, Jacobs R, Devlin H, Pavitt S, Bleyen E, Yan B, et al. Osteoporosis detection using intraoral densitometry. DentoMaxillo Facial Radiol 2008;37(5):282–7.

[113] Kim JY, Nah KS, Jung YH.Comparison of panorama radiomorphometric indices of the mandible in normal and osteoporotic women. Kor J Oral Maxillofacial Radiol 2004;34:69–74.

[114] Hua Y, Nackaerts O, Duyck J, Maes F, Jacobs R. Bone quality assessment based on cone beam computed tomography imaging. Clin Oral Implants Res 2009;20(8):767–71.

[115] Makker A, Singh MM, Mishra G, Singh BP, Jain GK, Jadhav S. Relationship between bone turnover biomarkers, mandibular bone mineral density, and systemic skeletal bone mineral density in premenopausal and postmenopausal Indian women. Menopause 2012;19(6):642–9.

[116] Jonasson G, Sundh V, Ahlqwist M, Hakeberg M, Björkelund C, Lissner L. A prospective study of mandibular trabecular bone to predict fracture incidence in women: a low-cost screening tool in the dental clinic. Bone 2011;49(4):873–9.

10

Intra-Articular Autologous Platelet Concentrate (APC) in the Treatment of Induced Knee Osteoarthritis (OA) in Rabbits — An Arthroscopic Evaluation

Cleuza Maria de Faria Rezende, Fabíola Paes Leme, Gilcinea Santana, Esteban Osório Carmona and Jessica Alejandra Castro Varón

Abstract

The treatment of osteoarthritis is a constant challenge in veterinary and human medicine. It is a disabling disease of widespread occurrence, whose primary purpose of treatment has been the relief of pain and improvement or maintenance of joint function. New therapeutic alternatives are continuously researched around the world. Among the alternatives is the use of autologous platelet concentrate (APC) or platelet rich plasma (PRP) intra-articular. CAP may have an important role in modifying therapy of osteoarthritis. It is easy to use and relatively low cost, which has led to research interest and to a wide clinical application. Clinical use has shown positive results, but standardized scientific studies and continued evaluation of the treatment are lacking. Many questions remain unanswered. Arthroscopy is a diagnostic and therapeutic method that can help to understand the action of this therapy. Experimental studies show marked reduction of synovitis, which explains the improvement observed in clinical cases.

Keywords: Arthroscopy, cellular therapy, regenerative medicine, cranial cruciate ligament, osteoarthritis, rabbit

1. Introduction

Osteoarthritis (OA) is a progressive disease that is painful and disabling. The available treatments for OA are unsatisfactory. The early diagnosis and monitoring of OA progression and treatment persist as challenges. Joint injuries represent a large percentage of cases in the treatment routines of veterinary hospitals. Such injuries may be due to trauma or diseases such as hip or elbow dysplasia, or they may have an immune-mediated origin. All species may be affected, but due to their greater contact with humans, dogs and cats are the animals most often referred for treatment. However, treatment is often given late, which reduces the chances of effectively controlling the problem and makes these animals candidates for prosthesis or even euthanasia.

One of the most common causes of lameness in dogs is the complete or partial rupture of the cranial cruciate ligament (CCLr[1–3]), whereby joint instability induces inflammatory and cellular changes causing synovitis, osteoarthritis, meniscal injury, and joint dysfunction.[2] OA results from a complex interaction between biochemical and biomechanical factors and possible changes involving all tissues such as the articular capsule and the subchondral bone and ligaments, resulting in the destruction of articular cartilage.[4–7] Changes in the articular surface are the most well documented histologically and biochemically.[8]

Although it is a constant topic of constant studies, OA research remains challenging. The primary goal of treatment has been pain relief to maintain or improve joint function[9] using, among others, polysulfated glycosaminoglycan, chondroitin sulfate, and intra-articular hyaluronic acid, which can reduce pain and inflammation and restore the articular environment.[2] Although these substances are employed frequently in treatment routines, they do not always have the desired effect and they do not satisfactorily control the development of the injury. NSAIDs are also used in an attempt to decrease inflammation and pain, but these drugs usually offer little benefit in the control of the disease and may have deleterious effects on joints and other body systems.[10–12]

In the absence of effective control of the degenerative process, new alternative therapies have been proposed based on the intra-articular application of different types of autologous cells obtained from different sources, whose action is the improvement of the recovery of damaged tissues. These cells contain growth factors that have the ability to proliferate and differentiate into different cell types that can modulate tissue recovery. These new therapies are known as regenerative therapy and tissue engineering.[13–15]

One type of cell therapy is autologous platelet concentrate (APC) or platelet-rich plasma (PRP). The literature[16–20] reports the benefit of its use in the repair and healing of sick or injured tissues. According to Everts et al.[21] autologous platelet concentrate is employed in different clinical situations, but scientific evidence supporting its action is lacking. The correct management technique of blood samples and the proper preparation of the APC are required to avoid inconsistent results. Factors such as blood collection, the quality of APC, the platelet count, the platelet activation, the methodology, and whether it is autologous or homologous may influence the results. Despite the lack of the standardization of the techniques employed, the literature reports promising clinical results in humans[22–24], horses[25–27], and dogs.[13,16,28,29]

Clinical studies have shown early recovery and pain relief, as observed in the evaluation of dogs after receiving treatment for a rupture of the cranial cruciate ligament[13,29] and the fragmented coronoid process.[13,28,29] Because APC stimulates the healing of tissue, it has been used to treat different joint injuries, such as osteoarthritis, osteochondrosis, hip and elbow dysplasia, chondral defects, tendinitis, bursitis, menisci injuries, muscle injuries, wounds, and fractures, and it has been used as an adjunct in the treatment of the rupture of the cruciate ligament.[22,16,28,29,25,30,18,31,32] The results may vary depending on the severity of the case[33] and the method for obtaining the APC.

Different in vitro and in vivo studies show the potential effect of the APC when associated with cartilage-repair techniques or the conservative treatment of OA. Autologous platelet concentrate increases chondrocyte synthesis capabilities including the regulation of gene expression, proteoglycan production, and the deposition of collagen type II.[34–37] When associated with chondrocyte transplantation, it induces repair tissue proliferation similar to hyaline tissue with increased proteoglycan and the deposition of collagen type II by chondrocytes.[38,39] In experimental osteochondral defects in rabbits, Sun et al.[36] reported increased regeneration of cartilage and increased production of glycosaminoglycans in the extracellular matrix in the rabbits that received intra-articular APC. Kwon et al.[33] showed that APC intra-articular injection influenced the regeneration of cartilage in all degrees of severity of OA in rabbits' knees but that the regenerative power was higher in moderate than in mild injuries. The use of intra-articular APC represents an alternative treatment that seems effective, easy to use, and relatively inexpensive, which has aroused the interest of researchers for clinical use.[40]

2. Autologous Platelet Concentrate (APC)

APC or platelet-rich plasma (PRP) is defined as a substrate that contains a platelet concentration above basal levels. Platelets are a source of important growth factors and other molecules that affect chemotaxis, differentiation, proliferation, and cell synthesis activity, thus regulating physiological remodeling and tissue repair.[41–44] The properties of APC are based on the production and release of multiple growth factors and cell differentiation. After platelet activation occurs, these growth factors are released, including a growth factor beta transformer (TGF-β), a growth factor derived from platelets (PDGF), a fibroblast growth factor (FGF), a vascular endothelial growth factor (VEGF), a growth factor for connective tissue (CTGF), and a hepatocyte growth factor (HGF).[40,13,42] These growth factors have various functions and operate in conjunction with other types of cells and pro-inflammatory substances to regenerate tissues. Studies have shown that PDGF promotes collagen synthesis and TGF-β stimulates chondrogenesis.[46,47] Based on this assumption, the autologous platelet concentrate has been employed in different clinical situations with satisfactory results.

In dogs, the APC is prepared from the whole blood of the patient, 8.5 mL of which is collected via venipuncture and placed into tubes containing 1.5 mL of sodium citrate. It is then subjected to centrifugation.[13] There are different ways to obtain APC.[48–50] It can be prepared by automated methods, semi-automated methods, or the simplest way, that is, the tube method with single[13,29,51] or double centrifugation.[42] The most important method to prepare platelet concentrate is to ensure that in addition to concentrating a high number of platelets, it allows for obtaining live and inactivated platelets.[25,52] The basic principle of the APC action is to mimic the natural way of healing by organizing the elements that influence healing and taking the place of injured molecules, thereby facilitating the functional recovery of tissues.[53]

3. Platelet activation

The substances most commonly used to activate platelets in APC for clinical purposes are thrombin and calcium salts.[22,54,55] In a study by Silva et al.[16, 56, 57] and Silva,[13] there was no difference between the concentrations of growth factors in APC supernatants activated with gluconate, calcium chloride, thrombin, or batroxobin, suggesting that the APC can be activated with any of these substances in dogs and cats. Considering the cost–benefit ratio, calcium gluconate is the best option. Platelet activation is performed with 10% calcium gluconate or chloride at a ratio of 1 mL of concentrate to 0.1 mL of activating substance.[16,25]

Although experimental studies have shown the positive effect of APC employment on the return of functioning after ligament injuries, traumatic injuries to the articular cartilage, and fractures, controversy remains regarding its action on articular tissues.[58,30,48] The objective of this study was to evaluate, through video-arthroscopy, the effect of APC in experimental OA in rabbits.

4. Materials and methods

The project was approved by the Ethics Committee on Animal Use (ECAU) of the Federal University of Minas Gerais under No. 63/2014. The study used 14 rabbits of the New Zealand breed. The rabbits were young adult males with a mean body weight of 3.0 kg. The inclusion criteria were an overall healthy state and no changes in the locomotor system. The animals were kept in individual 60 cm x 60 cm x 37 cm cages with access to water ad libitum and food twice daily, according to specific nutritional needs. The rabbits were subjected to a cranial cruciate ligament section guided by video-arthroscopy, and after 21 days, all rabbits underwent an intra-articular joint stabilization that was also guided by video-arthroscopy. Immediately after the stabilization, they were injected with APC or lactated Ringer solution in the joint. The animals were divided into two groups: the control group (I), which received 0.5 mL of lactated Ringer solution, and the treated group (II), which received 0.5 mL of APC activated with 10% calcium gluconate. The arthroscopic evaluation was performed at the time of the ligament section, 21 days and 15 days after stabilization and the intra-articular injection of lactated Ringer solution or APC. Postoperative analgesia was made with tramadol (Teuto-Cristalpharma, Brazil), at a dose of 1 mg/kg subcutaneously every 12 hours for three days, and anti-inflammatory therapy, with meloxicam (Ourofino, Brazil) at a dose of 0.2 mg/kg intramuscularly every 24 hours for three days after the section. The same treatment was made after joint stabilization at 21 days. Prophylactic therapy with cephalexin (Aspen-Pharma, Brazil) was given before joint stabilization.

During surgery, anesthesia consisted of pre-medicating the rabbits with midazolam (Cristália, Brazil) and methadone (Cristália, Brazil) at a dose of 1 mg/kg intramuscularly, 15 mg/kg ketamine, and an anesthetic blockade of the sciatic and femoral nerves with lidocaine (Cristália, Brazil) without vasoconstrictor at a dose of 5 mg/kg, maintained with isoflurane anesthesia. The heart rate, respiratory rate, blood pressure, and blood gases were monitored. The arthroscopic procedure was carried out in accordance with Beale et al.[59] After the suprapatellar recess was punctured and synovial fluid was harvested, the joint cavity was distended with 3 mL of lactated Ringer solution. A medial parapatellar stab skin incision was made, and the joint capsule was penetrated using a number 11 scalpel blade. Then, a blunt trocar locked in the arthroscopic sleeve penetrated the joint capsule. The blunt obturator was replaced by a 1.9 mm arthroscope (Storz, Germany) following the examination of the entire joint, including the evaluation of medial and lateral compartments, the intercondylar notch, cruciate ligaments, the synovial membrane, and the suprapatellar pouch. The same procedure was performed immediately using a 2.7 mm arthroscope (Storz, Germany).

Joint stabilization was carried out as described by Schawalder & Gitterle[60] after the arthroscopic evaluation at 21 days.

5. Collecting blood samples and APC preparation

We used the single-tube method of centrifugation, in accordance with Silva.[13] We modified the centrifugation time to 7 minutes to obtain a higher concentration of platelets in the rabbits. Plasma fractions with platelet concentrations between 1.5 and 2.5 times the baseline of the whole blood were considered APC. To perform the APC, 7 mL of blood was collected from the jugular vein of the rabbits in Group II and deposited in 8.5 mL tubes that contained ACD-A as an anticoagulant solution (trisodium citrate 22 g/L; citric acid 8 g/L; and dextrose 24.5 g/L). The samples were processed immediately after harvesting. CBC was performed to assess the baseline levels of the platelets in whole blood. The blood in ACD-A tubes was centrifuged at 191 g for 7 minutes at room temperature (Centribio- 80-2B, China). Using catheter number 22 and a 3 mL syringe, the first approximately 100 μL of the red fraction below the blood-plasma interface and the first 900 μL of plasma above the same interface were collected. The autologous preparations obtained were analyzed by automated blood count volumetric impedance. Each sample was analyzed three times, and the average was taken as a measurement sample. Additionally, 2 mL of whole blood in EDTA tubes was collected for CBC and biochemistry. In the prepared platelet and whole blood, the number of platelets; the hematocrit concentration; white blood cells; the absolute and relative values of lymphocytes, monocytes, granulocytes; the mean platelet volume; and the platelet distribution index were assessed. Just before the APC injection, it was activated with 10% calcium gluconate at a ratio of 0.1 mL to 1.0 mL of APC.

6. Results and discussion

Among the joint injuries observed in our clinical routine, the rupture of the cranial cruciate ligament is the most common, followed by elbow and hip dysplasia. The inevitable consequence of these changes is that OA, as reported in the literature,[2,11,12] is commonly treated continuously with so-called chondroprotective agents and analgesics. The emotional effect on the owner is considerable, and the financial costs are significant. Considering the actions of growth factors on tissues,[41,45,46,42,43] the purpose of using the APC is to promote joint recovery, heal tissues, and facilitate a painless functional recovery. Positive outcomes of APC use could be a sharp reduction in, or even the elimination of, the use of anti-inflammatory drugs, which have serious side effects. However, standardized studies on its action on tissues and the evolution of treatment are lacking. One of the great difficulties in the treatment of OA is the sequenced monitoring of their effects.

Although many studies on the degenerative process have been conducted, little is known about the molecular mechanisms that can be affected and modified by some type of therapy. Adding to this, the difficulty is the need for an early diagnosis and the evaluation of treatment.[61]

The changes associated with the degenerative process have a strong effect on patients by reducing their ability to use their joints due to pain. Unfortunately, when these changes are severe enough to be recognized clinically, they are irreversible with the treatments available today.

Joint changes can be monitored with minimally invasive surgery via arthroscopy.[62,63] Arthroscopy allows for a detailed evaluation of joint structures, for the identification of morphological changes, and, as a minimally invasive technique, for serial interventions.[64,65] It is therefore a way to track in vivo evolution of articular processes and their treatment. The limitations in second arthroscopic evaluation in clinical practice and the diversity of clinical situations[13,16,28,29] indicate the need for research that continuously assesses the process and treatment, as was performed in the first stage of this study. One of the difficulties encountered in this experimental model was the minimum quantity of synovial fluid in healthy joints, that is, 0.1 to 0.2 mL, which prevented the evaluation of the parameters. However, in the 21-day allotted time to start the evaluation of the degenerative process, joint effusion was observed in all animals with an average harvest of 0.55 mL. In the group treated with APC, effusion was reduced at 15 days after the intra-articular injection of APC, with an average harvest of 0.35 mL. In the control group, despite the joint stabilization, outpouring continued, with an average harvest of 0.62 mL.

Protein levels also showed a decrease after the intra-articular injection of APC. After 21 days, the average levels of protein were 3.7 g/dL (normal <2.5), and at 15 days after treatment, an average of 3.0 g/dL was observed. In the same observation period, the protein levels in the synovial fluid of the control group were 3.9 g/dL on average.

The protocol that was proposed by Silva[13] and modified in this research (1 minute was added in the centrifugation time) was effective in concentrating the platelets of rabbits. The concentration of platelets in the APC ranged from 1.5 to 2.5 times the baseline levels in whole blood with an average of 1.8 times (Tab.1).

However, the concentration proposed in the literature, that is, three to five times, was not reached.[66–68] A second spin could possibly elevate this concentration to the levels proposed in the literature, but the purpose of this study was to evaluate the action of this concentrate obtained simply and economically through monitoring by video-arthroscopy.

Baseline means values in total blood								
	WBC	RBC	HGB	PLT	MPV	%LYM	%MO	%GR
Average	6,16	5,28	9,48	169,85	5,85	43,97	5,94	50,1
Baseline means values in APC								
	WBC	RBC	HGB	PLT	MPV	%LYM	%MO	%GR
Average	0,39	0,03	0,11	312,85	5,88	***	***	***

WBC: leukocytes; RBC: erythrocytes; HGB: hemoglobin; PLT: platelets; MPV: mean platelet volume; LYM: lymphocytes; MO: monocytes; GR: granulocytes; ***= Value not detected by the device.

Table 1. Baseline total cell count in blood and APC in rabbits with femorotibiopatellar OA induced at 21 days after the rupture of CCLr

The role of leukocytes in APC is also a subject that requires further research, but their presence in a low concentration is considered favorable.[25] Clinical outcomes at 15 days after injection of the APC were also favorable in the experimental model, confirming owners' reports of clinical improvement in dogs after the first application of the APC. It is necessary, however, to conduct an assessment to track their in vivo effect, with the least possible morbidity.

Arthroscopy is a diagnostic tool that allows for tracking the evolution of an articular injury and the effect of treatment, but its clinical use for this purpose has limited application, leading to evaluation in an experimental model. The arthroscopic evaluation was initiated with a 1.9 mm arthroscope, but the 2.7 arthroscope enables a more detailed visualization of structures. Manipulation, however, was harder because of the instrument's size in relation to the rabbit's joints.

The arthroscopic evaluation showed different aspects between the groups, with a reduction of synovitis, a smooth synovial capsule, a lower degree of bleeding, less hypertrophy in the villi, smooth cartilage, and less evidence of fibrillation in the treated group than in the control group (Figs. 1, 2, 3, 4).

The results of the clinical evaluation showed that joint manipulation was painless during ambulation in the treated group. The arthroscopic evaluation showed the explanation for this result. A clinical response was observed in our routine in different situations, such as the relief of pain and the early recovery of limb function after rupture, CCLr treatment and functional limb return in cases of hip dysplasia, and joint pain of an unknown cause. Favorable results were also obtained in five cases of severe hip dysplasia, in which one joint was treated by triple pelvic osteotomy, and the other was subjected to treatment with three injections of APC at intervals of 15 days. The dogs recovered functional activity of the nonoperated limb, and it lasted one year. The owners reported improvement after the first injection.

It is important to consider how to obtain the APC and make sure that the concentrate has the required amount of platelets and that it is viable. The method used was the same standard as used in previous studies.[13,29]

The early diagnosis of joint injury is undoubtedly an important factor in controlling subsequent degenerative lesions, but this is not the clinical reality. Therefore, other forms of controlling or even inhibiting the degenerative process should be investigated. The monitoring of disease progression and the response to treatment requires knowledge about the disease to guide the conduct of treatment with more effective results.

Other studies on the use of autologous APC, APC banks, the influence of platelets concentration in the resolution of lesions, the range of applications, the need for repetition in the protocol, and APC's effect on fracture healing are future prospects of this research group.

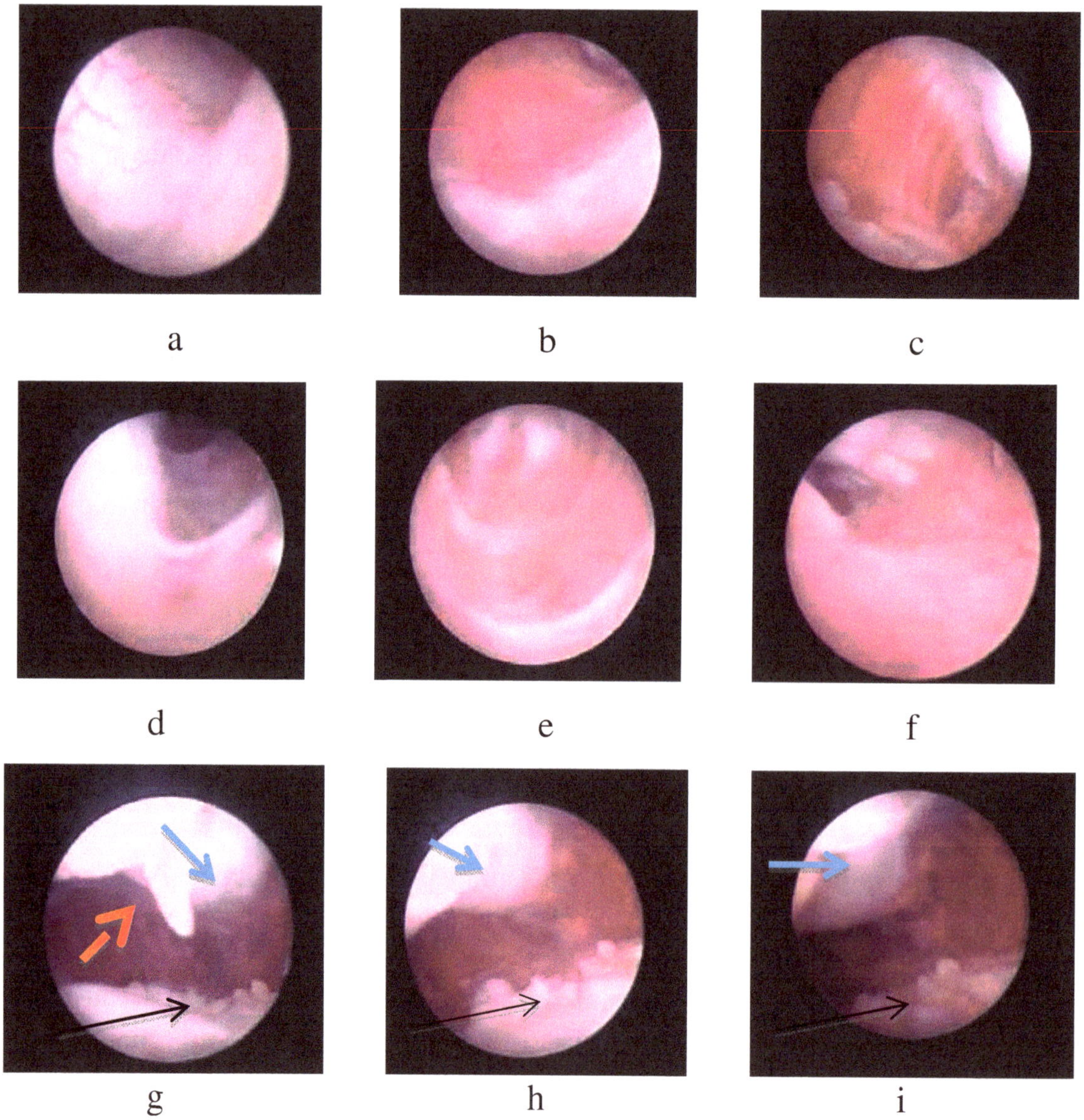

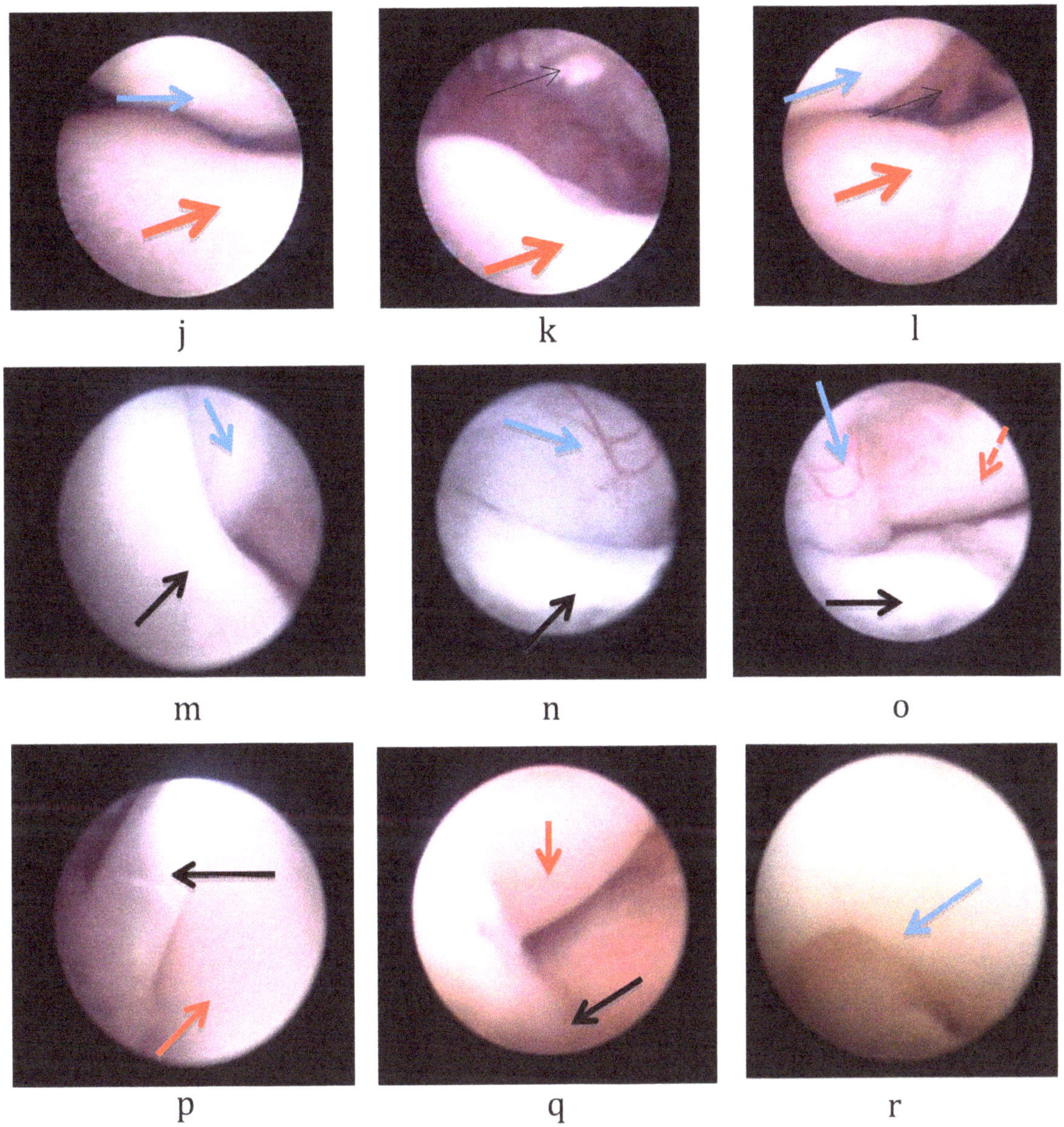

Figure 1. Arthroscopic aspects of the femorotibiopatellar joint of rabbits just before CCLr. a, b, c - the lateral compartment: smooth lateral synovial membrane, pink, with a slight vascularization and an absence of villi; d, e, f - medial compartment: smooth medial synovial membrane, pink, with slight vascularization and absence of villi; g, h, i - suprapatellar pouch: insertion of the patellar tendon (blue arrows), villus in the insertion of the patellar tendon (red arrow), presence of tissue in suprapatellar pouch (long arrow); j, k, l - patellofemoral joint: patella (blue arrow), trochlear surface (red arrow), villi in the insertion of the patellar tendon (thin black arrow); m, n, o - cranial cruciate ligament (black arrow), bright, without vascularization; m, n, o - cruciate caudal ligament (blue arrows) bright (m), with discrete vascularization (n, o), medial condyle (red dotted arrow); p - long extensor digital tendon (black arrow); lateral femoral condyle (red arrow); q - long extensor digital tendon - tibial insertion (black arrow); r- intercondylar notch, smooth and open (blue arrow).

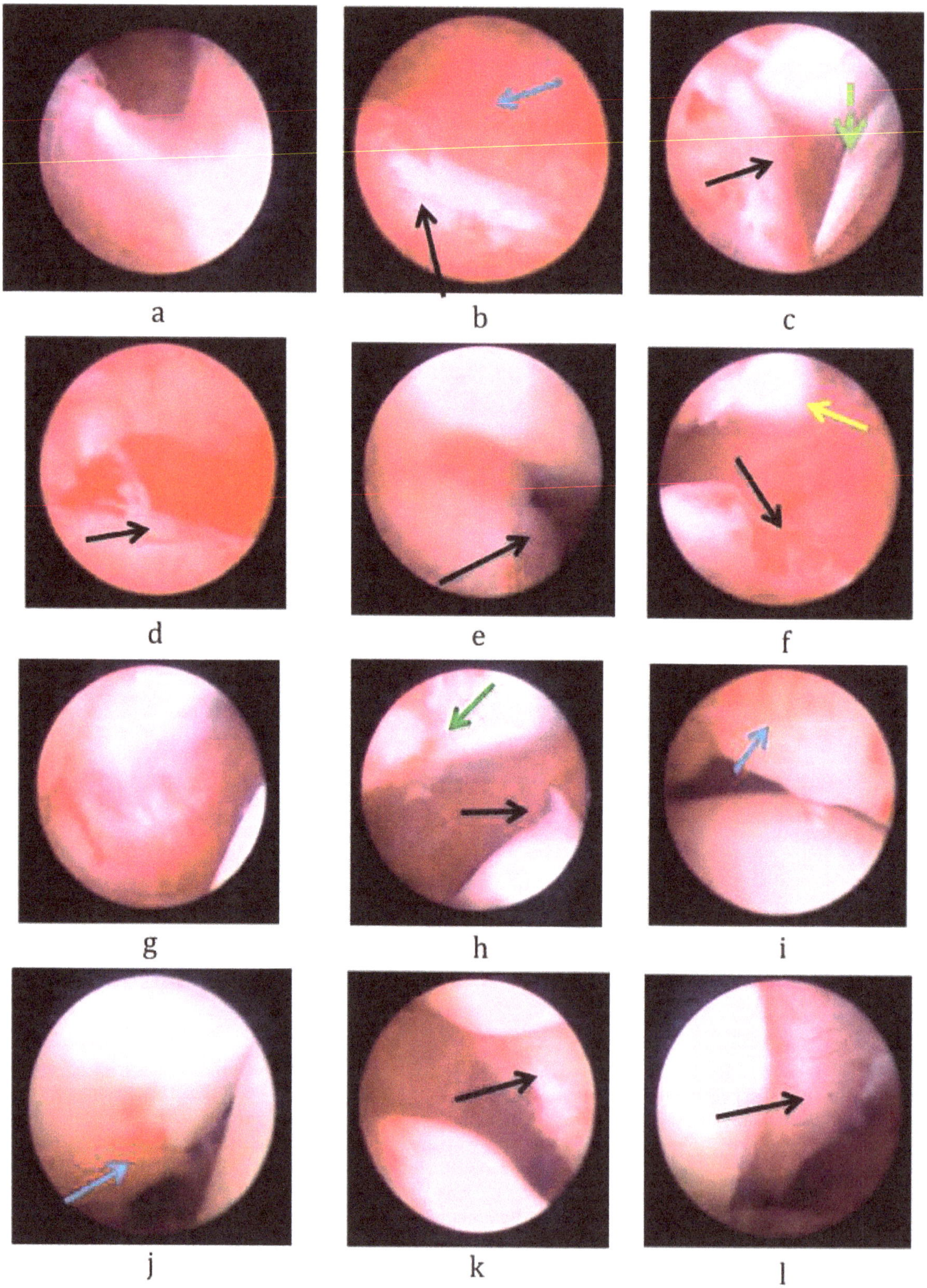

a b c d e f g h i j k l

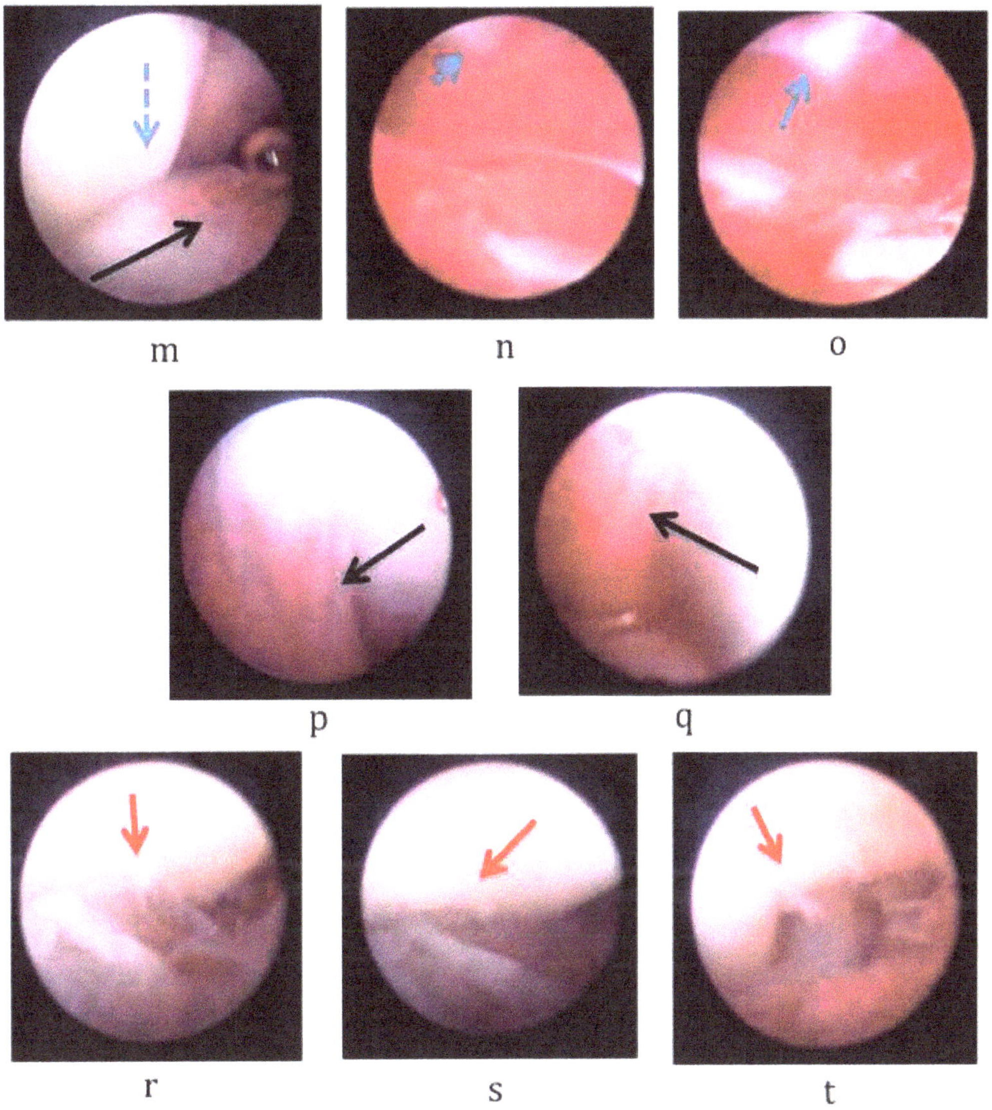

Figure 2. Arthroscopic aspects of the femorotibiopatellar joint of rabbits 21 days after the rupture of the cranial cruciate ligament. a, b, c - medial compartment: a - synovium, b- synovial membrane hyperemia (blue arrow), insertion of articular capsule - tissue formation (black arrow), c - villi, needle for drainage (dotted green arrow); d - suprapatellar pouch, clot presence, villus (black arrow); e - proximal medial condyle - villi and vascularization (black arrow); f - surface erosion of the proximal medial condyle (black arrow), insertion of the patellar tendon (yellow arrow); g - lateral compartment: hyperemic synovial membrane; h - proximal lateral condyle - tissue formation (black arrow), neovascularization in the patellar tendon insertion (green arrow); i, j - neovascularization in the patella (blue arrow); k, l - villi in the patellar insertion of the patellar tendon (black arrows); m - proximal medial condyle – vascularization (black arrow), patella (blue dotted arrow); n, o - suprapatellar pouch - neovascularization, patella (blue arrows); p, q - insertion of the long extensor digital tendon - neovascularization (black arrows); r, s, t - irregular intercondylar notch, fibrillation (red arrows).

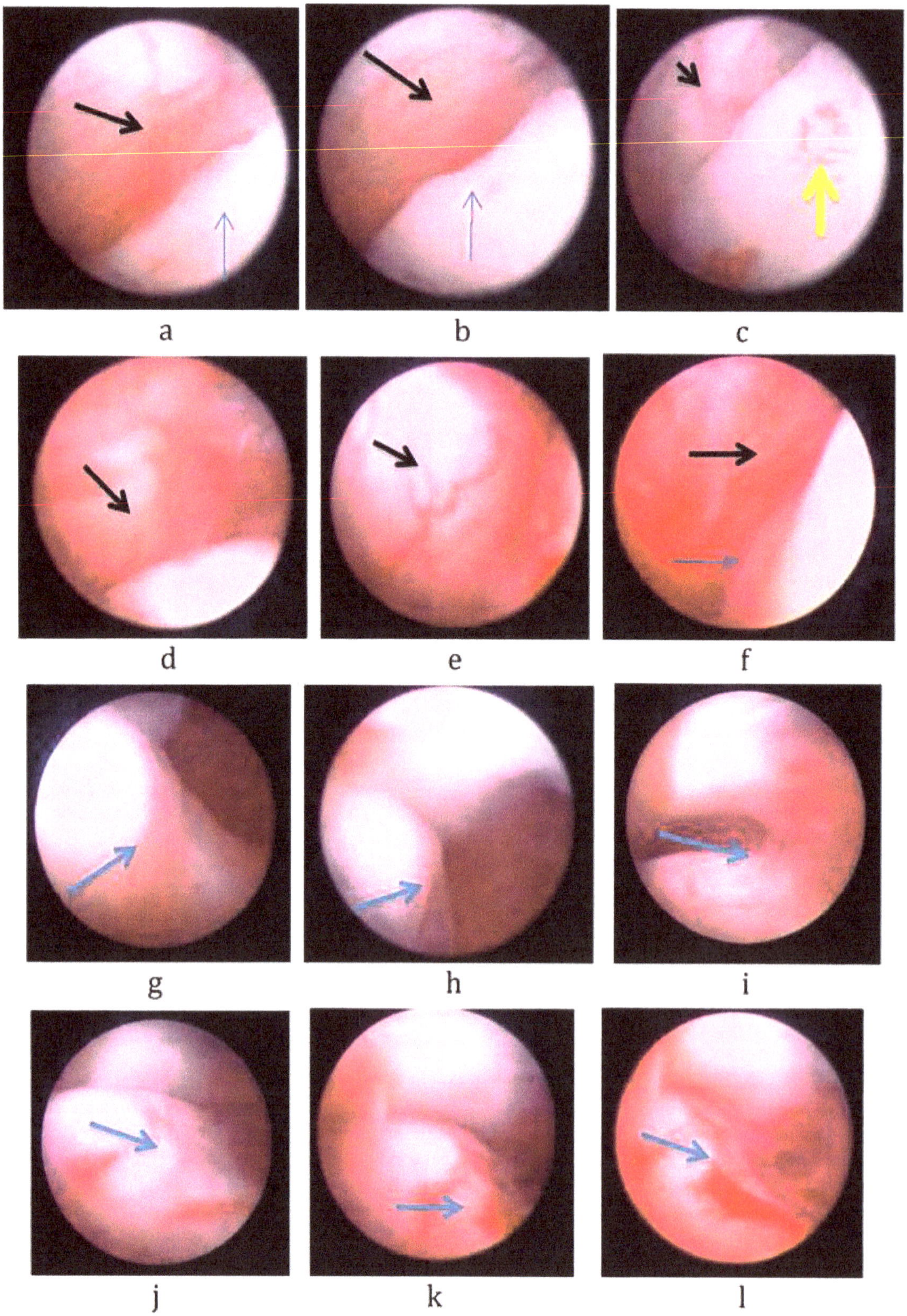

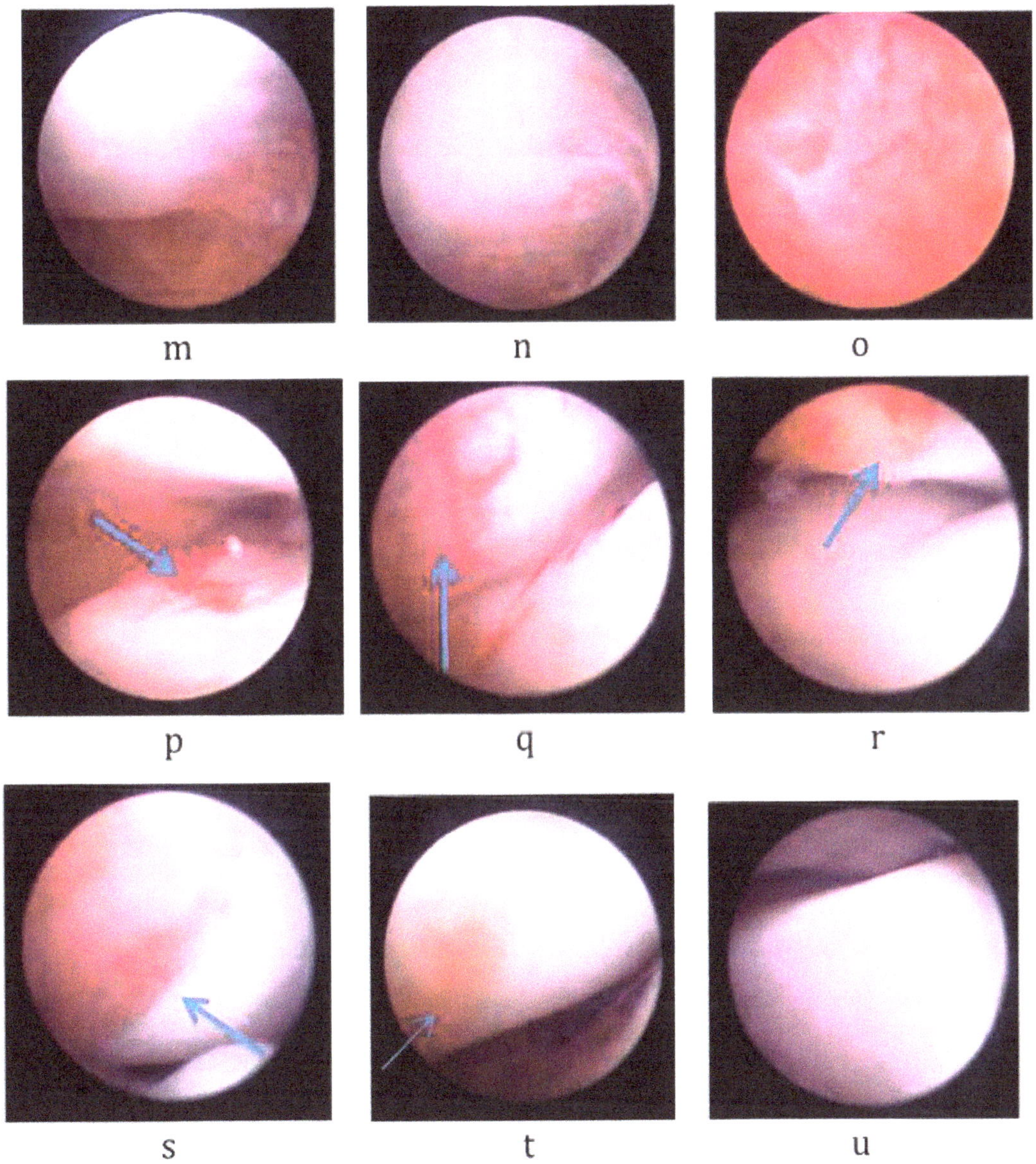
m
n
o
p
q
r
s
t
u

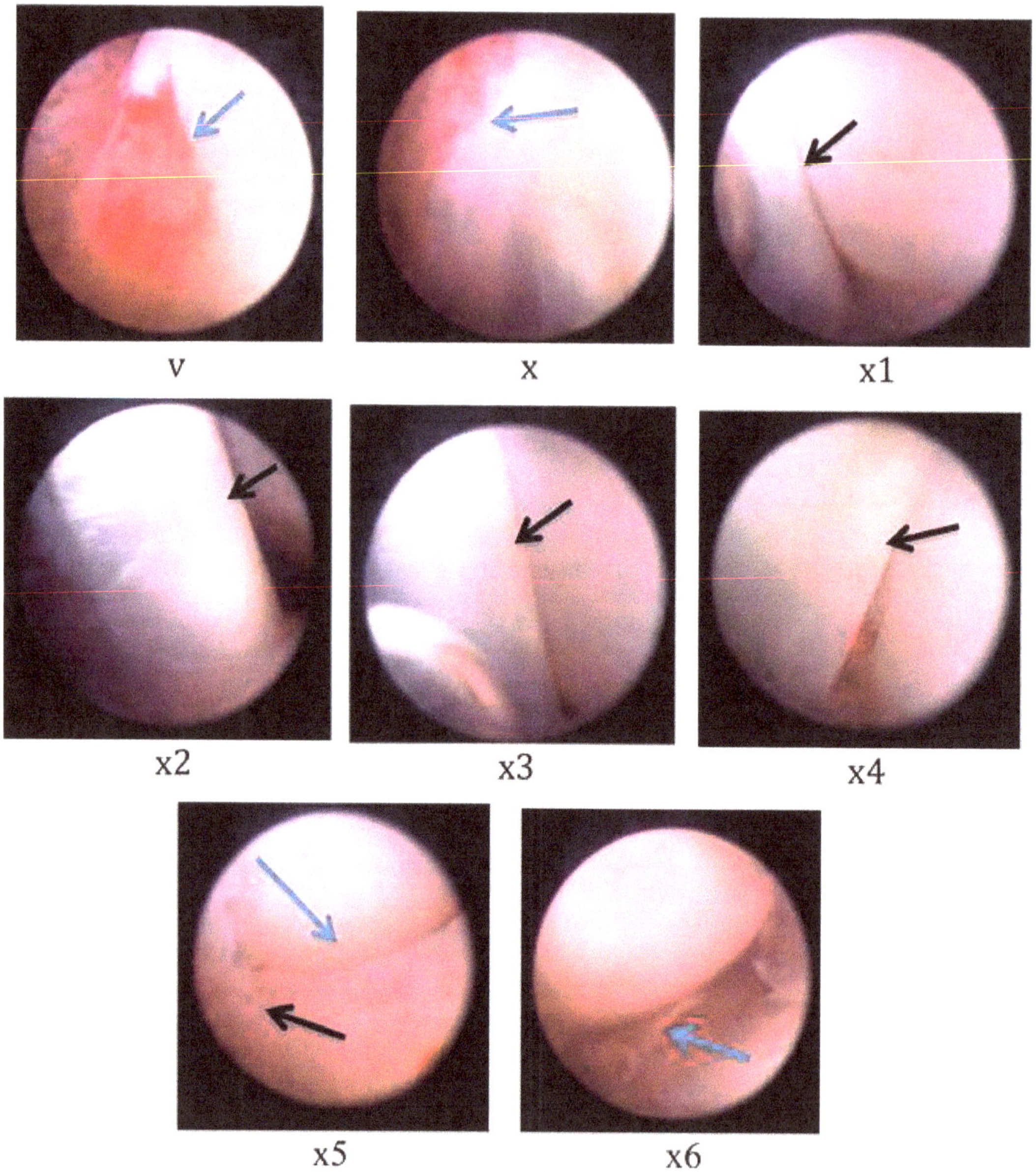

Figure 3. Arthroscopic aspects of femorotibiopatellar joint of rabbits 15 days after joint injection of autologous platelet concentrate. a, b, c, d, e, f - lateral compartment: synovial membrane (black arrows), lateral condyle, slight increase in the capsule insertion (blue arrows), neovascularization in the condyle (yellow arrow); d, e, f - lateral synovium (black arrows), lateral condyle, slight increase in the insertion of the capsule (blue arrow); g, h, i - medial compartment: g - slight irregularity in the medial condylar edge, h - capsule insertion (blue arrow), i - fibrillation in the proximal medial condyle; j, k, l - different aspects of the insertion of the capsule, fibrillation (blue arrow); m, n, o - different aspects of the medial synovial membrane; p - suprapatellar pouch; q, r, s, t - patellar neovascularization - different aspects; u - patellofemoral joint - smooth cartilage without change; v, x - neovascularization in the insertion of the long extensor digital tendon(blue arrow); x1, x2, x3 - long extensor digital tendon, middle-proximal third, bright (black arrows); x4 - long extensor digital tendon opaque (black arrow); x5 - smooth medial condyle (blue arrow), tissue formation, intercondylar notch (black arrow); x6 - partial projection of the medial horn meniscus (blue arrow).

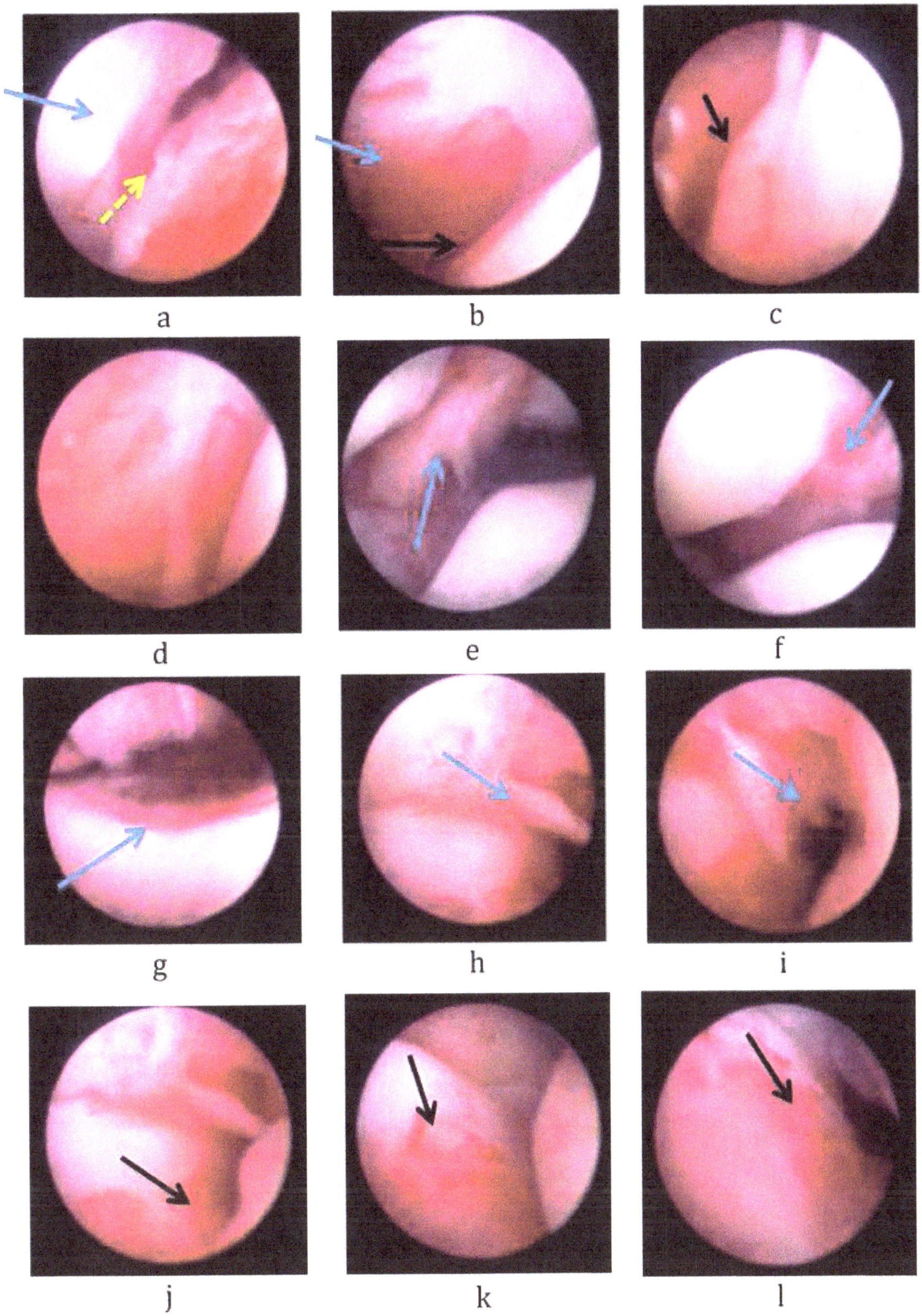
a
b
c
d
e
f
g
h
i
j
k
l

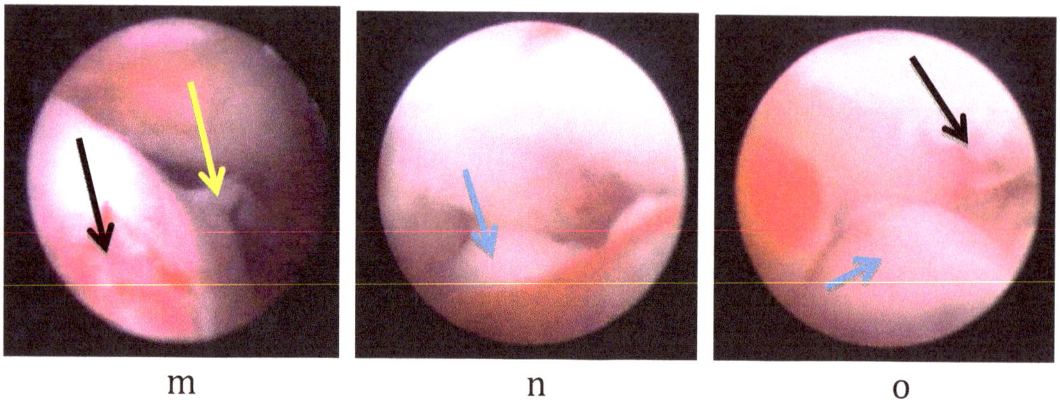

Figure 4. Arthroscopic aspects of femorotibiopatellar joint of rabbits 15 days after articular injection of lactated Ringer solution (control). a, b, c, d - lateral compartment: synovial membrane (blue arrows), lateral condyle - capsule insertion (yellow arrow), neovascularization, tissue formation; b - lateral femoral condyle, capsule insertion; c - osteophytes (black arrow); d - hyperemia of the synovial membrane; e, f - villi in the insertion of the patellar tendon (blue arrows); g - suprapatellar pouch – hyperemia (blue arrow); h, i, j, k, l, m - medial compartment: h, i - villi in the insertion of the patellar tendon (blue arrows); j, k, l, m - neovascularization in the capsule insertion (black arrows), tissue formation at the edge of the medial condyle (yellow arrow); n, o - intercondylar notch: fascia lata autograft (blue arrows), fibrillation in the intercondylar notch (black arrow).

Acknowledgements

This work was supported by CNPQ (Brazilian Council of Research and Development) and FAPEMIG (Foundation support to the Minas Gerais Research).

Author details

Cleuza Maria de Faria Rezende*, Fabíola Paes Leme, Gilcinea Santana,
Esteban Osório Carmona and Jessica Alejandra Castro Varón

*Address all correspondence to: cleuzaufmg@gmail.com

Department of Veterinary Medicine and Surgery, Veterinary School, Universidade Federal de Minas Gerais, Belo Horizonte, Minas Gerais, Brazil

References

[1] Doom, M.; De Bruin, T.; De Rooster, H. et al. Immunopathological mechanisms in dogs with rupture of the cranial cruciate ligament. Vet. Immunol. Immunopathol. 2008; 125: 143-161. DOI: 10.1016/j.vetimm.2008.05.023

[2] Canapp Jr., S.O. The canine stifle. Clin. Tech. Small Anim. Pract. 2007; 22: 195-205. DOI: 10.1053/s.ctsap. 2007.09.008

[3] Johnson, J.A.; Austin, C.; Breur G.J. Incidence of canine appendicular musculoskeletal disorders in 16 veterinary teaching hospitals from 1980 through 1989. Vet. Comp. Orthop. Traumatol. 1994; 7: 56-59. DOI: 10.1111/j.1532-950X.2006.00226.x

[4] Rayward, R.M.; Thomson, D.G.; Davies, J.V. et al. Progression of osteoarthritis following TPLO surgery: a prospective radiographic study of 40 dogs. J. Small Anim. Pract. 2004; v. 45: 92-97. DOI: 10.1111/j.1748-5827.2004.tb00208.x

[5] Innes, J.F.; Bacon, D.; Lynch, C. et al. Long-term outcome of surgery for dogs with cranial cruciate ligament deficiency. Vet. Rec. 2000; 147: 325-328. DOI: 10.1136/vr. 147.12.325.

[6] Johnston, S.A. Osteoarthritis: joint anatomy, physiology, and pathobiology. Vet. Clin. N. Am. Small Anim. Pract. 1997; 27: 699-723. DOI: 10.1016/j.cvsm.2015.06.

[7] Pond, M.J.; Nuki, G. Experimentally-induced osteoarthritis in the dog. Ann. Rheum. Dis. 1973; 387-388. DOI:10.1136/annrheumdis-2015-208300

[8] Fernandes, J.C.; Martel-Pelletier, J.; Pelletier, J.P. The role of cytokines in osteoarthritis pathophysiology. Biorheology. 2002. 30:237-246. DOI: 10.5435/JAAOS-22-01-29

[9] Rezende, U.M.; Gobbi, R.G. Tratamento medicamentoso da osteoartrose do joelho: drogas modificadoras da doença. Rev. Bras. Ortop. 2009; 44: 14-19. ISSN 0102-3616... http://dx.doi.org/10.1016/j.rbo.2012.08.006

[10] Filho, M.M.; Rahal, S.C. O uso de anti-inflamatórios inibidores cox-2 seletivos na osteoartrite canina. Veterinária e Zootecnia. 2008; 15: 407-415. ISSN 0102-5716

[11] Clark, T.P. The clinical pharmacology of ciclooxigenase-2-selective and dual inhibitors. Vet. Clin. N. Am. Small Anim. Pract. 2006; 36: 1061-1085. DOI: doi.org/10.1016/j.cvsm.2006.07.001

[12] Lees, P.; Landoni, M.F.; Giraudel, J. et al. Pharmacodynamics and pharmacokinetics of nonsteroidal anti-inflammatory drugs in species of veterinary interest. J. Vet. Pharmacol. Ther. 2004; 27: 479-490. DOI: 10.1111/jvp.12196. ISSN 0140-7783

[13] Silva, R.F. Caracterizações celular e ultra-estrutural do concentrado de plaquetas em cães e gatos e avaliação do seu efeito na osteoartrose em cães. 2012. 88f. Tese (Doutorado em ciência animal). Escola de Veterinária, Universidade Federal de Minas Gerais, Minas Gerais, 2012

[14] Huang, T.F.; Chen, Y.T.; Yang, T.H. et al. Isolation and characterization of mesenchymal stromal cells from human anterior cruciate ligament. Cytotherapy. 2008; 10: 806-814. DOI: http://dx.doi.org/10.1080/14653240802474323

[15] Petrigliano, F.P.; McAllister, D.R.; Wu, B.M. Tissue engineering for anterior cruciate ligament reconstruction: a review of current strategies. J. Arthrosc. Relat. Surg. 2006; 22: 441-451. ISSN 1526-3231

[16] Silva, R.F.; Rezende, C.M.F.; Carmona, J.U. Use of intra-articular autologous concentrates as coadjuvants in the surgical arthroscopy treatment of elbow dysplasia in a bitch. Arch. Med. Vet. 2013; 45: 213-217. DOI: ISSN 0301-732X/ISSN 0717-6201

[17] Stief, M.; Gottschalk, J.; Ionita, J.C.; Eispanier, A.; Oechtering, G.; Bötcher, P. Concentration of platelets and growth factors in canine autologous conditioned plasma. Vet. Comp. Orthop. Traumatol. 2011; 24:122-125. DOI: 10.3415/VCOT-14-12-0182

[18] Neumann, S.; Viefhues, G. Intraartikuläre Injection von autologem Thrombozytenkonzentrat bei der OCD. Veterinär Spiegel. 2010; 1: 22-26. DOI: 10.1055/s-004-28203

[19] Argüelles, D.; Carmona, J. U.; Climent F.; Munoz, E.; Prades, M. Autologous platelet concentrates as a treatment for musculoskeletal lesions in five horses. Vet. Rec. 2008; 81: 208-211. DOI: 10.1136/vr.h347

[20] Anitua, E.; Sanchez, M.; Nurden, A.T. et al. Platelet-released growth factors enhance the secretion of hyaluronic acid and induce hepatocyte growth factor production by synovial fibroblasts from arthritic patients. Rheumatology. 2007; 46: 1769-1772. DOI: 10.1093/rheumatology/keu484

[21] Everts, P.A.M.; Knape, J.T.A.; Weibrich, G.; Schönberger, J.P.A.M.; Hoffmann, J.; Overdevest, E.P.; Henk, A.M.; Van Zundert, A. Platelet-rich plasma and plasma gel: a review. J. Am. Soc. Extracorp. Technol. 2006; 38: 174-187. DOI: 10.3732/ajb.0900091

[22] Sánchez, M.; Delgado, D.; Sánchez, P.; Fiz, N.; Azofra, R.; Orive, G.; Anitua, E.; Padilla, S. Platelet rich plasma and knee surgery. BioMed Res. Int. 2014. Article ID 890630, 10 pages. DOI: 10.1155/2014/890630

[23] Rodriguez, J.; Palomar, M.A.; Torres, J. Plasma rico en plaquetas: fundamentos biológicos y aplicaciones en cirugía maxilofacial y estética facial. Rev. Esp. Cir. Oral Maxilofac. 2012; 34: 8-17. DOI: 10.1016/j.maxilo.2011.10.007

[24] Oates, T.W.; Rouse, C.A.; Cochram, D.L. Mitogenic effects of growth factors on human periodontal ligament cells in vitro. J. Periodontal. 1993; 64: 142-148. DOI: 10.1111/jre.12257

[25] Carmona, J.U.; López, C. Autologous platelet concentrates as a treatment for shoulder injury in a horse. J. Equine Vet. Sci. 2011; 31: 506-510. DOI: 10.1016/j.physletb.2010.09.059

[26] Carmona, J.U.; Argüelles, D.; Climent, F.; Prades M. Autologous platelet concentrates as a treatment of horses with osteoarthritis: a preliminary pilot clinical study. J. EquineVet. Sci. 2007; 27: 167-170. DOI: 10.1016/j.physletb.2010.09.059

[27] Carmona, J.U. Use of autologous platelet concentrates for the treatment of musculoskeletal injuries in the horse: preliminary clinical studies and cellular and molecular

evaluation of equine platelet concentrates obtained by single and double centrifugation tube methods. 2006. 100 f. Dissertação (Doutorado en Veterinaria) Faculty of Veterinary medicine, Universitat Autonoma de Barcelona, Barcelona, 2006

[28] Silva, R.F.; Carmona, J.U., Rezende, C.M.F. Uso de plasma rico em plaquetas intra-articular como tratamento pós-cirúrgico da ruptura do ligamento cruzado cranial num cão. Arq. Bras. Med. Vet. Zootec. 2012; 64: 847-852. DOI: 10.1590/s0102-09352012000200030

[29] Silva, R.F.; Rezende, C.M.F.; Carmona J.U. Uso de concentrados autólogos de plaquetas intrarticulares como coadyuvantes en el tratamiento quirúrgico de la rotura del ligamento cruzado anterior en una perra. Arch. Med. Vet. 2011; 43: 313-316. ISSN 0301-732X/ISSN 0717-6201

[30] Milano, G.; Sanna Passino, E.; Deriu, L. et al. The effect of platelet rich plasma combined with microfractures on the treatment of chondral defects: na experimental study in a sheep model. Osteoarthr. Cartil. 2010; 18: 971-980. DOI: 10.1016/j.joca.2010.03.013

[31] Murray, M.M.; Splinder, K.P.; Devin, C. et al. Use of collagen-platelet rich- plasma scaffold to stimulate healing of central defect in the canine ACL. J. Orthop. Res. 2006; 24: 820-830. DOI: 10.1002/(ISSN)1554-527X

[32] Zachos, T.A.; Bertone, A.L. Growth factors and their potential therapeutic applications for healing of musculoskeletal and other connective tissues. Am. J. Vet. Res. 2005; 66: 727-728. DOI: 10.1186/1297-9716-44-24

[33] Kwon, D.R.; Park, G.Y.; Lee, S.U. The effects of intra-articular platelet-rich plasma injection according to the severity of collagenase-induced knee osteoarthritis in a rabbit model. Ann. Rehabil. Med. 2012; 36: 458-465. DOI: 10.5535/arm.2012.36.4.458

[34] Park, S.I.; Lee, H.R.; Kim, S. et al. Time sequential modulation in expression of growth factors from platelet rich plasma (PRP) on the chondrocyte cultures. Mol. Cell Biochem. 2012; 361: 9-17. DOI: 10.1007/s11010-011-1081-1

[35] Saito, M.; Takahashi, K.; Aray, Y. et al. Intraarticular administration of platelet-rich plasma biodegradable gelatin hydrogel microspheres prevents osteoarthritis progression in the rabbit knee. Clin. Exp. Rheumatol. 2009; 27: 201-207. ISSN 0770-3198 (Print) 1434-9949 (Online)

[36] Sun, Y.; Feng, Y.; Zhang, C.Q. et al. The regenerative effect of platelet-rich plasma on healing in large osteochondral defects. Int. Orthop. 2010; 34: 589-597. DOI: 10.1007/s00264-009-0793-2

[37] Akeda, K.; An, H.; Okuma, M. et al. Platelet-rich plasma stimulates porcine articular chondrocyte proliferation and matrix biosynthesis. Osteoarthr. Cartil. 2006; 14: 1272-1280. DOI: 10.1016/j.joca.2006.05.008

[38] Filgueiras, R.R.; Del Carlo, R.J.; Alves, N.P. et al. Platelet rich plasma associated with heterologous fresh and thawed chondrocytes on osteochondral lesions of rabbits. Arq. Bras. Med. Vet. Zootec. 2014; 66: 177-184. ISSN 0103-0935

[39] Smyth, N.A.; Murawski, C.D.; Fortier. L.A. et al. Platelet-rich plasma in the pathologic process of cartilage: review of basic science evidence. Arthroscopy. 2013; 29: 1399-1409. DOI: 10.1016/j.arthro.2013.03.004

[40] Civinini, R.; Nistri, L.; Martini, C.; Redl, B.; Ristori, G.; Innocenti M. Growth factors in the treatment of early osteoarthritis. Clin. Case Miner. Bone Metab. 2013; 10: 26-29. DOI: 1138/ccmbm/2014.11.3.165

[41] Chung, R.; Foster, B.K.; Xian, C.J. Preclinical studies on mesenchymal stem cell-based therapy for growth plate cartilage injury repair. Stem Cells Int. 2011; 2011: 570125. DOI: 10.4061/2011/570125

[42] Argüelles, D.; Carmona, J.U.; Pastor, J.; Iborra, A.; Viñals, L.; Martínez P.; Bach, E.; Prades, M. Evaluation of single and double centrifugation tube methods for concentrating equine platelets. Res. Vet. Sci. 2006; 81: 237-245. DOI: 10.1016/j.physletb.2010.09.059

[43] Anitua, E.; Andia, I.; Ardanza, B. et al. Autologous platelets as a source of proteins for healing and tissue regeneration. Thromb. Haemost. 2004; 91: 4-15. DOI: 10.1111/jth.12857

[44] Carmona, J.U.; Argüelles, D.; Prades, M. Transforming growth factor beta-3 and nitric oxide levels in four autologous platelet concentrates and plasma derived from equine blood. Arch. Med. Vet. 2008; 40: 155-160. ISSN 0301-732X/ISSN 0717-6201

[45] Fortier, L.; Barker, J.; Strauss, E.; MacCarrel, T.; Cole, B. The role of growth factors in cartilage repair. Clin. Orthop. Relat. 2011; 469: 2706-2715. DOI: 10.1016/j.actbio.2015.01.010

[46] Fan, J.; Gong, I.; Ren, L. et al. In vitro engineered cartilage using synovium derived mesenchymal stem cells with injectable gellan hydrogels. Acta Biomater. 2010; 6: 1178-1185. DOI: 10.1016/j.actbio.2009.08.042

[47] Kurth, T.; Hedbom, E.; Shintani, N. et al. Chondrogenic potential of human synovial mesenchymal stem cells in alginate. Osteoarthr. Cartil. 2007; 15: 1178-1189. DOI: http://dx.doi.org/10.1016/j.joca.2007.03.015

[48] Weibrich, G.; Kleis, W.K.; Hitzler, W.E.; Hafner, G. Comparison of the platelet concentrate collection system with the plasma-rich in growth factors kit to produce platelet rich-plasma: a technical report. Int. J. Oral Maxillofac. Implants. 2005; 29: 118-123. DOI: 10.11607/jomi.2015.1

[49] Sutter, W.W.; Kaneps, A.J.; Bertone, A.L. et al. Comparison of hematologic values and transforming growth factor-β and insulin-like growth factor concentration in

platelet concentrates obtained by use of buffy coat and apheresis methods from equine blood. Am. J. Vet. Res. 2004; 65: 924-930. DOI: 10.1111/j.1939-1676.2009.0335.x

[50] Carter, C.A.; Jolly, D.J.; Worden, C.E. et al. Platelet rich-plasma gel promotes differentiation and regeneration during equine wound healing. Exp. Mol. Pathol. 2003; 74: 244-255. DOI: 10.1006/exmp.2001.2380

[51] Silva, R.F.; Rezende, C.M.F.; Paes-Leme, F.O.; Carmona, J.U. Evaluación del método del tubo para concentrar plaquetas caninas: estudo cellular. Arch. Med. Vet. 2011; 43: 95-98. ISSN 0301-732X/ISSN 0717-6201

[52] Marx, R.E. Platelet-rich plasma: evidence to support its usage. J. Oral Maxillofac. Surg. 2004; 62: 489-496. DOI: 10.1016/j.joms.2014.08.011

[53] Anitua, S.; Prado, R.; Sanchez, M. et al. Platelet-rich plasma: preparation and formulation. Oper. Tech. Orthop. 2012; 22: 25-32. DOI: 10.1053/j.oto.2012.01.004

[54] Mazzuco, L.; Balbo, V.; Cattana, E.; Borzini, P. Platelet-rich plasma and platelet gel preparation using platelex. Vox Sang. 2008; 94: 202-208. DOI: 0.1111/vox.12093

[55] Roberts, D.E.; Archibald, M.N.; Ratna, B. Mechanism of collagen activation in human platelets. J. Biol. Chem. 2004; 279: 19421-19430. DOI: 0.1074/jbc.P114.609743

[56] Silva, R.F.; Carmona, J. U.; Rezende, C.M.F. Comparison of the effect of calcium gluconate and batroxobin on the release of transforming growth factor beta1 in canine platelet concentrates. BMC Vet. Res. 2012; 8: 121-128. DOI: 10.1186/1746-6148-8-212

[57] Silva, R.F.; Álvarez, M.E.; Rios, D.L.; López, C.; Carmona, J.U.; Rezende, C.M.F. Evaluation of the effect of calcium gluconate and bovine thrombin on the temporal release of transforming growth factor beta 1 and platelet-derived growth factor isoform BB from feline platelet concentrates. BMC Vet. Res. 2012; 8: 212. DOI: 10.1186/1746-6148-8-212

[58] Patel, S.; Dhillon, M.S.; Aggarwal, S. et al. Treatment with platelet-rich plasma is more effective than placebo for knee osteoarthritis : a prospective, double-blind, randomized trial. Am. J. Sports Med. 2013; 41: 356-364. DOI: 10.1177/0363546514537991

[59] Beale, S.B.; Hulse, A.D.; Schultz, K.S. et al. Small animal arthroscopy. Philadelphia: Saunders; 2003. pp. 117-157. ISBN 0-7216-8969-8

[60] Schawalder, P.; Gitterle, E. Eigene methoden zur operativen rekonstruktion bei rupturen des vorderen und hinteren kreuzbandes. Kleintierpraxis. 1989; 7: 323-330. ISSN 0023-2076

[61] Zhai, G.; Eshghi, E.A. Biomarkers for osteoarthritis: investigation, identification and prognosis. Curr Biomark. Find. 2012; 2: 19-28. DOI: 10.2147/CBF.S27901

[62] Borges, N.F.; Rezende, C.M.F.; Melo, E.G.; Malm, C.; Gheller V.A.; Doretto, J.V. Video-artroscopia da articulação fêmoro-tibio-patelar em cães após secção do ligamento

cruzado cranial guiada por artroscopia. Arq. Bras. Med. Vet. Zootec. 2008; 60: 1035-1044. DOI: 10.1590/S0102-09352013000300013

[63] Rezende, C.M.F.; Melo, E.G.; Malm, C.; Gheller, V.A. Tratamento artroscópico da fragmentação do processo coronóide da ulna/Arthroscopical treatment of fragmented medial coronoid process (FCP) of the ulna. Arq. Bras. Med. Vet. Zootec. 2012; 64: 09-14. ISSN 1678-4162

[64] Van Ryssen, B.; Van Bree, H. Diagnostic and surgical arthroscopy in small animals. In: Bloomberg, M.S.; Dee, J.F.; Taylor, R.A., editors. Canine sports medicine and surgery. Philadelphia: Saunders; 1998. pp. 250-254. DOI: ISBN 0-7216 5022-8

[65] Rezende, C.M.F.; Melo, E.G.; Madureira, N.G.; Freitas, P.M. Artroscopia da articulação fêmoro-tíbiopatelar de cão. Arq. Bras. Med. Vet. Zootec. 2006; 58: 841-848. DOI: 10.1590/S0102- 09352013000300013

[66] Kon, E.; Filardo, G.; Di Matteo, B. et al. Platelet-rich plasma in sports medicine: new treatment for tendon and cartilage lesions. Oper. Tech. Orthop. 2012; 22: 78-85. ISSN 1048-6666 (Print); 1558-3848 (Electronic)

[67] Flores, J.R.; Gallego, M.A.P.; García-Denche, J.T. Plasma rico en plaquetas: fundamentos biológicos y aplicaciones en cirugía maxilofacial y estética facial. Rev. Esp. Cir. Oral Maxilofac. 2012; 34: 8-17. DOI: 10.1016/j.maxilo.2011.10.007

[68] Carrasco, J.; Bonnete, D.; Gomar, R. Plasma Rico en Plaquetas vs. Plasma rico en factores de crecimiento. Rev. Esp. Cir. Osteoartic. 2009; 46: 127-140. ISSN 0304-5056

Permissions

All chapters in this book were first published in ARTHROPLASTY, by InTech Open; hereby published with permission under the Creative Commons Attribution License or equivalent. Every chapter published in this book has been scrutinized by our experts. Their significance has been extensively debated. The topics covered herein carry significant findings which will fuel the growth of the discipline. They may even be implemented as practical applications or may be referred to as a beginning point for another development.

The contributors of this book come from diverse backgrounds, making this book a truly international effort. This book will bring forth new frontiers with its revolutionizing research information and detailed analysis of the nascent developments around the world.

We would like to thank all the contributing authors for lending their expertise to make the book truly unique. They have played a crucial role in the development of this book. Without their invaluable contributions this book wouldn't have been possible. They have made vital efforts to compile up to date information on the varied aspects of this subject to make this book a valuable addition to the collection of many professionals and students.

This book was conceptualized with the vision of imparting up-to-date information and advanced data in this field. To ensure the same, a matchless editorial board was set up. Every individual on the board went through rigorous rounds of assessment to prove their worth. After which they invested a large part of their time researching and compiling the most relevant data for our readers.

The editorial board has been involved in producing this book since its inception. They have spent rigorous hours researching and exploring the diverse topics which have resulted in the successful publishing of this book. They have passed on their knowledge of decades through this book. To expedite this challenging task, the publisher supported the team at every step. A small team of assistant editors was also appointed to further simplify the editing procedure and attain best results for the readers.

Apart from the editorial board, the designing team has also invested a significant amount of their time in understanding the subject and creating the most relevant covers. They scrutinized every image to scout for the most suitable representation of the subject and create an appropriate cover for the book.

The publishing team has been an ardent support to the editorial, designing and production team. Their endless efforts to recruit the best for this project, has resulted in the accomplishment of this book. They are a veteran in the field of academics and their pool of knowledge is as vast as their experience in printing. Their expertise and guidance has proved useful at every step. Their uncompromising quality standards have made this book an exceptional effort. Their encouragement from time to time has been an inspiration for everyone.

The publisher and the editorial board hope that this book will prove to be a valuable piece of knowledge for researchers, students, practitioners and scholars across the globe.

List of Contributors

Ulrich Bechler, Bernhard Springer and Friedrich Boettner
Adult Reconstruction and Joint Replacement Division, Hospital for Special Surgery, New York, NY, USA

Binghua Zhou and Kanglai Tang
Department of Orthopedic Surgery, China

Stefan Cristea, Vlad Predescu, Serban Dragosloveanu, Stefan Cuculici and Nicholas Mărăndici
Emergency Hospital of Saint Pantelimon, Carol Davila University of Medicine and Pharmacy, Bucharest, Romania

Satish B. Sonar
Sports Med-Joint Care Centre, Nagpur, India

Christopher Paul O'Boynick and Bruce V. Darden II
OrthoCarolina Spine Center, Charlotte, USA

Hiran Wimal Amarasekera
Neville Fernando Teaching Hospital and South Asian Institute of Medicine, Colombo , Sri Lanka
Warwick Orthopaedics, University of Warwick,Coventry, United Kingdom

Hamid Reza Seyyed Hosseinzadeh, Alisina Shahi, Mohamad Qoreishy and Mehrnoush Hassas Yeganeh
Thomas Jefferson University, USA

Tsutomu Gomi
School of Allied Health Sciences, Kitasato University, Japan

Oksana Ivask and Ülle Voog-Oras
Department of Stomatology, University of Tartu, Estonia

Edvitar Leibur
Departments of Stomatology and InternalMedicine, University of Tartu, Estonia

Cleuza Maria de Faria Rezende, Fabíola Paes Leme, Gilcinea Santana, Esteban Osório Carmona and Jessica Alejandra Castro Varón
Department of Veterinary Medicine and Surgery, Veterinary School, Universidade Federal de Minas Gerais, Belo Horizonte, Minas Gerais, Brazil

Index

www.ingramcontent.com/pod-product-compliance
Lightning Source LLC
LaVergne TN
LVHW060555210926
848485LV00005B/1318
* 9 7 8 1 6 3 9 8 7 0 5 8 5 *